Pocket Consultant

OCCUPATIONAL HEALTH

Sixth Edition

Professor Kerry Gardiner
Professor of Occupational Health, School of Public Health, University of the Witwatersrand, Johannesburg, South Africa

Professor David Rees
Emeritus Professor, School of Public Health, University of the Witwatersrand; National Institute for Occupational Health, Johannesburg, South Africa

Professor Anil Adisesh
Associate Professor and Division Director, Occupational Medicine, Department of Medicine, University of Toronto, Ontario, Canada; Canadian Health Solutions, Saint John, New Brunswick, Canada

Professor David Zalk
Director of Occupational Hygiene, University of Illinois at Chicago, Chicago, Illinois; School of Public Health, Global Program on Occupational Health Practice Online, San Jose, California, USA

Professor Malcolm Harrington CBE
Emeritus Professor of Occupational Medicine, University of Birmingham, UK

With contributions from

Dr Roxane Gervais (Chapter 11)
Director, Practical Psychology Consultancy Ltd, Hull, UK

Professor Joan Saary (Chapters 9.5 and 18.17)
Associate Professor, Department of Medicine, Division of Occupational Medicine, University of Toronto, Toronto, Ontario, Canada

WILEY Blackwell

Registered Office(s)
John Wiley & Sons, Inc., 111 River Street, Hoboken, NJ 07030, USA
John Wiley & Sons Ltd, The Atrium, Southern Gate, Chichester, West Sussex, PO19 8SQ, UK

Editorial Office
9600 Garsington Road, Oxford, OX4 2DQ, UK

For details of our global editorial offices, customer services, and more information about Wiley products visit us at www.wiley.com.

Wiley also publishes its books in a variety of electronic formats and by print-on-demand. Some content that appears in standard print versions of this book may not be available in other formats.

Library of Congress Cataloging-in-Publication Data
Names: Gardiner, K., author. | Rees, David, 1954- author. | Adisesh, Anil, author. | Zalk, David, author. | Harrington, J. M. (John Malcolm), author.
Title: Occupational health / Kerry Gardiner, Professor of Occupational Health, School of Public Health, University of the Witwatersrand, Johannesburg, South Africa, David Rees, Emeritus Professor, School of Public Health, University of the Witwatersrand, National Institute for Occupational Health, Johannesburg, South Africa, Anil Adisesh, Associate Professor and Division Director Occupational Medicine, University of Toronto, Toronto, Ontario, Canada, Head of Division Occupational Medicine, St. Michael's Hospital, Toronto, Ontario, Canada, David Zalk, Director of Occupational Hygiene; University of Illinois at Chicago, School of Public Health, Global Program on Occupational Health Practice Onlline, San Jose, California, USA, Malcolm Harrington, John Malcolm Harrington CBE, Emeritus Professor of Occupational Medicine, University of Birmingham, UK ; with contributions from Dr. Roxane Gervais, (Chapter 11) Director, Practical Psychology Consultancy Ltd, Hull, UKJoan Saary.
Description: Sixth edition. | Hoboken, NJ : Wiley-Blackwell, 2022. | Series: Pocket consultant | Includes index.
Identifiers: LCCN 2021049300 (print) | LCCN 2021049301 (ebook) | ISBN 9781119718611 (paperback) | ISBN 9781119718635 (adobe pdf) | ISBN 9781119718628 (epub)
Subjects: LCSH: Industrial hygiene–Handbooks, manuals, etc. | Occupational diseases–Handbooks, manuals, etc.
Classification: LCC RC967 .H33 2022 (print) | LCC RC967 (ebook) | DDC 613.6/2–dc23/eng/20211109
LC record available at https://lccn.loc.gov/2021049300
LC ebook record available at https://lccn.loc.gov/2021049301

Cover Design: Wiley
Cover Images: © Anna/Adobe Stock Photos, PRASANNAPIX/ Adobe Stock Photos, Максим Слепухинv/ Adobe Stock Photos, BGStock72/Adobe Stock Photos, deagreez/Adobe Stock Photos, Shinji Toyama/Adobe Stock, motorradcbr/Adobe Stock Photos

Set in 10/12pt STIXTwoText by Straive, Pondicherry, India

CONTENTS

FOREWORD

When a text such as *Pocket Consultant: Occupational Health* has survived over six iterations, the authorship has most likely changed. This is certainly the case here: the first version was authored by Malcolm Harington and Frank Gill – with just Malcolm Harrington remaining in this the sixth edition. What has enabled this book to be (hopefully) so comprehensive and coherent yet retain its 'pocket consultant' format is that every edition has been written by colleagues in the same academic department. However, it is with deep sadness we report that, since the fifth edition (2006) was published, both Frank Gill and Tar Ching Aw have passed away – it is to them that this book is dedicated.

With deliberate intent, it was decided to utilise the profound knowledge and experience of some of our friends and colleagues from further afield geographically to make the text less parochially British and reflect a more global perspective. In addition, there have been significant developments in various aspects of occupational health, and the structure and content of the book have been chosen to reflect this, particularly the new chapters on clinical evaluations, control banding, tertiary prevention and the legal and ethical aspects of occupational health. The chapter on special issues has also been expanded greatly.

We hope that you enjoy and learn from this text as much as we have had fun writing it – and, ultimately, that it resides as a fitting testament to Frank and Ching.

Malcolm Harrington and Kerry Gardiner
2021

CHAPTER 1

Introduction

1.1 What is occupational health?

Occupational health is a multifaceted and multidisciplinary activity concerned with the prevention of ill health in working populations. This involves a consideration of the two-way relationship between work and health, wherein it is as much about the effects of the working environment on the health of workers as it is about the influence of the workers' state of health on their ability to perform the tasks for which they were engaged. The main aim of occupational health is to **prevent**, rather than **cure**, ill health from wherever it arises in the working environment.

$$\boxed{\text{Health} \leftrightarrow \text{Work}}$$

A joint International Labour Organization/World Health Organization (ILO/WHO) Committee defined the subject back in 1950 as: 'the promotion and

Pocket Consultant: Occupational Health, Sixth Edition. Kerry Gardiner, David Rees, Anil Adisesh, David Zalk, and Malcolm Harrington.
© 2022 John Wiley & Sons Ltd. Published 2022 by John Wiley & Sons Ltd.

maintenance of the highest degree of physical, mental and social wellbeing of workers in all occupations'.

The relationship between the worker and the world of work is, necessarily, complex (Figure 1.1). The worker brings to the place of work a pre-existent health status influenced by many factors – only some of which are under the worker's direct control; hence, any disease/illness/outcome that manifests in the individual has to be viewed in this context. The health outcome could be caused by work, modulated by work or completely unrelated to it. Such a view of occupational health is, however, predominantly a medical model; albeit now the situation was and has been realised to be very much more complex.

1.2 Who is involved in occupational health?

Historically, occupational health has been viewed as a clinical subject, implying that the dominant roles in prevention should be played by the physician and the nurse. The ILO/WHO definition from 70 years ago is explicit that a broader and fully integrated perspective is essential.

Thus, the list of professionals involved is extensive and includes:

- occupational/industrial hygienists
- physicians
- nurses
- sociologists
- toxicologists
- psychologists
- health physicists
- microbiologists
- epidemiologists
- ergonomists
- engineers (including ventilation)
- safety practitioners and safety engineers
- work organisation specialists
- acousticians
- lawyers.

Yet, the ultimate responsibility for maintaining the health of the workforce rests with the employer and, to a lesser extent, with the employee. This is the way most health and safety law is formulated. On the basis of this model, one can begin to view those involved as an even broader group. The 'stakeholders' would thus include a number of groups who, although they may not be professionally responsible for ensuring the wellbeing of the workers, do have a crucial interest in the outcome (Figure 1.2).

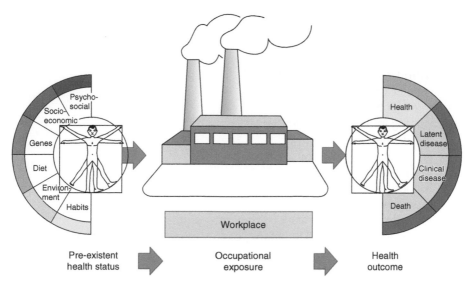

FIGURE 1.1 The problems facing the occupational health practitioner attempting to establish a link between work and health. The new employee brings a legacy of genetic, social, dietary and environmental factors affecting health to the new workplace, which may influence their response to workplace hazards.

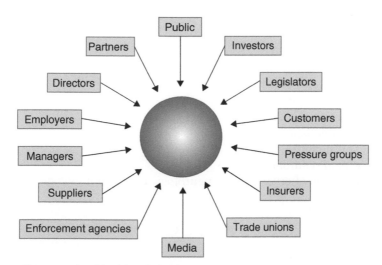

FIGURE 1.2 The occupational health stakeholders.

1.3 The world of work

The changing patterns of employment in the 'world of work' will have important and significant implications for the future make-up and expertise of occupational health, as well as for the competence needed to deliver the goods. Across the world, the days of full-time long-term employment in one industry for a worker with one set of skills are rapidly disappearing. The main features for the future seem to be:

- fragmented industry (with materials sourced globally)
- hybrid working - work and home
- smaller workforces
- more mobile employees
- waning influence of 'organised labour'
- multiskilled workers
- greater use of subcontracted tasks
- less job stability
- less job security
- more part-time work
- more flexible hours of work (zero hours contracts)
- more mechanised (and therefore possibly more dehumanised) workplaces.

1.4 The world of people at work

Today, certainly in high-income and some middle-income countries, occupational physicians see more illness but less disease. Although musculoskeletal disorders and stress-related complaints dominate the scene, they too are interrelated, and both are subject to 'somatising tendencies' (presenting as physical symptoms related to different target organ systems). Thus, the new 'age of existentialism' is dominated by such conditions as:

- stress-related disorders
- non-specific effect modifiers
- post-traumatic stress disorder
- chronic fatigue syndrome
- chronic somatising disorders
- multiple chemical sensitivity
- diffuse pain syndromes
- a combination of psychological, neurological and immunological issues.

1.5 The roles of the occupational health professional

In high-income and some upper middle-income countries, many of the 'classic' occupational diseases have been controlled or, at least, the means for controlling them are known. In fact, for many, the industries themselves have been closed and hence the incident cases have stopped – proof, if ever it were needed, of the relationship between exposure and disease. In such settings, the delivery of an effective occupational health service to employed people will become more complex and more difficult in the future; although, with greater emphasis on control, there should be less to do in dealing with the injured or sick. These, by definition, represent the 'failings' of an effective preventive programme.

Moreover, the influences of the stakeholder and the complexities of the employment scene have shifted the traditional emphasis away from the structure of 'see the health effect, diagnose the illness, find the cause' to the more proactive stance of 'control the exposure and monitor the effects'. In this model, the roles of the occupational/industrial hygienist become central and should sit as the primary or at least equal lead to the clinical aspects rather than being secondary to them. One further aspect of occupational health services is worth mentioning: in the market economies, there has been a shift towards demonstrating to employers the economic value to them of such a service (Figure 1.3).

To exemplify how the European perspective of the more clinical aspects of occupational health have changed, a brochure produced by the UK's Faculty of Occupational Medicine listed the ways in which occupational physicians can

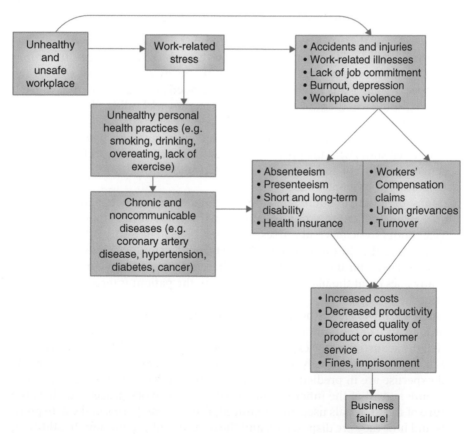

FIGURE 1.3 The business case in a nutshell. Source: Joan Burton, *WHO Healthy Workplace Framework and Model: Background and Supporting Literature and Practices*. https://www.who.int/occupational_health/healthy_workplace_framework.pdf.

help employers to 'meet their obligations' under European health and safety legislation. These included:

- helping with company compliance with the law
- advising on health and safety policy
- assisting in the control of sickness absence
- reviewing the fitness of employees following sickness absence
- managing rehabilitation
- advising on fitness to work
- managing access to first aid services
- organising health promotion initiatives
- designing and managing substance abuse programmes at work
- advising on the management and alleviation of stress
- advising employees about overseas travel on company business
- assessing employees' eligibility for long-term disability benefits or retirement on health grounds
- advising on work accommodation of employees with chronic illnesses; this is a prominent role, especially in countries with ageing workforces.

The order of these functions is probably not random, and many might dispute the contents of this list and certainly the order. Nevertheless, it demonstrates the move towards delivering an economically attractive package to the employer. Whether this is what the employee **needs** is another matter. Indeed, one can dispute whether this medical model has any real validity for the twenty-first century.

In low-income and some middle-income countries, an occupational health service often starts with the provision of medical care for the workforce (akin to a general practice at the worksite, and often with provision for the workers' dependants) (see Chapter 2).

Many of these functions are often performed by an occupational health nurse, who frequently works in isolation from any form of direct medical advice. Both physicians and nurses, however, have to be aware of their clinical limitations (either by training or by the fact that the employee is another physician's patient), and both also must see the workplace in the context of what actually goes on at the place of work and how the patient interacts with it (see Section 1.6).

Such a knowledge of the activities and processes at the place of work is a central feature of the work of the occupational/industrial hygienist, the ergonomist, the acoustician, the expert in work organisation, etc. These professionals are in short supply globally and few businesses employ their own. Their role and expertise are in predicting, recognising and understanding the sources of exposure and all of the inherent complexities of the work process, such as the nature of the materials used and produced, the intermediaries and waste products and how they are disposed of, and the methods of production. In addition, the hygienist is also an expert in measuring the concentrations and emissions of workplace contaminants/agents (and particularly the context) to assist in decision-making – particularly 'control'. It is often said that the only real responsibility of an occupational/industrial hygienist is to effect change in the workplace – to fail to do so renders any efforts in measurement and so on as moribund.

The investigation of a putative link between a hazard and health effect requires a study of the populations exposed (a task for the epidemiologist), as well as a knowledge of the toxicological effects (a task for the toxicologist) with the necessary accompaniment of a risk assessment (a task for the occupational health and safety professional with experience in risk assessment/management).

Often, safety is not only considered separately from health but also corporately located in a separate part of the organisation. This is inappropriate and counterproductive to the development and execution of an integrated health and safety strategy to protect health in the workplace.

Who does what then comes down to the resources available to the company, as well as the hazards and risks inherent in the process. As industry becomes more fragmented, the large, company-financed, multidisciplinary teams will disappear as well. The role of independent consultant advisers will then come to the fore, but the integrated activity of several professional groups working together to achieve long-term goals could be lost. In this context, the corporate control of the company may need to take the coordinating role.

Every professional providing occupational health advice and service must ensure that they have had the relevant training; the syllabus and standards are usually set/monitored by the professional bodies of their specialty that are responsible for overseeing competence. Training and education schemes are available for the main groups listed in Section 1.2. Furthermore, many of these bodies now insist upon programmes of continuing professional development for the career lifetime after successful completion of the examinations for competence.

Whatever the workplace activity and whoever is responsible for managing health and safety, the means of protecting the workforce from workplace hazards can be summarised as:

- hazard identification
- risk assessment
- management intervention
- control procedures
- review and audit effectiveness.

1.6 Occupational health in modernity

Such an ideal of the total 'ownership' of health and safety by all – managers and managed alike – may be some time distant, if it is achieved at all. Nevertheless, occupational health professionals need to be looking for the newer emphases that will emerge in the next few decades as these will influence the content and style of their work. Apart from the shifts in workforce size, skills and structure

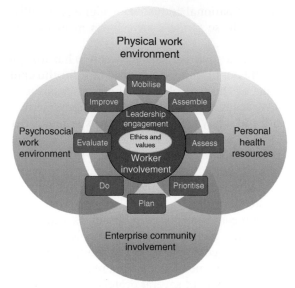

FIGURE 1.4 The World Health Organization's Healthy Workplace Model: Avenues of Influence, Process and Core Principles. *Source:* Joan Burton, *WHO Healthy Workplace Framework and Model: Background and Supporting Literature and Practices.* https://www.who.int/occupational_health/healthy_workplace_framework.pdf.

mentioned in Section 1.3, several other influences have emerged, which necessitate yet more shifts in the job content of the occupational health practitioner. These are some to think about:

- public safety/consumer protection
- public risk perceptions (and effective public risk communication)
- environmental impact of workplace process
- leisure industry risks
- hybrid working
- a drive towards the concept of 'healthy workplaces' (Figure 1.4) and 'wellbeing at work'
- being an employer of choice because of effective health-promoting programmes.

1.7 Summary

The health of the employee at a place of work is the concern of many professional groups. There is a need to identify hazards, be they physical (agents + motion), chemical, biological or psychosocial, and even those unrelated to work hazards in sufficiently resourced settings. Once identified, the risks to the workforce must be assessed and measures to control these risks must be implemented. Measuring the effectiveness of this process involves the monitoring of the workplace environment, the health status of the employees and risks to health from lifestyle factors. Auditing the effectiveness of these measures and improving the control are never-ending processes.

The absolute requirement remains the health of the worker. This is what both the workers and employers desire – a healthy high-performing workforce at work. It follows that the culture of good health and safety policy and practice must pass from the professionals – and the management – to the workforce. When everyone at the workplace believes that such policies and practice are part of their responsibility, occupational health can be considered to have achieved its main goal.

CHAPTER 2

Occupational Health Services – An International Perspective

2.1 Delivery of occupational health services

Only about 15–25% of the global workforce is covered by occupational health services. Even in developed countries provision is incomplete. Delivery is particularly low in the informal economy, agriculture and micro- and small-sized enterprises and for migrant and short-term contract workers. These work arrangements and sectors predominate in low-income and some middle-income countries but they occur in all nations. The widespread informalisation of work arrangements has probably reduced occupational health service coverage. General health services have a substantial role in the delivery of occupational health services: workers presenting to these facilities include those underserved by their enterprises or with an unrecognised

Pocket Consultant: Occupational Health, Sixth Edition. Kerry Gardiner, David Rees, Anil Adisesh, David Zalk, and Malcolm Harrington.
© 2022 John Wiley & Sons Ltd. Published 2022 by John Wiley & Sons Ltd.

work-related condition; the unemployed; and patients with diseases of long latency (cancers for instance) who have long left employment in the causative work. Many non-occupational conditions impact on work ability and require accommodation at work; the treating doctors and workplace practitioners need to work together to manage the situation optimally. The generally low level of occupational health service coverage and the interfaces between general and more specialised worker-orientated services mean that a national system should ensure that the services are complementary and that there is a goal to make at least basic occupational health services (BOHSs) universally available.

Different models exist for the provision of occupational health in various countries, with the differences lying in the mix of occupational health professionals that make up the occupational health team, the range of services that they provide, the legislative requirements and framework and the perceived needs by workers and their employers. Some of the legislative and preventive activities are performed by government departments, whereas the provision of occupational health services for groups of workers is often organised by employers. The training of occupational health professionals is usually offered by academic centres or training institutes.

An important difference between countries lies in the method used to pay for occupational health services. For those countries where there is an insurance-based workers' compensation system in place, or national legislation that requires employers to ensure that workers have access to an occupational health service, the services are often not provided by an in-house service directly connected with the company, but instead by a commercial provider from a site distant from the workplace. The range of services that can be provided in these systems is often clearly defined but restricted to what the insurance system allows or national legislation requires the employer to provide. In these types of systems the occupational health services often enjoy a degree of independence from the employer, but they may have more limited influence over workplace conditions than in other systems. In those countries where the occupational health services are paid for directly by the employer – either via an in-house service based on the company premises or purchased from an external supplier – there is the potential for services to be provided that are restricted only to what the employer wishes to purchase or provide to its staff. However, an in-house service working closely with the employer may be in the best position to identify workplace risks and influence the employer to improve working conditions in a more proactive manner.

2.2 Low- and middle-income countries

In many low- and middle-income countries (LMICs), such as in parts of Africa, South America and Asia, occupational health provision is extremely low at the enterprise or worksite level. Statutory compulsion is unlikely to extend coverage because employers (or the self-employed) do not have the resources or knowledge to provide services. International and regional agencies have, therefore, encouraged using primary care services as vehicles to deliver basic occupational health, including preventive activities. Training on the safer use of organophosphate pesticides in small-scale farming and monitoring of exposed sprayers are examples of services that can be provided through primary care.

Where occupational health services are provided, they are typically delivered as part of the general medical care for the workforce. In-house medical services are usually only available for larger companies, especially those belonging to multinational organisations. Larger companies that employ more workers have the resources to provide medical facilities for their workforce and often have occupational health policies and standards that apply to all their member companies worldwide. For LMICs, this model often places emphasis on the treatment of illnesses, whether occupational or non-occupational in origin, with fewer resources for occupational health prevention. Some companies even have their own private clinics and hospitals to care for local workers and their families. These clinical facilities also cater for the medical needs of overseas expatriate staff and their families. One reason why companies often concentrate on treatment services is the limited availability and access to medical facilities in these countries and the improved relationships with government. Another is the importance attached to dealing with the immediate health problems as they present at that time, and the often longer term health problems that arise out of hazardous occupational exposures.

Preventive occupational health functions are often organised as a separate safety (or health and safety) department, which increasingly includes environmental aspects in its remit. The model, which relies on the availability of doctors, dentists, nurses, care assistants and other clinical staff, has been described as providing 'family medicine in industry', rather than providing occupational health cover. Treatment-orientated medical services are the rule in some countries where occupational physicians focus on the recognition and treatment of occupational disease, with less emphasis on workplace visits and assessments to identify potential hazards and to recommend corrective action.

2.3 Rapidly industrialising countries

In countries such as Thailand, Malaysia, Vietnam and Indonesia (part of the group of countries referred to as the 'tiger cub economies'), there has been rapid economic and industrial development. In these countries, increasing attention is being paid to occupational and environmental health issues. In recent decades, many parts of South East Asia (particularly Malaysia, Singapore and Indonesia) have been affected by episodes of environmental haze, which enveloped the major cities. This haze was accompanied by an increase in respiratory, eye and other health effects. Historically, the source of this haze was thought to be primarily the burning of biomass material during the clearing of tropical forest areas for shifting agriculture, forestry or land development. Other contributors include traffic exhaust fumes, industrial activity and the El Niño weather phenomenon.

Occupational health professionals in these countries are increasingly involved in advising on such matters of environmental and health concern. Governmental and quasi-governmental organisations have been formed to coordinate activity on occupational and environmental health.

The developments in occupational health in Malaysia can be used as an example of how occupational health services may be provided in an industrialising country. In Malaysia, the National Council for Occupational Safety and Health (in the Ministry of Human Resources) is responsible for determining the direction and policy on occupational safety and health for the country. Several entities give effect to the Council's determinations. The Department of Occupational Safety and Health of the Ministry of Human Resources develops and enforces occupational health and safety legislation. A goal is to develop a culture of prevention in the country. The Occupational Health Unit, Institute for Medical Research, Ministry of Health, Malaysia, is a central government source of advice and information, with satellite government occupational health clinics operating in different parts of the country to provide services to health workers. A National Institute of Occupational Safety and Health (NIOSH) provides training, consultation services and information and conducts research in the field of occupational safety and health. The Malaysian Social Security Organisation has offices throughout the country and, among other responsibilities, operates workers' compensation and rehabilitation. There are several avenues for training physicians in occupational medicine. These include local academic institutions, some of which have links with training establishments in other countries. The Academy of Occupational and Environmental Medicine Malaysia represents physicians in the field of occupational and environmental medicine and aims to improve practice in these disciplines. Historically occupational hygiene lagged behind the medical disciplines, but this has improved. The Malaysian Industrial Hygiene Association promotes the discipline and supports the development of hygienists. Private clinics with occupational health doctors and more specialised multidisciplinary occupational health clinics service some larger enterprises. The country has adopted a programme to develop BOHSs in line with the recommendations put forward by the World Health Organization (WHO) and International Labour Organization to cover underserved workplaces, with small- to medium-sized enterprises a focus. With the development of notification schemes for occupational diseases, and the agreement of uniform criteria for diagnosing such diseases, the preventive aspects of occupational health services have been emphasised.

2.4 High-income countries

High-income countries usually have some legal requirement for the provision of occupational health services. The situation in Europe varies from country to country, although the directives issued by the European Commission attempt to harmonise occupational exposure standards and the requirements for occupational health provisions across the European Union (EU). The approach specifies minimum standards for compliance but allows individual flexibility and higher standards to be promulgated if desired by EU member states. In 1994, the EU established the European Agency for Safety & Health at Work (EU-OSHA), which coordinates partnership activities, communications and research. The European Risk Observatory is one of the forward-looking functions provided by EU-OSHA. The European Foundation for the Improvement of Living and Working Conditions (Eurofound) looks more towards helping to develop social, employment and work-related policies. It also conducts the well-known European Quality of Life Survey, European Working Conditions Survey and European Company Survey.

In Austria, there is a legal requirement to appoint company occupational physicians for companies with more than 50 employees to undertake health surveillance, whereas for employers with fewer staff workplace inspections that include an occupational physician should be undertaken. The staffing of occupational medical centres specifies medical management by a physician with occupational medicine training who provides at least 20 hours a week of occupational healthcare. Health surveillance is mandated for a wide range of specified substances, exposures and work activities. The Netherlands has legislation that requires active management of sickness absence in the first six weeks with the input of occupational health professionals. Other requirements are the review of a company's occupational health and safety risk assessments and the provision of health surveillance for workers identified to be at occupational risk.

In the UK, occupational health nurses and safety practitioners are among the biggest professional groups in the provision of occupational health. Specialist occupational physicians are accessible to perhaps 13% of workers while the coverage for occupational health services is around 38% of employees; for those in the public sector, in theory, coverage approaches 100%. There is however no legal requirement for the provision of occupational health services. The enforcement of health and safety legislation is the responsibility of a government agency – the Health and Safety Executive (HSE) – which is part of the Department for Work & Pensions. It employs hygienists, engineers, nurses, various scientists and a few physicians. The HSE maintains a Science and Research Centre, which provides scientific and technical advice to support government and private sector companies as well as training. The regulatory regime requires employers to appoint 'competent persons' to assist them in their health and safety duties. Doctors have to be appointed by the HSE for companies with workers exposed to some specified workplace hazards such as lead, asbestos, ionising radiation, compressed air and certain chemicals listed in the Control of Substances Hazardous to Health Regulations 2002 (as amended in 2004). Where provided, occupational health services may be an in-house facility or employers may rely on external contracted providers of occupational healthcare. Independent providers of occupational health services are organised on a regional or national level. All hospitals in the UK's National Health Service (NHS) have some form of occupational health cover, which is typically managed by human resources departments and may be in-house or contracted, or some mixture such as the physician services being a contracted element. NHS occupational health services often provide services on a commercial basis for local employers both to increase the availability of provision and to generate income for the NHS. The activities focus on preplacement fitness, collaboration with infection prevention and control for healthcare, absence management, which is a major function, and health surveillance. A particular emphasis on wellbeing has developed with an NHS Health and Wellbeing Framework that identifies 'organisational enablers' and 'health interventions'. Invariably the former are more difficult to address than the latter.

In France and Germany, the model used places emphasis on the requirement for the workforce to have periodic access to an occupational health service. The rationale is to allow a review of the health status of the workers, with the aim of early detection of ill health. If there is any indication that illness may be related to workplace factors, investigations and preventive action can follow. The French Labour Code requires employers to utilise either an intercompany occupational health service funded by participating companies or, for companies with more than 500 employees, they may establish their own integrated occupational health service (an in-house provision). The role of the occupational physician is specified in the French Labour Code, including that the occupational physician is responsible for directing a multidisciplinary team. German law provides an Act on Occupational Physicians, Safety Engineers and Other Occupational Safety Specialists, which requires employers to appoint occupational physicians and occupational safety specialists to support them in occupational safety and health as well as accident prevention. The Act lays out the duties of these professionals and requires paid continuing professional development. For smaller enterprises of less than 50 employees (varies by industry) they may not require an occupational physician. The concept of 'workplace health management' has evolved in recent years and parallels in many respects the US NIOSH's 'Total Worker Health' approach (see Section 18.8).

The Scandinavian countries, for example Finland and Sweden, have systems for occupational health cover that are much admired. In Finland, the Occupational Health Care Act obliges the employer to arrange preventive occupational healthcare services for its employees when there are one or more employees. Occupational health services can be obtained from a municipal service provider or a private medical centre. The Finnish Institute of Occupational Health (FIOH) is a national resource based in Helsinki, with satellite departments in other cities providing services for private and public organisations. FIOH is also a research and training provider with advisory functions for government, similar to the UK's HSE Science and Research Centre.

In the USA, there is variation between states in the provision of occupational health services. In New York State, private occupational and environmental medicine services predominate, including mobile clinics, multispecialty clinics and other services, invariably paid for by employers. The New York State Occupational Health Clinic Network has been developed as centres for the diagnosis of occupational disease, some with industrial hygienists attached. The hygienists are in a position to investigate the workplace with the cooperation of the employer and the unions. There is a wider network of clinics across the USA – the Association of Occupational and Environmental Clinics – but the funding and resource models vary and meeting criteria for membership is required. The diagnosis of a case of occupational disease is treated as a sentinel health event, which indicates a need to assess co-workers exposed to similar workplace factors. The main government agency for enforcing occupational health and safety legislation in the USA is the Occupational Safety and Health Administration (OSHA) – part of the Department of Labor. Another such agency is the Mine Safety and Health Administration, which oversees mining operations. Responsibility for research and health hazard evaluations lies with NIOSH in the USA. This is one of the centres within the Centers for Disease Control and Prevention (CDC) – a service as part of the Public Health Service belonging to the Department of Health and Human Services. Occupational exposure standards in the USA are produced by several organisations, including NIOSH and OSHA. However, the best known standards are the threshold limit values and biological exposure indices produced by the American Conference of Governmental Industrial Hygienists (ACGIH) – a non-governmental independent professional organisation (despite its name). The standards are reviewed annually and revised as necessary. They are used by many countries outside the USA.

In Canada the provincial and territorial ministries of labour are responsible for ensuring compliance with the Canada Labour Code and there is no national enforcing body. There is an exception for some federal employees and a range of industries that are interprovincial or international, e.g. rail and road transportation, marine shipping and banking, where the federal government takes jurisdiction. There is no mandated provision of occupational health services, although certain aspects of provincial legislation may require some provision, such as the Ontario Designated Substances Act, which has a code for medical surveillance. This requires the periodic recording of a medical history, physical examination and clinical tests as specified, and is conducted at the employer's expense. Although not all physicians would perhaps have familiarity with the substances listed, it is accepted, and not uncommon, that employees choose to see their family physician for these purposes. An unusual model of provision is the Occupational Health Clinics for Ontario Workers, which arose from union sponsorship and now has seven clinics with funding from the provincial Ministry of Labour. Large employers and public sector organisations tend to have occupational health provision that may be in-house, private sector or a mixture of provision. A common driver for the use of occupational health is what is termed 'disability management', which is the approach to managing return to work for ill or injured employees. For occupational exposure standards these can vary between provinces and territories that follow ACGIH standards, but not necessarily the current version.

Australia has a federal structure with six states and two territories and 10 statutes relating to work health and safety with a Commonwealth Act for employees and another for maritime and offshore operations. There is no requirement to promote the use of specialist work health and safety services by 'persons conducting businesses or undertakings' (PCBU) – this term encompasses employers and subcontractors. Guidance from Safe Work Australia requires that where a relevant exposure exists the PCBU engages a 'health monitoring doctor' who is a registered medical practitioner with experience in health monitoring. New Zealand also uses the PCBU terminology in its updated Health and Safety at Work Act (2015). There is a similar requirement for health monitoring, although it is clarified that this is carried out or supervised by an occupational health practitioner (a medical doctor, registered nurse or nurse practitioner) with knowledge, skills and experience in health monitoring.

2.5 From occupational health to healthy workplaces

Successful measures have been introduced to reduce workplace exposures and prevent occupational disease in some industries. These have mainly occurred in high-income countries and have resulted in occupational health attention being directed at more difficult targets for achieving better health; for example, the reduction of stress, retaining workers with chronic diseases in employment and activities aimed at strengthening the health status of workers. Occupational health services in these countries may also place emphasis on general health improvement measures in addition to workplace assessment and health surveillance. Health promotion activities include the provision of facilities for regular exercise at the workplace, campaigns to reduce cigarette smoking and advice on the consumption of alcohol in moderation, safe driving and healthy diet. The rationale proposed for this approach is that, once traditional occupational diseases are prevented, the focus should shift to the improvement of the general health status of the workforce. Unfortunately, in some workplaces general health activities have been emphasised at the expense of efforts towards the reduction and control of workplace hazards. In many instances these activities are not considered in relation to the hazards faced by workers, e.g. cholesterol testing of welders rather than a more beneficial smoking cessation programme for this group.

The WHO has given encouragement for this more comprehensive approach to health and work through its *Healthy Workplace Framework and Model: Background and Supporting Literature and Practice*. The Framework identifies four main avenues of influence on health: the physical work environment (the part of the workplace facility that can be detected by human or electronic senses); the psychosocial work environment (which includes the organisation of work and the workplace stressors that may cause emotional or mental stress to workers); personal health resources (efforts to improve or maintain healthy personal lifestyle practices, as well as to monitor and support their ongoing physical and mental health); and enterprise community involvement (the activities and other resources that an enterprise engages in or provides to the community in which it operates). There is an evidence-based case given for the Framework and guidance on its implementation.

2.6 Functions of occupational health services

The range of functions provided by occupational health services is given below.

Clinical occupational health activities

Preplacement assessments
Preplacement assessments vary from the use of a self-completed questionnaire to a general 'hands-on' clinical examination by a physician. The argument against the use of a questionnaire is that job applicants wanting to be employed may be somewhat economical with the truth when answering questions on the state of their health. This is especially the case when the denial of ever experiencing specific health problems is difficult to check and confirm. General clinical examinations are, however, time-consuming and have a low detection rate for relevant abnormalities. A compromise approach is to use an initial screening questionnaire focused on bona fide health requirements and the expected work activities with a staged evaluation, first by an occupational health technician or nurse and then by an occupational physician where indicated (further details of health assessments are discussed in Chapter 5). With promulgation of human rights legislation that prohibits discrimination on the grounds of protected characteristics such as sex, gender and disability, preplacement assessment and its use needs to be aligned with jurisdictional requirements.

Periodic medical examinations (including health surveillance)
These may be performed because of statutory requirements or when clinically indicated for groups of workers exposed to specific hazards. In many countries, examples of statutory medical examinations include clinical examination of professional drivers and examination and blood lead determination for workers exposed to lead compounds. Periodic examinations have also been advocated in health surveillance schemes for workers exposed to respiratory sensitisers, such as isocyanates. The health surveillance of specific groups, for example executives, is often in demand from employers and the executives themselves. This is based on the following assumptions: executive staff are expensive to employ, they make critical decisions that can affect the success of the company, they are time-consuming to train and they are difficult to replace; therefore, employers often choose to place executives in a system where there is periodic confirmation that they are in good health. Despite this, executive medical examinations are of questionable economic value and some practices are ethically questionable, leading to spurious findings. They are costly to perform, with a low detection rate of significant clinical abnormalities. It has also been argued that, if there is clinical value in such periodic assessments, they should be made available to other categories of staff.

Post-sickness absence review
The rationale behind reviewing individuals with long-term sickness absence is to ensure that the cause of the illness has not affected their capacity to continue in

their present job. It also allows any necessary adjustments to the workplace to be made to accommodate the individual temporarily or permanently on his/her return to work. For food industries, occupational health services often have the responsibility to ensure that workers are non-infectious before returning to handling food products, especially after a spell of gastrointestinal illness.

Key questions that are often asked of the clinician include the following.

- Can you confirm that there is an underlying medical condition causing the absence and that the length of absence is consistent with that condition?
- Can you estimate the length of time the employee is likely to be absent with this condition?
- Can you indicate whether on return to work the employee is likely to be able to resume his or her normal duties?
- Are there likely to be any significant implications for the health and safety of the employee, or others, on his or her return to work?
- Should restricted duties, redeployment or retirement on the grounds of ill health be considered at this stage?
- Are there any legal implications for the management of this case?

The answers to these questions allow the employer to actively manage and plan ahead for the employee's return to work. It is not necessary for the manager to know confidential medical information in order to manage the employee. Occupational health professionals may also add value to these reports by identifying workplace factors that may have aggravated or incited the condition, suggesting ways of protecting this employee and others who may be similarly exposed, offering advice on rehabilitation and reintegration strategies and, where appropriate, helping the employee to address the occupational factors that may lead to protracted sickness absence. Absence from work is itself a risk factor for developing other conditions, through social exclusion, isolation and deteriorating physical condition. It is generally accepted that good work is therapeutic and that an early, safe, sustainable return to work is beneficial.

Immunisation

This is provided by occupational health departments for healthcare workers (see Section 4.2) and laboratory and research staff, when the workforce includes many employees travelling abroad as part of their job duties or when specific vaccine-preventable infections are encountered in the course of work. Travel to many locations requires that the necessary immunisations against communicable diseases are provided (see Sections 4.3 and 4.5). When this is performed by occupational health departments, it also involves general health advice for other infectious diseases, for example sexually transmitted diseases and foodborne infections.

Health education and counselling

The encouragement of workers to look after their health in terms of healthy lifestyles, proper diets, avoidance of smoking, consumption of alcohol in moderation, adequate exercise and reduction of cardiovascular risk factors has been incorporated into the activities of many occupational health services. These efforts are aimed at using access to the workforce to reduce risk factors for diseases in general, in part driven by reduced employer health insurance costs, and to introduce measures to prevent occupational disorders. These efforts must take into consideration the context of the workplace culture and work activities to be effective.

Treatment

The functions of occupational health services may include provision of services from first aid and treatment of minor injuries to the provision of full curative medicine facilities. The extent of clinical services within occupational health services varies from non-existent to the availability of dentists, chiropodists and opticians. The provision is dependent upon the local operating circumstances and the nature of the industry.

Rehabilitation

Occupational health staff can liaise with treating clinicians and workplace managers for the facilitation of rehabilitation and return to work. Familiarity with the workplace and job alternatives and an understanding of the illness or disability stand the occupational health staff in good stead for this activity.

Workplace assessments

It follows that, without exposure, there is no effect. Therefore, the evaluation of the workplace to eliminate or reduce exposure is critical in achieving the aims of the occupational health service. These tasks are usually carried out by occupational hygienists, who structure their work in terms of recognition, evaluation and control as follows.

Recognition

This is not really a function, but includes the understanding of the toxicology of contaminants or disease aetiology, the industrial process itself (and all of its hazards) and the law.

Evaluation

This often starts at the point of a walk-through survey, where knowledge of the process/contaminant means that decisions can be made without recourse to measurements, and extends to situations in which sophisticated measurements and/or analytical techniques are necessary to quantify the contaminant with the required accuracy/precision.

Control

The most important attribute of any occupational health professional, but specifically an occupational hygienist, is to be able to improve the work environment. Occupational hygienists use their knowledge of disciplines, such as industrial chemistry, chemical engineering and ventilation design, to try to ensure that the putative agent is either eliminated or controlled.

General advice and support

Advice on compensation
When an occupational disease has been diagnosed, or is considered likely, occupational health services are able to advise the patient on obtaining benefits through workers' compensation schemes or industrial injuries and diseases benefit.

Disaster planning and advice on dealing with chemical incidents
Planning committees for the development of procedures to deal with chemical spills, road and rail accidents with the discharge of chemicals into the environment, emissions from industrial sites or pandemic preparedness often include staff from occupational health services. Occupational health professionals can facilitate communication with managers of industrial sites and advise on the nature and extent of exposure, possible health effects and appropriate personal protective equipment for rescue and emergency crew.

Food hygiene
The provision of advice to food handlers and on precautions for the safe handling of food is an important role for occupational health services in the food industry (see Section 4.5). In addition to the need to ensure the health of the workforce, there is the additional requirement to ensure the safety of the food product.

Advice on environmental issues
Occupational health services are increasingly covering safety and environmental issues, such that some departments are now organised as safety, health and environment (SHE) services. The activities under this umbrella are often to be found in organisational corporate social responsibility reports.

Other activities

Audit, quality assurance and evaluation
Part of the work of occupational health services involves compliance with internal and external quality standards. An audit or systematic, critical review of the structure, process and outcome can lead to steps to improve the quality of the service; as such, the term quality improvement is commonly used (see Section 18.5).

Worker protection and business protection
The challenge for occupational health services is to provide a balance of functions: to detect and control workplace hazards early; to recognise occupational

disease without missing non-occupational illness; to provide effective health surveillance; to facilitate treatment, rehabilitation and return to work; and to ensure that the business of the employer can be conducted safely without detriment to the health of the workforce while contributing to corporate goals for community engagement.

Further Reading

World Health Organization and Burton, J. (2010). *WHO Healthy Workplace Framework and Model: Background and Supporting Literature and Practices*. World Health Organization https://apps.who.int/iris/handle/10665/113144.

CHAPTER 3

Occupational Diseases

3.1 Historical perspective

People were subject to hazards in their daily life long before the Industrial Revolution and the advent of industrial workplaces. True occupational exposures must have arrived by the time of the Stone Age – the knapping of flints resulting in silica exposure, for example. This task, however, produces only small clouds of silica dust and our ancestors are unlikely to have lived long enough to die of silicosis. The fashioning of iron tools and the development of mining and smelting are more likely to have increased the dangers for those so engaged.

Indeed, mining was recognised in ancient Egyptian times as being so hazardous that the job was reserved for slaves and criminals. It was not until Agricola (1494–1555) and Paracelsus (1493–1541) formally recorded these risks to employed mediaeval

Pocket Consultant: Occupational Health, Sixth Edition. Kerry Gardiner, David Rees, Anil Adisesh, David Zalk, and Malcolm Harrington.
© 2022 John Wiley & Sons Ltd. Published 2022 by John Wiley & Sons Ltd.

artisans that any real attention was paid to their plight. By the sixteenth century, mining had become a skilled occupation, and Agricola not only described the hazards but also prescribed some remedies, such as improvements to ventilation and mine shaft design, which were necessary to diminish the staggering death rate in the mines of Joachimsthal and Schneeberg in the Carpathians. The same Carpathian Mountains are still mined today, but, instead of silver (used to make the Joachimsthaler = thaler = dollar), the main ore extracted is uranium. Recent studies in these mining areas have identified high risks of lung cancer in workers and residents. This may explain the rampant 'consumption' and 'an angel choking old miners to death' noted by Agricola, which was possibly lung cancer caused by radioactive gases and dusts.

Nevertheless, the first general and authoritative treatise on diseases related to occupations was written by Bernardino Ramazzini (1633–1714), the physician to the D'Este family in Modena, Italy. His book *De Morbis Artificum* is still unparalleled as a source of classic descriptions of many occupational diseases, ranging from those of cesspit workers to those of the mirror silverers of Murano, Italy. His work was largely unread until the Industrial Revolution in Britain brought occupational diseases to the attention of large numbers of people. Child labour and the atrocious working conditions in the cotton mills of Lancashire shocked many late Georgians and early Victorians, and the first factory legislation was pushed through by philanthropic factory owners, such as Robert Owen, Michael Sadler, Anthony Astley Cooper (Earl of Shaftesbury) and Robert Peel, despite some stiff opposition.

In the UK, the first occupational health law, the Health and Morals of Apprentices Act of 1802, was greatly weakened by amendments in Parliament, but it started the process of legislation to protect workers that culminated in the Health and Safety at Work, etc. Act of 1974. In between these dates, successive Acts reduced the hours of work, particularly of women and young children, and the Factory Act of 1833 established the factory inspectorate. Four inspectors were appointed to cover the whole country. Eleven years later, the inspectors were given the additional power to appoint certifying surgeons in each district to decide on the age of children. The advent of birth certification in 1836 eventually made that role redundant, but an embryonic industrial medical service had been born. Later Acts gave these surgeons other duties, including the investigation of industrial accidents and the certification of fitness for work.

In the USA, the first child labour law was passed in the State of Massachusetts in 1836, requiring that employed children aged under 15 years must have at least 3 months in school per year. Similar legislation followed in most European countries as the Industrial Revolution proceeded apace. By the turn of the twentieth century, the toxic effect of certain materials in widespread use in industry was sufficiently well recognised in Europe and North America to warrant their notification. This provided the power to investigate cases of suspected occupational diseases, with a view to prevention.

Initiatives to protect workers were not confined to the most industrialised parts of the world. South Africa's response to a crisis of occupational disease in gold mining is illustrative. South Africa became the first state to compensate silicosis (1911) and tuberculosis (1916) as occupational diseases. The Witwatersrand mines were among the first globally to invest heavily in dust control technologies, and the Miners' Phthisis Acts of 1911, 1916 and 1919 were among the first to introduce a statutory system of medical surveillance. The system mandated pre-employment examinations to evaluate fitness of men to work in mining and exit medicals to identify those eligible for compensation claims. Traumatic injury received less attention and rates remained high.

In the UK, the first agents to become notifiable (in 1895) were lead, phosphorus, arsenic and anthrax. The list later extended to some 16 diseases. The flood of notifications that emanated from the print factories, match works, smelters and slaughterhouses in the nineteenth century necessitated the appointment in 1898 of the first medical inspector of factories, Sir Thomas Legge (1863–1932). Legge is famous for many things, not least the furore over his resignation in 1919 due to the government's refusal to ratify an international convention prohibiting the use of white lead for the inside painting of buildings. His aphorisms, although sounding a little paternalistic to twenty-first century ears, are still worth citing.

1. Unless and until the employer has done everything (and everything is a lot), the workman can do little to protect himself.
2. If you bring an influence to bear external to the workman (i.e. one over which he can exercise no control), you will be successful and if you do not, or cannot, you will not be successful.
3. Practically all lead poisoning is due to inhalation.
4. All workers should be told something of the hazards of the materials they work with – if they find out for themselves it may cost them their lives.
5. Influences, useful up to a point but not completely effective when not external but dependent on the will or whim of workers, include respirators, goggles, gloves, etc.

Today, the task of providing occupational health services for all workers is still an unattained ideal, even in developed countries. Furthermore, although many of the older occupational diseases are controlled, new ones continue to surface. The need for continued control is essential, but the registration of occupational diseases and injuries is an imprecise tool, even in the most developed of countries.

3.2 The toll of occupational injuries and disease

Occupational injuries

Accidental injuries at work are common, but the precise numbers are unclear as under-reporting is also common, especially in low- and middle-income countries and in the informal economy (both the informal sector and informal work arrangements in the formal economy such as casual work and seasonal migrancy). A great deal of data on workplace injuries (and diseases) are available from the International Labour Organization (ILO) through its ILOSTAT website (https://ilostat.ilo.org/topics/safety-and-health-at-work). The ILO estimates that there are 340 million occupational accidents annually, 360 000 of them fatal. Economic sectors with the highest injury fatality rates vary by country but construction; agriculture, forestry and fishing; mining; and transport are prominent in many localities.

Occupational diseases

Extent of occupational ill health

Occupational ill-health rates are imprecise in most of the world partly because the work-relatedness of these maladies is unrecognised or, when it is, not reported, because of more urgent demands on clinicians or scarcity of reporting systems. Nevertheless, estimates of the Global Burden of Occupational Disease (GBD) have been published. Notably, a 2020 publication by the GBD 2016 Risk Factors Collaborators presents information on several risk factors (determinants of ill health) for men and women and by world regions. Selected GBD 2016 data are shown in Table 3.1. Disability-adjusted life years (DALYs) are essentially the years of disability experienced by the population as a consequence of the factor; and the population attributable fraction (PAF) is the percentage of disease in a population that would be avoided had the risk factor been absent.

The DALYs show a negative impact on the quality of life of millions of people and support the GBD 2016 Risk Factors Collaborators' conclusion that 'Occupational exposures continue to cause an important health burden world-wide, justifying the need for ongoing prevention and control initiatives.'

At country level, there are great variations in the quality and style of the reporting of occupational diseases, with reported incidences varying by one or even two orders of magnitude. Some of this reflects true differences, but it is possible that most of the variance is due to shortcomings in the reporting procedures

---

TABLE 3.1

Global deaths, disability-adjusted life years (DALYs) and population attributable fractions (PAFs) for PMGF + SHS[a], ergonomic risk factors and noise for 2016.

Risk factor	Deaths	DALYs (years)	PAF (%)
PMGF + SHS	460 000	10 687 953	16.9
Ergonomic risk factors	0	15 479 932	26.8
Noise	0	7 108 277	19.6

[a] PMGF + SHS = particulate matter, gases and fumes and second-hand smoke causing chronic obstructive pulmonary disease.
Source: Data from GBD 2016 Occupational Risk Factors Collaborators (2020).

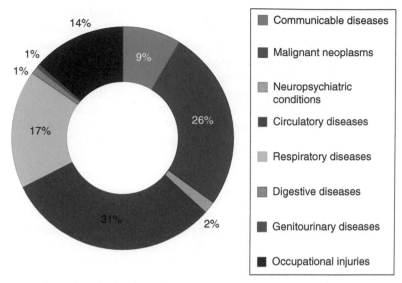

14%

1%

1%

9%

26%

17%

31%

2%

- Communicable diseases
- Malignant neoplasms
- Neuropsychiatric conditions
- Circulatory diseases
- Respiratory diseases
- Digestive diseases
- Genitourinary diseases
- Occupational injuries

FIGURE 3.1 Estimated work-related mortality by cause for 2015. *Source:* Hämäläinen et al. (2017).

or to poorer systems for prevention of occupational ill health. Countries with good registration systems report average rates of occupational disease at a level of 4–12 cases per 1000 employed, but there is great disparity between the lists of registrable occupational diseases between countries.

Occupational mortality

In 2017, the Workplace Safety and Health Institute, Singapore (www.wshi.gov.sg) published estimates of the proportions of worldwide work-related mortality by cause. The estimates are surprising, as shown in Figure 3.1: fatal diseases combined far outweighed occupational injuries (14%). The main cause of work-related death was circulatory diseases (31%), and cancers made a substantial contribution (26%). Communicable diseases caused only 9% of fatalities but the proportion was higher in low-income countries.

3.3 The ILO List of Occupational Diseases (Revised 2010)

To help recognise occupational diseases, to improve consistency in reporting and to enhance workers' compensation systems, the ILO in 2010 produced an updated list of occupational diseases. The list is organised into four categories: (i) occupational diseases caused by exposure to agents arising from work activities, with sub-categories of chemical, physical and biological agents and infections or parasitic diseases; (ii) target organ systems; (iii) occupational cancers; and

(iv) other diseases. This listing covers 41 chemicals, 7 physical agents, 9 biological agents, 12 respiratory diseases, 4 skin diseases, 8 musculoskeletal diseases, 2 mental and behavioural disorders, 21 carcinogens and 2 other diseases. Each of these categories also includes an 'open category' that allows for any other diseases not mentioned in the preceding items, meaning the list can be customised for jurisdictional use. Member countries are urged to use the list for several purposes, including recording and reporting of occupational diseases and workers' compensation   (https://www.ilo.org/wcmsp5/groups/public/---ed_protect/----protrav/---safework/documents/publication/wcms:125137.pdf).

3.4 Diagnosis of occupational diseases

The rigour applied in deciding on attribution of a disease to occupational exposures or workplace conditions varies according to its purpose. In most workers' compensation jurisdictions, attribution is on the balance of probability, meaning greater than 50% probability that the condition arose from work. Thus, there can be quite a lot of uncertainty about the aetiology, but work attribution would still be reasonable. If removal from further exposure to a putative causative agent is relatively easy to arrange without loss of benefits to the worker, a precautionary approach is sensible, even in the face of quite substantial diagnostic uncertainty. But, if attribution of a disease to work may result in job loss, especially in settings of scant social security benefits, more stringent diagnostic criteria are necessary. Criteria more demanding than on the balance of probability are also commonly required in some legal proceedings, for example if negligence by an employer is at issue, the association between the disease and work usually needs to be firmly established.

Nevertheless, the key diagnostic criteria are common to all settings. Notably, the identification of an occupational disease may be considered a 'sentinel event' signalling the potential need to examine co-workers and strategies to reduce workplace exposures at the causative workplaces.

The key criteria for diagnosing an occupational disease are:

- clinical effects that fit those known to be associated with the agent
- evidence of sufficient workplace exposure to the agent
- an interval of time between exposure and effect that fits in with the pathophysiology
- a consideration of other diseases that can cause similar effects. If other non-occupational determinants exist, then a clinical decision may be made regarding causation on the basis of probable contribution of each cause (apportionment) or else it may be accepted that it is not realistic to reliably distinguish between the relative importance of competing causes but that work was on balance probably a material contributor to the disease.

The above criteria are especially useful for agents where a threshold level of exposure can be determined below which health effects are unlikely to occur. Attribution of ill health to exposure to an agent is more difficult for allergens and some carcinogens. Genotoxic carcinogens do not appear to have an easily determined threshold for safety. Allergens may require considerable exposure for sensitisation, but, once sensitised, individuals can react to molecular amounts of the agent.

The European Commission publishes information on a list of occupational diseases (https://osha.europa.eu/en/legislation/guidelines/information-notices-on-occupational-diseases-a-guide-to-diagnosis). The list includes many diseases and information on each condition, including a description of the causative agent, the known acute, chronic, local and systemic clinical effects and a statement on the required:

- minimum intensity of exposure – the minimum amount of exposure necessary to produce disease
- minimum duration of exposure – the minimum length of exposure time for disease to result
- maximum latent period – the maximum length of time following cessation of exposure, beyond which it is unlikely that the link between clinical effects and exposure is causal
- induction period – the minimum time necessary between initial exposure and the development of clinical effects.

Other problems in attributing aetiology include the additive or synergistic effect from mixed exposures and 'low' levels of exposure that are associated with health effects. Pre-existing disease, although not caused by work, may be 'work aggravated' or 'exacerbated'. Employees with work aggravated or exacerbated conditions may be eligible for workers' compensation and their occurrence emphasises the importance of protecting vulnerable workers from workplace exposures.

3.5 Target organs

Introduction

In this section, consideration is given to the organs of the body and the way they respond to insult and assault from occupationally related agents. Toxicological information on most agents cited is given in Chapter 6. However, it is the organ's response to injury that will usually herald the onset of ill health. This is what brings the worker to the attention of physicians. Chronic lead poisoning, for example, may present itself in a variety of system dysfunctions, and the physician will have to unravel the differential diagnosis: it is a rare event indeed for a patient to complain of over-exposure to inorganic lead!

The target organ systems included in this section are:

- respiratory system
- central and peripheral nervous system
- genitourinary system

- cardiovascular system
- skin
- liver
- reproductive system
- bone marrow.

Respiratory System

Structure
The upper and lower respiratory tracts are particularly vulnerable to occupationally related noxious agents. Over 80% of these agents gain access to the body through the respiratory system. The effects of such exposure may also be felt in other organ systems, but the brunt of the damage frequently occurs in the air passages and lungs.

The system is composed of several anatomically discrete sections:

- the mouth, nasal sinuses, pharynx and larynx
- the trachea, main and segmental bronchi
- the bronchioli
- the alveoli
- the alveolar–capillary interface.

The repeated branching of the airways from tracheal bifurcation to alveoli has the effect of greatly increasing the surface area of the respiratory mucosae, while reducing the rate of air flow. Thus, the 300 million alveoli offer a surface area of some $70\,m^2$ for gas exchange, but no alveolus exceeds 0.1 mm in diameter. The thickness of the alveolar epithelial wall, together with the endothelial cell layer of the pulmonary capillaries, is, in health, rarely greater than 0.001 mm and constitutes the blood–gas interface.

Testing function
The main function of the lungs is to supply oxygen for uptake by the pulmonary capillaries and to provide the means for removing carbon dioxide diffusing in the opposite direction. The successful achievement of this gas exchange requires three main system functions:

- ventilation
- gas transfer
- blood–gas transport.

Lung function tests can be similarly grouped.

Ventilatory function is commonly measured by a variety of portable instruments, the most common of which are the peak flow meter and the spirometer. Developments in microcomputer analysis have been of great benefit in providing rapid digital and graphical read-outs of ventilatory function. Computerised data can also be stored and compared with pre-programmed normal values. The main indices determined are:

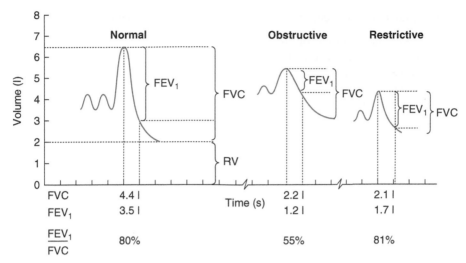

FIGURE 3.2 Spirograms to illustrate the difference in forced expiratory volume in 1 s (FEV$_1$) and forced vital capacity (FVC) in health, airways obstruction and restrictive defects (such as diffuse lung fibrosis or severe spinal deformity). Inspiration is upwards and expiration downwards. Although the vital capacity is reduced in both obstructive and restrictive lung disease, the proportion expired in 1 s shows considerable differences. RV is residual volume.

- forced expiratory volume in one second (FEV1)
- forced mid-expiratory flow rate (FEF25–75%)
- forced vital capacity (FVC)
- vital capacity (VC)
- FEV$_1$/FVC ratio
- flow/volume patterns.

Figure 3.2 illustrates these indices.

Gas transfer and transport measurements require less portable apparatus and are a means of assessing:

- ventilation/perfusion ratios – mainly involving the use of radioactive gases
- gas diffusion – usually transfer of carbon monoxide (TL$_{co}$ or DL$_{co}$)
- red cell gas uptake and transport – usually blood gas levels and pH.
  Lung function is altered by a number of non-occupational factors and tables of 'normal' values take some of these variables into account, including
  - age
  - sex
  - height
  - ethnic group, which is also required by some prediction equations.

The Global Lung Function Initiative (https://www.ers-education.org/guide-lines/global-lung-function-initiative) has produced reference equations for spirometry across a wide age range that are suitable for many populations. These are particularly useful where local reference equations are unavailable or outdated.

Other factors that affect the results of lung function tests include:

- smoking habits or use of bronchodilators
- a heavy meal or a recent chest infection
- exercise tolerance
- observer error
- instrument error
- diurnal variation
- ambient temperature.

Chest imaging

The chest radiograph remains the most important imaging tool for surveillance – and diagnosis in most settings – but computed tomography is a common diagnostic tool in high-income countries.

The chest radiograph can show structural lung damage from workplace exposures and infections and is thus useful for diagnosis and surveillance. Nevertheless, frequent routine surveillance should be avoided unless there is clear benefit. In high-burden tuberculosis settings, the chest radiograph is a useful part of the set of screening tools for workers exposed to respirable crystalline silica.

A classification of chest radiographs has been agreed internationally for use in standardising the coding of radiological features of pneumoconioses. This ILO classification requires a chest radiograph to be taken in a standard fashion, read and classified to a standard format in comparison with reference radiographs. A version with digital images has been produced. The main features of this format are listed in Table 3.2.

- Profusion relates to the area of spread across the lung fields, with 0 being none and 3 very extensive.
- Type relates to the size and shape of the opacities.
- Extent relates to the zones affected.

The 0, 1, 2 and 3 profusion groups can be extended to a 12-point system: 0/−, 0/0, 0/1, 1/0, 1/1, 1/2, 2/1, 2/2, 2/3, 3/2, 3/3, 3/+.

Pathology
Occupational lung disorders
Harmful effects to the lung produced by noxious agents can be grouped into the following categories:

- acute inflammation
- work-related asthma and chronic obstructive pulmonary disease (COPD)
- pneumoconiosis
- hypersensitivity pneumonitis (extrinsic allergic alveolitis)
- malignancy (see Chapter 7)
- infections (see Chapter 4).

Acute inflammation This is primarily caused by the irritant gases and fumes. Their solubility determines whether their effects are most noticeable in the upper or lower respiratory tracts.

TABLE **3.2**	

International Labour Organization classification of pneumoconioses.

Feature	Classification
No pneumoconiosis	0
Pneumoconiosis	
Rounded small opacities	
Profusion	1, 2, 3
Type	p, q, r
Extent	Zones: upper, middle and lower
Irregular small opacities	
Profusion	1, 2, 3
Type	s, t, u
Extent	Zones: upper, middle and lower
Large opacities (≥ 1 cm)	
Size	A, B, C
Pleural plaques	By site, extent and calcification
Pleural thickening	By site and extent
Other features	Many abnormalities unrelated to pneumoconioses

Soluble gases that irritate the upper respiratory tract will cause affected individuals to move away from the source of the gas (a protective mechanism). Examples of such gases are:

- ammonia
- chlorine
- sulphur dioxide.

Some irritant gases can also cause a delayed pulmonary oedema, with respiratory distress occurring 24–72 hours after exposure. Examples are:

- nitric oxide
- phosgene
- fluorine
- ozone.

Work-related asthma This type of asthma is either exacerbated by work or caused by workplace exposures, i.e. occupational. Work exacerbation is the triggering of bronchospasm or worsening of *pre-existing* asthma as a result of exposure while working. Almost all workplaces have exposures that can exacerbate asthma – cold air, cleaning materials, irritants, physical exertion, smoke – so work exacerbation is common. Occupational asthma is of two types: irritant induced; and immunologically mediated following a period of sensitisation. Irritant-induced asthma occurs after a short intense encounter with an irritant, or after more prolonged exposure but still at fairly high levels. Sensitiser-induced asthma may be caused by a variety of materials, which, once a worker is sensitised, produce an immediate reaction or a late (non-immediate) type. The former may develop within minutes of exposure; the latter may take four to eight hours to develop. It is in this latter group that the suspicion of a work-related cause may be missed as the effects of the allergenic material may not be noticed until the night of the day of exposure, when the individual is away from the workplace. Some affected individuals experience a combination of immediate and late effects, and others may have repeated episodes of asthma attacks. The two main types of occupational asthma due to agents of different molecular weight are contrasted in Table 3.3.

TABLE 3.3

Occupational asthma due to high- and low-molecular-weight agents.

Agent	Examples	IgE	Specific inhalation challenge
High-molecular-weight protein antigen (>10 kDa)	Flour/cereals Enzymes especially proteases Rodent urine Seafood Latex Insects and mites (nearly 400 agents identified) Wood dusts	Typically elicited by skin prick or specific IgE blood test	Immediate type most often
Low-molecular-weight chemicals (<10 kDa)	Toluene di-isocyanate Acid anhydrides Epoxy resins Metal salts, e.g. platinum salts Plicatic acid (woods) Abietic acid (colophony)	Uncommonly identifiable	Late-type reaction more common

IgE, immunoglobulin E.

Occupational asthma has been estimated as causing around 15% of all adult-onset asthmas, but it is important to realise that atopy is not a strongly predisposing state. Although a good occupational and medical history is important to the diagnosis, some cases are exceedingly difficult to unravel. In these rare cases, it may be necessary to resort to bronchial challenge testing, which should only be performed by trained, competent staff and in hospital facilities with full clinical back-up. Skin prick testing and serology for immunoglobulin E (IgE) levels are more readily available and may also be of value. Serial peak expiratory flow (PEF) recordings while the worker is still present in the workplace during periods at and off work for at least three weeks with a minimum of four daily readings are useful confirmatory tests. They require careful plotting and interpretation; this can be assisted by computerised software such as the free Oasys (http://www.occupationalasthma.com/default.aspx). Pre- and post-workplace exposure measurement of sputum eosinophils can increase the specificity of serial PEF while fractional expired nitric oxide is an emerging diagnostic tool.

Treatment ideally involves the removal of the sensitised subject from exposure (in some cases, this may necessitate a change in job) and non-specific treatment for the asthmatic symptoms.

Prevention involves several factors:

- elimination of the causative agent
- substitution with less allergenic materials
- process enclosure or segregation
- local and general ventilation
- efficient and rigorous hygiene control in the workplace, e.g. cleaning practices
- effective personal respiratory protection for the worker for specific unavoidable tasks where exposure is anticipated
- identification of workers at risk – not an easy task; determining atopic individuals is of limited use as up to 30% of the population have atopic characteristics and atopy is not necessarily a prognostic feature for occupational asthma
- health surveillance, with pre- and post-shift ventilatory capacity measurements (secondary prevention).

Byssinosis There is some debate over whether byssinosis should be classified as a type of occupational asthma. The condition is, however, broader and more complex than other forms of asthma. In susceptible individuals, exposure to the dusts of cotton, sisal, hemp or flax can produce acute dyspnoea, with cough and reversible obstruction of the airways. It is noticed initially on the first day of the working week and then subsides on subsequent days. Later, with continued exposure, symptoms also occur on subsequent days of the week, until even weekends and holidays are not free of symptoms.

The effects are greatest where the dust concentrations are highest and are more noticeable with coarser cotton. This has led to the suggestion that the condition is (in part) due to organic contaminants of the cotton boll, such as bracts, and Gram-negative bacterial endotoxin. Smoking exacerbates the condition and, although irreversible obstruction of the airways may eventually supervene, with possible resulting fatality, no specific pathological features have been identified in the lungs at post-mortem. Chest radiography is unhelpful and treatment is symptomatic.

Studies of Ulster flax workers and Lancashire cotton workers have cast doubt on the ability of this condition to influence mortality rates. Byssinosis, as described today, is probably a mixture of conditions ranging from true asthma to exacerbated chronic bronchitis.

Chronic obstructive pulmonary disease COPD is defined by the Global Initiative for Chronic Obstructive Lung Disease (GOLD) as being characterised by 'persistent respiratory symptoms and airflow limitation that is due to airway and/or alveolar abnormalities usually caused by significant exposure to noxious particles or gases and influenced by host factors including abnormal lung development'. Work-related COPD is clinically indistinguishable from the disease caused by other inhaled toxins, smoking of course being the most common. Consequently, the diagnostic criteria and treatment are the same irrespective of the cause. The GOLD publications are comprehensive and reliable references for prevention, diagnosis and treatment (https://goldcopd.org). To make a diagnosis the post-bronchodilator spirometry (FEV_1/FVC ratio <70%) is required; the 5th percentile lower limit of normal (LLN) of the ratio of FEV_1 to VC may be preferred. Where there is repeated longitudinal spirometry, a 15% annual decline plus that expected from ageing in FEV_1 is considered excessive.

COPD is now firmly associated with work exposures and around 30% of COPD cases in non-smokers might be attributed to work. Early studies linked the condition to specific agents such as silica, coal mine dust and cadmium, but more recent population-based investigations have found associations with less specific exposures generally termed vapours, gases, dusts and fumes (VGDF). About 15% of COPD cases would be prevented if workplace causes were avoided.

Work attribution in individual workers is often complex. One reason for this is that the disease has multiple non-occupational causes – smoking, general environmental pollution and burning of fossil fuels for heating and cooking being the most widespread. Another is that there is great variation in individual responses to respiratory toxins: only approximately 20% of long-term smokers get COPD, for instance. The effect of significant occupational exposure to VGDF in causation of COPD appears to be more than a simple additive effect to that of smoking. For diseases such as COPD due to cumulative tissue injury and gradual disease onset attribution to work is possible on the balance of probabilities. It may also be reasonable to infer causation by work irrespective of whether other identifiable causes, such as smoking, may also have had a role.

Asthma–chronic obstructive pulmonary disease overlap syndrome (ACOS) describes the group of patients who present with concomitant asthma and COPD characteristics. The prevalence of ACOS in subjects with airway disease ranges between 15% and 60%, indicating variations in the age group, populations and definitions used for asthma and COPD. Around 39% of patients with COPD actually show significant reversibility in response to bronchodilators. Workplace exposure may also be relevant in the onset of either the asthmatic or COPD component.

Pneumoconioses The term 'pneumoconiosis' literally means 'dusty lungs'. It is the accumulation of dust in the lungs and the tissue reaction to its presence. For practical purposes, pneumoconiosis is usually restricted to those conditions that cause a permanent alteration in lung architecture following the inhalation of mineral dusts. These dusts include:

- silica (most commonly in the form of quartz)
- coal
- asbestos.

The clinical and radiographic features of silicosis, coal workers' pneumoconiosis and asbestosis are summarised in Figure 3.3.

Silicosis occurs following the inhalation of 'free' silica and is most common among workers involved in quarrying, mining and tunnelling through quartz-bearing rock, for example during gold mining. Silica is cheap and abundant; new uses thus arise from time to time and they can result in uncontrolled exposure and severe disease: sandblasting denim and artificial stone work are recent examples. The more traditional processes in which silica is also a recognised hazard are:

- use of abrasives
- sand blasting
- glass manufacture
- stone cutting and dressing
- foundry work
- ceramic manufacture
- cutting and grinding of siliceous materials in construction.

Silicosis may present as one of four main clinical types:

1. chronic nodular, with hyaline and collagenous lesions in the lungs
2. progressive massive fibrosis with lesions greater than 1 cm
3. 'acute' – a rapidly developing alveolar lipoproteinosis
4. silico-tuberculosis – the occurrence of tuberculosis in siliceous lungs, a common complication in high-burden tuberculosis countries.

The fibrotic lung lesions may calcify and characteristic 'eggshell' calcification of lymph nodes may be seen on chest radiographs.

Recent epidemiological studies have shown that silica is a lung carcinogen. The International Agency for Research on Cancer (IARC) in 2012 classified silica as an established human carcinogen. The lung cancer association is stronger in subjects with radiological silicosis than in those with exposure but without radiological disease. Many workers' compensation jurisdictions therefore include radiological silicosis as a criterion for certification.

Coal dust produces a somewhat different picture, and frequently has less severe sequelae and is less aggressively fibrotic. Indeed, the distinction between 'simple' and 'complicated' coal pneumoconiosis is often marked, with only a minority of the former progressing to the latter. The factors that predispose to this serious turn of events are unknown.

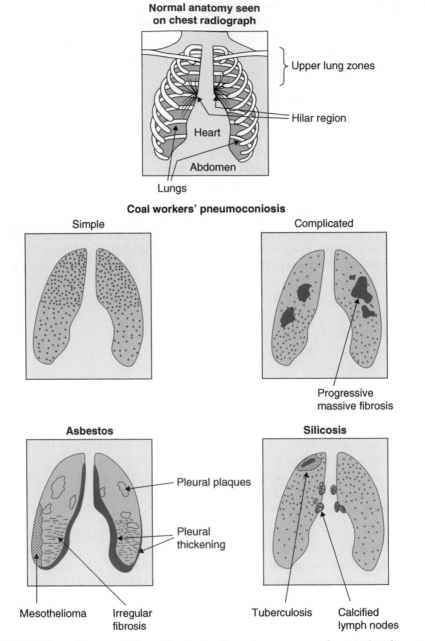

Normal anatomy seen on chest radiograph

Upper lung zones

Hilar region

Heart

Abdomen

Lungs

Coal workers' pneumoconiosis

Simple

Complicated

Progressive massive fibrosis

Asbestos

Pleural plaques

Pleural thickening

Mesothelioma   Irregular fibrosis

Silicosis

Tuberculosis   Calcified lymph nodes

FIGURE 3.3 Schematic representation of the chest radiograph appearances of certain dust diseases.

In the UK, the prevalence of all categories of coal pneumoconiosis had fallen to less than 5%, with a prevalence of the complicated form (progressive massive fibrosis) of 0.4% by the latter part of the twentieth century. The probability of developing ILO category 2 or 3 chronic pneumoconiosis over a working lifetime in British mines stood at between 2% and 12% if dust levels were maintained at concentrations below the occupational exposure limits of $3\,mg\,m^{-3}$ for operations where the average level exceeded $0.45–7\,mg\,m^{-3}$ for long wall, coal face operations. Of concern, though, is the resurgence of coal mine dust pneumoconiosis in the USA. Severe pneumoconiosis after relatively short exposure has been documented in US coal miners, presumably because seams of coal in silicarich country rock are being mined more frequently as the mines age. In China it is estimated that 6% of coal miners had coal mine dust lung disease but accurate prevalence data, especially after long follow-up, are scant.

Asbestos fibres produce pleural plaques (typically of minor clinical significance), diffuse pleural thickening and more irregular and more florid fibrotic changes in the lung. The disease is progressive in a proportion of cases, and death from restrictive lung disease may occur. Clinically, the disease may first present as dyspnoea, non-productive cough or weight loss. The presence of persistent chest pain frequently heralds a recognised complication of asbestos exposure, namely malignant disease – usually a bronchogenic carcinoma but occasionally a pleural mesothelioma. There is a synergistic effect between asbestos compounds and cigarette smoking in terms of the risk of developing lung cancer.

For completeness, it is worth noting that some dusts seem to produce disturbingly florid lung mottling on chest radiographs, but with little or no evidence of clinical effect or progression. These so-called 'benign pneumoconioses' are associated with the dusts of:

- barium sulphate – causing baritosis
- tin – causing stannosis
- iron – causing siderosis (although haematite mining is associated with lung cancer, which is thought to be due to radon gas in the mines)
- antimony, zirconium and the rare earth metals.

Hypersensitivity pneumonitis (extrinsic allergic alveolitis) As noted above, the inhalation of organic materials can give rise to asthma. However, other organic dusts produce alveolitis, either non-fibrotic or fibrotic, with the resultant lowering of gas transfer across the blood–gas interface. Most of the agents capable of producing this effect are fungal spores, and the most common clinical condition in the UK is farmer's lung. These diseases frequently have acute, influenza-like episodes, malaise, sometimes weight loss, chest tightness and wheezing. If exposure is continued, a fibrotic disease with an usual interstitial pneumonia (UIP)-like pattern is more likely. The diagnosis is challenging and requires identification of exposure, chest high-resolution computed tomography scan, and possibly bronchoscopic and histopathological findings. Serum immunoglobulin G testing against potential antigens and/or specific inhalation challenge can be

TABLE 3.4

Types of hypersensitivity pneumonitis (extrinsic allergic alveolitis).

Type	Exposure to	Allergen
Farmer's lung	Mouldy hay	*Saccharopolyspora rectivirgula, Thermoactinomyces vulgaris*
Bagassosis	Mouldy sugar cane	*Thermoactinomyces sacchari*
Suberosis	Mouldy cork	*Penicillium frequentans*
Bird fancier's lung	Droppings and feathers	Avian protein
Malt worker's lung	Mouldy barley	*Aspergillus clavatus*
Humidifier fever	Dust or mist	*Thymus vulgaris, T. sacchari, Thermoactinomyces thalpophilus* and amoebae (various)
Cheese worker's lung	Mould dust	*Piophila casei*
Wheat weevil lung	Mouldy grain or flour	*Sitophilus granarius*
Animal handler's lung	Dander, dried rodent urine	Serum, epithelial and urine proteins

helpful, the latter being carried out in carefully controlled facilities. Examples of types of hypersensitivity pneumonitis are summarised in Table 3.4.

Nervous system

The basic unit of the nervous system is the neuron, which has four components as follows, with the nerve impulse passing from the first to the last:

- the dendrites
- the cell body itself
- the axon
- the synaptic terminal.

The axon is one long nerve fibre with or without myelin sheathing, the presence of which speeds nerve conduction. In the normal resting state, the axonal membrane has a resting potential of about $-85\,\mathrm{mV}$; this *outside* positive charge is maintained by an active sodium pump mechanism. A nerve impulse is a wave of depolarisation and repolarisation that runs along the nerve fibre as the membrane permeability to sodium increases, allowing a rapid reversal of polarity, followed by a recovery period as 'normal' permeability is restored. Conduction along the axon is all or nothing, but along the dendrites it is incremental. At the synapse, the electrical energy is transformed into chemical energy by the release of a neurotransmitter, such as acetylcholine. These neurotransmitters may be excitatory or inhibitory.

Occupationally Related Disorders Of Peripheral Nerves

Occupationally related disorders of peripheral nerves may be motor or sensory nerve effects, and commonly both. Sensory disturbances are usually distal; motor dysfunction may be proximal or distal. Most toxic substances cause axonal degeneration, usually by a mechanism that is largely unknown. The damage may be limited and reversible or severe and permanent, depending on the agent, the dose and the duration of exposure. In the case of n-hexane and methyl-n-butylketone (MnBK), the effect seems to be due to a common metabolite, 2,5-hexanedione, and leads to giant axonal swelling in the proximal parts of the axon, with peripheral 'dying back'. Apart from the clinical features of peripheral neuropathy, subclinical effects may be detected by nerve conduction studies, which can be useful in the detection of early effects in workers exposed to known neurotoxins.

The most well-recognised peripheral neurotoxins from occupational or environmental exposure are:

- acrylamide and/or dimethyl-aminoproprionitrile
- antimony
- arsenic
- carbamate pesticides
- carbon disulphide
- lead and its compounds (inorganic)
- mercury compounds (inorganic and organic)
- methyl-n-butylketone (MnBK)
- n-hexane
- organophosphate pesticides
- thallium
- triorthocresyl-phosphate.

Occupationally Related Disorders of the Central Nervous System

Disordered brain function can be acute or chronic. Acute effects typically arise after inhalation of toxicants such as vapours of solvents or gases. The primary change is one of disordered consciousness, varying from mild disorientation through to profound coma. Chronic central nervous system (CNS) changes are more complex and agent specific; for example, manganese produces parkinsonism whereas excessive mercury uptake may result in erethism, which manifests with irritability, excitability, excessive shyness and insomnia.

Occupational toxins affecting the CNS include organic solvents, heavy metals and CNS depressants, such as anaesthetic gases. Examples are:

- gases, e.g. carbon disulphide
- chlorinated hydrocarbons, e.g. trichloroethylene, perchloroethylene, 1,1,1-trichloroethane, methylene chloride

- halothane
- metals, e.g. lead, mercury, manganese
- non-halogenated aromatic organic compounds, e.g. toluene, styrene
- organic lead compounds
- pesticides such as dieldrin
- white spirit.

Screening for CNS effects is not easy and involves a battery of behavioural tests, including cognitive and perceptual psychomotor assessments. International meetings have shown that an agreed battery of psychological tests can be formulated, but findings need to be interpreted by experienced practitioners, usually psychologists. Examples of such test procedures are available in the larger texts referenced in Chapter 11.

Chronic exposure to various organic solvents can cause organic psychosis (chronic solvent-induced encephalopathy; CSE). The prevalence of the disorder varies among countries, having been highest in Scandinavia and infrequently diagnosed in the UK. Long-term exposure to fairly high concentrations of solvents is required to cause the disease – 10 TLV-years or more has been suggested as a measure of the requisite exposure (Threshold Limit Value [TLV]-years is a measure of cumulative exposure combining duration [years] with intensity [the TLV, an occupational exposure limit of the ACGIH]). The condition is now diagnosed infrequently in developed countries along with the decline in the use of organic solvents. CSE results in some tests of higher cerebral function showing a decremental change following occupational exposure. The diagnosis is difficult, costly and established deficiencies are irreversible. Prevention through reduction of levels of solvent vapour is thus warranted.

Alcohol abuse may exacerbate the effects of the occupational neurotoxin, but these effects are, nevertheless, relatively rare. In normal clinical practice, diabetes is a more probable diagnosis for patients with a nervous system disorders.

Genitourinary system

The kidney has a crucial role in the excretory and detoxification mechanisms of the body. When a toxic substance is absorbed, the liver will frequently alter its chemical structure. Although it is naive to imagine that the liver 'knows' how to detoxify such foreign material, it is nevertheless a fact that the liver frequently succeeds in increasing the toxin's polarity and/or acidity. Both of these changes will render the material more water soluble, and hence more readily excretable through the kidney. Some toxic substances reach the kidney unchanged; others reach the kidney in the form of a more toxic metabolite; yet others are able to cause damage either by being sequestered in the renal cortex (e.g. cadmium) or by being present in the bladder long enough to cause malignant change (e.g. some of the arylamines, such as 2-naphthylamine and its metabolites).

Common forms of disordered function resulting from occupationally related substances include tubular dysfunction leading to aminoaciduria, proteinuria and glycosuria (e.g. mercury) or acute renal failure due to tubular necrosis (e.g.

thallium), hypovolaemic shock (arsenic) or tubular blockage by crystalluria (oxalic acid). Cortical necrosis, while a rare cause of acute renal failure, occurs more commonly with the toxic nephropathies than with other causes of kidney damage. Furthermore, severe liver damage, due to, for example, organic solvents, may induce renal failure as a complication; it is worth remembering that renal damage caused by drug-induced hypersensitivity can occur not only in those taking the drug therapeutically but also in those making the drug occupationally. The nephrotic syndrome can be occupationally induced if the proteinuria is of sufficient severity. This can occur following exposure to mercury, gold and bismuth.

Epidemic chronic kidney disease of unknown cause (CKDu) occurs among agricultural workers, notably sugar cane cutters doing heavy manual work in hot tropical environments in Mesoamerica. Occupational heat stress from strenuous work in high environmental temperatures is one postulated cause. Decrements in kidney function have been found after a part or whole of a season of agricultural work, but, more importantly, frank kidney failure requiring renal replacement therapy occurs in a proportion of these workers and thousands of deaths have been attributed to CKDu. The condition may extend to other industries with heavy manual labour in heat, but this has not been convincingly documented yet.

Renal tract malignancy of occupational origin is an important condition, primarily affecting that part of the genitourinary system in contact with the agent for longest and at the highest concentration, namely the bladder. Agents linked to an excess risk of bladder cancer include chemicals such as 2-naphthylamine and dichlorobenzidine and infectious agents, for example schistosomiasis (an occupational risk for those who have to work in endemic areas).

Although the prostate possesses the curious ability to concentrate (and excrete) heavy metals, little incontrovertible evidence exists of occupationally induced prostatic disease in workers exposed to heavy metals. The putative link between cadmium exposure and prostatic cancer has not been corroborated by more recent, careful studies.

A short list of the more important occupational factors in nephrotoxicity is given in Table 3.5.

Cardiovascular system

The cardiovascular system is not front-of-mind for most occupational health practitioners; nevertheless, work may be a risk factor in the pathogenesis of cardiovascular disease. The main risk factors for cardiovascular disease include:

- age
- sex
- weight
- ethnic background
- smoking
- blood pressure

TABLE 3.5

Occupational and non-occupational exposures with nephrotoxic effects.

Inorganic	Organic	Miscellaneous
Arsenic	Aniline	Antimicrobials
Bismuth	Carbon tetrachloride	Chlorinated hydrocarbon insecticides
Boron	Chloroform	
Cadmium	Dimethyl sulphate	Electric shock
Gold	Dioxan	Fungi
Iron salts (in overdose)	Ethylene glycol	Horse serum
	EDTA	Trauma
Lead	Methoxyflurane	Radiographic contrast media
Mercury	Methyl alcohol	
Phosphorus	Methyl chloride	
Potassium chlorate	Paraquat	
Thallium	Pentachlorophenol	
Uranium	Phenol	
	Turpentine	
	Toluene	

EDTA, ethylenediaminetetra-acetic acid.

- serum cholesterol and diet
- exercise levels
- stress
- oral contraceptive use
- family history
- medical history (e.g. diabetes)
- harmful use of alcohol.

Hazards directly emanating from the workplace tend to have a secondary effect on the cardiovascular system. For example, lead can cause nephropathy, which, in turn, can cause hypertension. Cadmium causes emphysema, which can lead to cor pulmonale; cobalt can cause cardiomyopathy; and arsenic is thought to be a factor in peripheral vascular disease.

Certain organic solvents, e.g. trichloroethylene and 1,1,1-trichloroethane, are thought to be capable of inducing cardiac arrhythmias, and vinyl chloride exposure has been linked with Raynaud's phenomenon. Methylene chloride (dichloromethane) produces carbon monoxide as a metabolite, while carbon disulphide seems to cause a direct atherogenic effect. Certain gases, e.g. carbon monoxide and hydrogen cyanide, can cause hypoxia, directly or at a cellular level, and physical factors, such as vibration, can induce vasospastic disease in the small arteries of the hand.

The list of specific chemical and physical occupationally related factors that can cause, induce or exacerbate cardiovascular disease is considerable and includes:

- anaesthetic gases, e.g. chloroform and halothane
- metals, e.g. antimony, arsenic, cadmium, cobalt, lead, manganese, mercury
- gases, e.g. carbon disulphide, carbon monoxide, carbon tetrachloride, fluorocarbons
- electric shock
- low atmospheric pressures
- noise
- glyceryl trinitrate and trinitrotoluene (encountered in the explosives industry)
- methylene chloride
- extremes of temperature
- trichloroethylene
- 1,1,1-trichloroethane
- vibration.

Probably more important than specific chemical and physical agents are factors commonly encountered in working life. Long working hours, shift work and work stress have all been linked to cardiovascular diseases. The mechanisms resulting in the increased risk are not conclusive but disruption of metabolic processes and lifestyle factors such as reduced physical activity, smoking and poor diet have been posited. Ultrafine airborne particulate matter is commonly encountered at work, and this too has been associated with increased incidence and mortality for cardiovascular diseases.

Skin

The area of skin covering an adult human is approximately 1.8 m^2. The skin consists of two basic elements: an outer epidermis, which acts as a protective covering and is non-wettable, and a dermis, which provides the inherent strength of the skin, largely through its collagen content. The skin has a quadruple defensive structure: biological – the skin microbiome; chemical – pH and natural moisturising factor; physical – the integrity of the structure and composition principally of the stratum corneum; and immunological – epidermal Langerhans cells and T cells with other dermal elements. The waterproofing capability of the epidermis is, in occupational health terms, a potential problem as its greasy surface aids the absorption of fat-soluble materials and is thus a ready route of entry for many organic chemicals.

Skin disease may be characterised by rashes that often bear a limited topographical resemblance to the area of initial contact. Scratching a rash because of an itch can lead to the extension of the area affected. The use of combination ointments without a clear diagnosis may worsen rather than alleviate the symptoms. The use of gloves may protect against further contact with the causative chemicals, but the inappropriate use of gloves may cause chemicals to be trapped between the gloves and the skin of the hands. This can worsen contact dermatitis. Some individuals are also allergic to latex and other components in gloves and the prolonged use of impermeable gloves causes hyperhydration of the epidermis and maceration followed by dermatitis.

Occupational dermatoses may be broadly divided into two groups:

1. primary irritant contact dermatitis
2. allergic contact dermatitis.

Primary Irritant Contact Dermatitis

Nearly three-quarters of all occupational dermatoses are of this type. The irritants produce a direct effect on the skin with which they come into contact, and the effect will be more dependent on the dose and duration of exposure than on any inherent response emanating from the individual. For example, concentrated sulphuric acid splashed onto the face of anybody will produce a skin reaction. Soap and water are more variable, but these seemingly harmless materials can cause irritation in non-allergic subjects who carry out frequent handwashing. The degree of effect depends on factors such as:

- skin dryness
- sweating
- pigmentation
- integrity of the epidermis (i.e. whether damaged by trauma)
- presence of hair
- presence of dirt
- concurrent or pre-existent skin disease
- environmental factors, such as temperature, humidity and friction.

Furthermore, some chemicals, such as arsenicals and mercurials, can combine with skin protein and cause skin damage. Hydrofluoric acid and hexavalent chromium compounds can cause deep skin ulcers. Acneiform conditions can also arise from work exposure to cutting oils and semisynthetic coolants, which cause a follicular hyperkeratosis with comedones, folliculitis, papules and pustules. Frictional effects and humidity can also induce acne. A rare acne variant can arise from exposure to polyhalogenated naphthalenes, polyhalogenated biphenyls and related chemicals. It was originally termed 'chloracne' owing to the original descriptions occurring with chlorinated compounds; it is now called MADISH – metabolising acquired dioxin-induced skin hamartomas. This new description better reflects the skin pathology in which the sebaceous glands become cystic and do not show typical acneiform features.

Allergic Contact Dermatitis

Allergic contact dermatitis accounts for 15–20% of all occupational dermatoses. The initial clinically inapparent sensitising episode may require substantial concentrations, repeated and/or prolonged contact or presentation with a mixture of other allergens or microbes. Subsequently reactions can be provoked by shorter and/or smaller exposures. The response is usually specific to one agent and the skin reaction after contact may be delayed for a week or more. Occasionally the responsible substance is an airborne dust or vapour leading to a rash distribution on the exposed skin of the face and eyelids.

The mechanism of the response is a delayed hypersensitivity reaction. The allergen acts as a hapten to combine with protein in the living epidermis to provoke a cell-mediated type IV immune reaction. The acute effect is itching, erythema, papular eruption, vesiculation, sometimes bullae, oozing and desquamation. In a chronic form, this leads to thickened, fissured skin.

Common occupational contact allergens include:

- acrylates
- cobalt and its salts
- dichromates
- dyes, such as paraphenylenediamine
- epoxy resins
- formaldehyde
- preservatives and biocides, such as isothiazolinones
- natural rubber latex
- nickel and its salts
- rubber accelerators and antioxidants.

Diagnosis by patch tests

Patch testing is a type of provocation test used to confirm a diagnosis of allergic contact dermatitis. This involves the epicutaneous application of a series of compounds to the skin of the back in circular Finn or square IQ chambers, followed by assessment of the skin reaction when the patches are removed, usually at 48 hours, and a further reading seven days after application. Readings determine negative reactions, doubtful reactions, three gradations of positive reactions and irritant reactions. Interpretation means that the clinical relevance is considered with respect to exposure to the allergen and the presenting dermatitis. A contact allergy may be elicited but be of past, current or unknown relevance. Advice then needs to be given to the patient which will need to include identification and avoidance of substances containing relevant allergens. Hence the need for dermatological expertise. There is a standard series of test materials that may have to be supplemented by additional test substances for specific occupational exposures. In the case of occupational allergic contact dermatitis, familiarity with the work processes and chemicals used is an essential adjunct to patch testing.

Photodermatitis

Exposure to certain agents through skin contact or following ingestion can result in a rash after exposure to ultraviolet light. This includes occupational exposure to tar, pitch and acrylates, for example those used in ultraviolet-cured inks, augmented by subsequent exposure to sunlight. Pharmaceutical agents known to cause photodermatitis following ingestion include griseofulvin and thiazides.

The 'strimmer's dermatitis' is a phytophotodermatitis due to skin contact with the sap of furocoumarin-containing plants, e.g. Umbelliferae, and sun exposure. The non-occupational use of some perfumes and sun creams may lead to photodermatitis.

Occupational Leucoderma

Contact with chemicals can lead to depigmentation of the skin. This usually occurs at the site of contact but in predisposed individuals other areas may be involved. Examples include hydroquinones and certain substituted phenols and catechols. Hydroquinone is used as an intermediate in the synthesis of antioxidants for rubber; *p*-tertbutylphenol is present in adhesives, coating products, resins, plasticisers and inks. Hydroquinone is also an agent found in cosmetic products used for skin lightening. The reversibility of the depigmentation depends on the extent of damage to the melanocytes.

The industries with a recognised risk of occupationally related skin disease are many, including:

- cleaning
- construction
- making leather goods
- food processing and packing
- use of adhesives and sealants
- boat building and repair
- use of abrasive products
- agriculture and horticulture
- mining
- healthcare.

Some of these agents are also encountered in the course of hobbies.

Liver

The liver is the largest visceral organ. Its mass of parenchymal cells, portal tracts and abundant blood supply is witness to its crucial role as the body's main metabolic factory. The functional unit resides in the lobule and consists of a group of sinusoids running between a terminal portal tract and a few terminal hepatic venules. The liver cells nearest the hepatic venules differ from those near the portal tracts, in that the former receive blood lower in oxygen content. These centrilobular hepatocytes are therefore more vulnerable to toxic (and anoxic) conditions than the periportal cells.

Disordered hepatic function has two main aspects. First, the hepatocytes may be damaged and, second, the transport mechanism to, through or from the hepatocytes may be blocked. Both dysfunctions will, sooner or later, lead to jaundice. The liver's remarkable capacity for hepatocyte regeneration following assault is not matched by its ability to reproduce, faithfully, the basic liver architecture. Thus, major hepatic damage can lead to florid cellular regeneration in a disrupted lobular pattern.

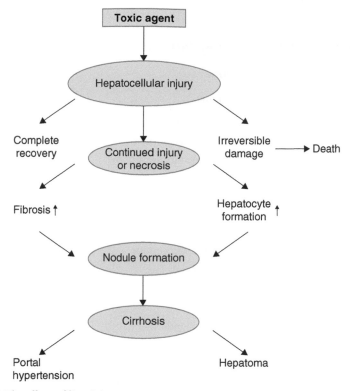

FIGURE 3.4 The effects of liver injury.

The effects of liver injury are shown in Figure 3.4.

Pre-existent liver disease may enhance the effects of a new toxic onslaught, and the liver is thus particularly vulnerable to the effects of organic solvents if already subject to excessive ethyl alcohol intake or with non-alcoholic fatty liver disease, which affects about 20% of the global population. Furthermore, it is worth noting that hepatic enzyme induction may alter the liver's ability to handle certain toxins, and the organ itself is occasionally subject to hypersensitivity reactions. The effects of hepatotoxins of occupational origin may be sub-classified as shown in Table 3.6.

Reproductive system

It has been noted that in the early twentieth century there was a competing tension between workplace discrimination against women and the emergence of industrial health and safety with concerns for women's child-bearing capacity and the health of their unborn and infant children. Early regulations in the pottery industry applied specifically to women and could see them suspended without pay. Only relatively recently has serious attention been paid to the possibility that occupational factors could disrupt the normal functioning of the male and female reproductive systems (Table 3.7).

TABLE 3.6

Effects of occupationally related hepatotoxins.

Effect	Substance	
	Organic	Inorganic
Hepatocel-lular injury	Acrylonitrile	Antimony
	Carbon tetrachloride	Arsenic
	Chlorinated hydrocarbon insecticides	Boranes
	Chlorinated naphthalenes	Phospho-rus (yellow)
	Dimethyl formamide	Selenium
	Dimethyl hydrazine	Thallium
	Dimethyl nitrosamine	
	Dinitrophenol	
	Ethyl alcohol	
	Halothane	
	Methyl chloride	
	Nitrobenzene	
	Phenol	
	Polychlorinated biphenyls	
	Tetrachloroethylene	
	1,1,1-Trichloroethane	
	Trichloroethylene	
	Trinitrotoluene	
	Toluene	
	Vinyl chloride	
Hepatic infections	Viral hepatitis (A, B, C)	
	Leptospirosis	
	Q fever	
	Schistosomiasis	
	Amoebiasis	
Cholestatic, cholangiolitic	Methylene dianiline	
	Organic arsenicals	
	Toluene diamine	
	4,4-Diaminodiphenylmethane	

TABLE 3.7

Examples of suspected female and male reproductive effects of occupational exposures.

Agent	Fertility	Spontaneous abortion	Prematurity	Congenital disorders
Anaesthetic gases	–	?	–	–
Cadmium	+	–	–	–
Carbon disulphide	+	?	–	?
Chlordecone	+	–	–	–
Cytotoxic drugs	+	+	–	–
Dibromochloropropane	+	–	–	–
Diesel exhaust	+	–	–	+
N,N-dimethylformamide	+	?	?	?
Ethylene oxide	–	?	–	–
Ethylene glycol ethers	+	?	–	+
Fenvalerate	+	?	?	?
Heat	+	–	–	–
Heavy work	–	+	?	–
Infectious agents, e.g. rubella, cytomegalovirus	?	+	+	+
Laboratory work	–	?	–	?
Lead	+	?	–	?
Ionising radiation	+	–	+	+
Mercury	?	?	–	+ (methyl mercury)
Non-ionising radiation	–	?	–	?
Oral contraceptives	+	–	–	–
Organic solvents	?	–	–	+
Polychlorinated biphenyls	?	–	–	+
Shift work	–	?	?	–
Vinyl chloride	?	?	?	?

+, probable or established effect; –, no effect shown, either not investigated or not found; ?, questionable effect, confirmation required.

Now, considerable attention is being paid to the possibility that the health of off-spring may be affected by parental exposure. Effects have been reported in children of a male parent who smokes, and parental exposure to ionising radiation has been suggested as a cause of childhood malignancy, although the evidence is conflicting.

Animal studies have indicated a wide range of chemicals that can disrupt reproductive capacity. For the male, these endocrine disruptors include steroidal hormones, alkylating agents, anti-metabolites, diuretics, psychopharmacological agents, anaesthetics, oral hypoglycaemics, ethyl alcohol, heavy metals, insecticides, herbicides, fungicides, cyclamates, organic solvents, radiation and heat. For female animals, the list is shorter but contains many of the same chemicals.

It is important to remember that an abnormal pregnancy outcome spans a wide range of events in the timetable from ovum/sperm to live birth. These include:

- normal gonadal function
- union of ovum and sperm
- placental implantation
- embryonic organogenesis (one to three months in utero)
- fetal development (three to nine months in utero)
- normal birth
- healthy childhood (absence of health effects such as cancers).

The many events in producing a healthy child mean that adverse effects of work exposures can have many manifestations. Among them are reduced male and female fertility, resulting in prolonged time to pregnancy or failure to conceive; effects during pregnancy such as low birth weight, spontaneous abortion and congenital defects; and ill health in offspring which manifest after birth.

Furthermore, at least 15–20% of normal conceptions fail to reach full growth and normal delivery. These could be termed 'normal' spontaneous abortions, although most that have been analysed show gross genetic abnormalities. Congenital malformations have been reported in about 3% of all newborn children, with a further 3% reported during postnatal or later development. Some childhood cancers are traceable to maternal exposure during pregnancy, for example vaginal carcinoma resulting from mothers treated during pregnancy with diethylstilboestrol. Most abnormal pregnancy outcomes, however, have no known obvious cause.

Bone marrow

The bone marrow contains several important constituents. For the purpose of a review of target organs, two components are of particular note:

- haematopoietic stem cells
- bone marrow fat.

The stem cell is a remarkable structure that is capable of differentiating into most of the major cellular components of the blood. The marrow fat deposits are toxicologically important because of their inherent ability to absorb fat-soluble compounds, and thereby store these potentially toxic compounds in close proximity to the stem cells.

While some agents are capable of damaging mature red cells (arsenic) or of altering haem synthesis (lead), the most serious effect on the bone marrow is stem cell death (aplastic anaemia) or abnormal division (leukaemia). The two occupational exposures most likely to achieve these disastrous outcomes are:

- benzene
- ionising radiation.

Benzene exposure has been associated with aplastic anaemia and leukaemia, notably acute myelogenous leukaemia. There is little doubt that high doses of benzene can cause these effects. What is in dispute is where to place the lower limit of exposure for (relatively) safe working conditions. Ionising radiation can cause many leukaemia cell types, but notably the myeloid series. Chronic lymphatic leukaemia seems not to be radiation induced. Multiple myeloma and other lymphomas have, however, been implicated.

The IARC lists carcinogenic agents by cancer site (https://monographs.iarc. who.int/wp-content/uploads/2019/07/Classifications_by_cancer_site.pdf). The list contains 28 carcinogenic agents with sufficient evidence in humans for leukaemia and/or lymphoma; many can be encountered at work.

Finally, cytotoxic therapeutic agents, by their very nature, destroy or damage bone marrow cells. These agents are a theoretical risk in pharmaceutical manufacture and in hospital staff who have to prepare and dispose of these agents, and a measurable risk in those patients who receive these drugs. Evidence of such effects from other agents encountered in industry, such as ethylene glycol ethers, trinitrotoluene and arsenic, is tenuous and disputed.

3.6 Prescribed diseases in the UK

Many workers' compensation jurisdictions have a list of diseases for which there is a presumption of occupational origin, typically in stipulated exposure situations. These are known as prescribed diseases. The UK's list of these diseases and exposure situations is of interest despite its local applicability because the list is extensive and the type of work leading to exposure is informative for attribution (https://www.gov.uk/government/publications/industrial-injuries-disablement-benefits-technical-guidance/industrial-injuries-disablement-benefits-technical-guidance#appendix-1-list-of-diseases-covered-by-industrial-injuries-disablement-benefit).

The UK's list of prescribed diseases has four groups of causes:

- A for a physical cause, 15 diseases
- B for a biological cause, 15 diseases
- C for a chemical cause, 34 diseases
- D for any other cause, 13 diseases.

Examples from each category with type of job or activity for which they are prescribed are shown in Table 3.8.

TABLE 3.8

Examples from the list of diseases covered by Industrial Injuries Disablement Benefit in the UK.

Disease number	Name of disease or injury	Type of job – Any job involving:
A12	Carpal tunnel syndrome	(a) The use, at the time the symptoms first develop, of hand-held powered tools whose internal parts vibrate so as to transmit that vibration to the hand, but excluding those tools which are solely powered by hand; or
		(b) Repeated palmar flexion and dorsiflexion of the wrist for at least 20 hours per week for a period or periods amounting in aggregate to at least 12 months in the 24 months prior to the onset of symptoms. We use 'repeated' to mean once or more often in every 30 s.
B10(a)	Avian chlamydiosis	Contact with birds infected with *Chlamydia psittaci*, or with the remains or untreated products of such birds. For example, duck farm workers, feather processing workers, abattoir workers, poultry meat inspectors, pet shop owners and assistants.
C23	Primary neoplasm of the epithelial lining of the urinary tract	(a) The manufacture of 1-naphthylamine, 2-naphthylamine, benzidine, auramine, magenta or 4-aminobiphenyl (also called biphenyl-4-ylamine);
		(b) Work in the process of manufacturing methylene-bisorthochloroaniline (also called MbOCA) for a period of, or periods which amount in aggregate to, 12 months or more;
		(c) Exposure to 2-naphthylamine, benzidine, 4-aminobiphenyl (also called biphenyl-4-ylamine) or salts of those compounds otherwise than in the manufacture of those compounds;
		(d) Exposure to orthotoluidine, 4-chloro-2-methylaniline or salts of those compounds; or

TABLE 3.8 (Continued)

Examples from the list of diseases covered by Industrial Injuries Disablement Benefit in the UK.

Disease number	Name of disease or injury	Type of job – Any job involving:
		(e) Exposure for a period of, or periods which amount in aggregate to, 5 years or more, to coal tar pitch volatiles produced in aluminium smelting involving the Soderberg process (that is to say, the method of producing aluminium by electrolysis in which the anode consists of a paste of petroleum coke and mineral oil which is baked in situ).
D7	Asthma which is due to exposure to any of the following agents: (a) isocyanates (b) platinum salts (c) fumes or dusts arising from the manufacture, transport or use of hardening agents (including epoxy resin curing agents) based on phthalic anhydride, tetrachlorophthalic anhydride, trimellitic anhydride or triethylenetetramine (d) fumes arising from the use of rosin as a soldering flux (e) proteolytic enzymes (f) animals including insects and other arthropods used for the purposes of research or education or in laboratories (g) dusts arising from the sowing, cultivation, harvesting, drying, handling, milling, transport or storage of barley, oats, rye, wheat or maize, or the handling, milling, transport or storage of meal or flour made therefrom	Exposure to any of the agents set out in column 2 of this paragraph.

TABLE 3.8 (Continued)

Examples from the list of diseases covered by Industrial Injuries Disablement Benefit in the UK.

Disease number	Name of disease or injury	Type of job – Any job involving:
(h)	antibiotics	
(i)	cimetidine	
(j)	wood dust	
(k)	ispaghula	
(l)	castor bean dust	
(m)	ipecacuanha	
(n)	azodicarbonamide	
(o)	animals including insects and other arthropods or their larval forms, used for the purposes of pest control or fruit cultivation, or the larval forms of animals used for the purposes of research, education or in laboratories	
(p)	glutaraldehyde	
(q)	persulphate salts or henna	
(r)	crustaceans or fish or products arising from these in the food processing industry	
(s)	reactive dyes	
(t)	soya bean	
(u)	tea dust	
(v)	green coffee bean dust	
(w)	fumes from stainless steel welding	
(wa)	products made with natural rubber latex	
(x)	any other sensitising agent. (Occupational asthma)	
(y)	products made with natural rubber latex	

References

GBD 2016 Occupational Risk Factors Collaborators (2020). Global and regional burden of disease and injury in 2016 arising from occupational exposures: a systematic analysis for the Global Burden of Disease Study 2016. *Occupational and Environmental Medicine* **77**: 133–141. https://doi.org/10.1136/oemed-2019-106008.

Hämäläinen, P., Takala, J., and Tan, B.K. (2017). *Global Estimates of Occupational Injuries and Work-Related Illnesses*. Singapore: Workplace Safety and Health Institute www.wshi.gov.sg.

CHAPTER 4

Occupational Infections

4.1 Introduction

Occupation has long been recognised as an important association for infectious disease. Anthrax – otherwise known as wool-sorter's disease because of its occurrence at the time in the textile industry – was one of the first occupational diseases listed by the International Labour Organization in 1919. This is an example of a zoonosis, which is an infection that is naturally transmissible from vertebrate animals to humans. Occupationally acquired infections can be caused by a variety of infectious agents – from viruses and bacteria to rickettsiae, parasites and possibly prions.

Certain work activities are associated with an increased risk of contracting infections. This may be because the work brings an individual into contact with large numbers of people with infections, for example healthcare workers; or materials that contain infectious agents, for example pathological or laboratory

Pocket Consultant: Occupational Health, Sixth Edition. Kerry Gardiner, David Rees,
Anil Adisesh, David Zalk, and Malcolm Harrington.
© 2022 John Wiley & Sons Ltd. Published 2022 by John Wiley & Sons Ltd.

samples; or infected animals, as in zoonotic infections. Others affected include those who have to travel to endemic areas during the course of their work. In addition to considering the risk of acquiring infections from work activities, there is also a need to ensure that infected individuals do not transmit infection to others during their work, for example healthcare workers to patients or food handlers to consumers.

Occupational exposures to infection will vary according to their geographical prevalence. In many countries there will be a system to notify and report occupational injuries and diseases to the Ministry of Labour or its equivalent; there may also be requirements for reporting under public health legislation of specific contagious infections. Additionally workers' compensation systems may have criteria for recognising occupationally acquired infections. Table 4.1 describes well-recognised associations between occupations, activities and infections. This chapter discusses healthcare workers as a specific group, and other occupational infections.

TABLE 4.1

Occupational infections showing route of transmission with some associated infections and jobs.

Occupation	Route of transmission	Infection
Abattoir/slaughter-house worker Animal handler Butcher and meat handler Conservation officer/ranger Construction worker Demolition worker Farm worker Military personnel Pest control worker Poultry worker Sewage worker Wool and leather worker Veterinary surgeons Zoo worker	**Zoonotic:** respiratory, oral, mucous membrane, inoculation, bite or scratch.	**Bacterial:** anthrax, brucellosis, *Campylobacter, Capnocytophaga,* cat-scratch fever, erysipeloid, *Escherichia coli* O157, glanders, infectious diarrhoea, leptospirosis, *Mycobacterium bovis, Mycobacterium marinum, Mycobacterium tuberculosis,* ornithosis, pasteurellosis, Q fever, rat bite fever, *Streptococcus suis* meningitis, tularaemia, *Yersinia* **Viral:** arenaviral haemorrhagic fever, avian influenza, B virus, hantavirus, *Hendra,* lymphocytic choriomeningitis, monkeypox, Newcastle disease, Nipah, orf, rabies, vesicular stomatitis **Parasitic:** cryptosporidiosis, *Echinococcus,* toxoplasmosis **Fungal:** ringworm, histoplasmosis

(Continued)

TABLE 4.1 (Continued)

Occupational infections showing route of transmission with some associated infections and jobs.

Occupation	Route of transmission	Infection
Conservation officer/ranger Farm worker Forestry worker Landscape gardener Military personnel Pest control worker Rail track/highway maintenance	**Vector borne**: tick, flea, louse or mite bite, midges, mosquitoes, sandflies	**Bacterial:** anaplasmosis, babesiosis, *Borrelia* infections (Lyme disease, relapsing fever), ehrlichiosis, Rocky Mountain spotted fever, tularaemia, scrub typhus, typhus, *Yersinia*, tick-borne rickettsial infections, *Bartonella* infection **Viral:** chikungunya, Colorado tick fever, dengue, Eastern equine encephalitis, Mayaro, Powassan, sandfly fever, West Nile, yellow fever
Dental worker Embalmer Healthcare worker Housekeeper Janitor Laboratory worker Tattooist Recycling plant worker Waste worker	**Blood borne**: mucous membrane, inoculation	**Viral:** HIV, hepatitis B, hepatitis C, Ebola, Lassa, Marburg
Abattoir/slaughterhouse worker Animal handler Butcher and meat handler Daycare provider Dental worker Embalmer Farm worker Food handler Healthcare worker Oyster shucker or fisherman Pest control worker Plumber Teacher Veterinary surgeon	**Skin**: direct contact with another person, or contaminated object (fomite), ingress through damaged or intact skin	**Bacterial:** anthrax, staphylococcal infection, e.g. meticillin-sensitive (MSSA) or resistant *Staphylococcus aureus* (MRSA), *Vibrio vulnificus* **Viral:** herpetic whitlow, varicella, viral warts **Fungal:** *Candida* paronychia, chromomycosis, sporotrichosis **Parasitic:** cutaneous larva migrans **Mite:** scabies

TABLE 4.1 (Continued)

Occupational infections showing route of transmission with some associated infections and jobs.

Occupation	Route of transmission	Infection
Daycare provider Dental worker Embalmer Healthcare worker Teacher	**Faecal–oral:** exposure to human excreta	**Bacterial:** typhoid/paratyphoid **Viral:** cytomegalovirus, hepatitis A, norovirus **Parasitic:** cryptosporidiosis
Archaeologist Building cleaning worker Conservation officer/ranger Construction worker Daycare provider Dental worker Embalmer Farm worker Forestry worker Healthcare worker Laboratory worker Miner Prison staff Stoneworker Teacher Welder	**Respiratory:** aerosol exposure (suspended particulate <100 μm)	**Bacterial:** diphtheria, meningococcus, *Mycoplasma* infection, pneumococcus, tuberculosis **Viral:** influenza, measles, mumps, parvovirus, pertussis, rubella, severe acute respiratory syndrome virus (SARS-CoV-1 and SARS-CoV-2) **Fungal:** histoplasmosis, coccidioidomycosis, paracoccidioidomycosis, blastomycosis

Note: there is not a one-to-one correspondence between either the example occupations or the infections listed, and some are one to many.
HIV, human immunodeficiency virus.

4.2 Healthcare workers

Even before the establishment of 'fever hospitals' in the nineteenth century, healthcare work has been an occupation long associated with a risk of infection. The nature of the work entails close proximity to patients with known, suspected and sometimes unrecognised infectious disease as well as potential contact with their blood and body fluids.

The main occupational bloodborne infections of concern are hepatitis B, hepatitis C, and human immunodeficiency virus (HIV). Infection control risk management is often framed in terms of preventing risk to patients from infected healthcare workers when in fact the reverse risk is much greater. Prior to the advent of hepatitis B vaccination the seroprevalence of hepatitis B in the 1970s was more than 10 times that of the general population for US surgeons and health-care workers in renal dialysis units. Non-occupational risks of transmission for these diseases, for example from unprotected sexual activity, are far more common than occupational factors. Some of the general concerns are a result of media publicity, public reaction, the nature of the illness and the previous lack of effective treatment for these infections. Needlestick injuries involving hollow-bore used needles pose a significant risk of transmission, as does implantation of spiculated bone. Prevention includes sharp instrument avoidance; use of safety-engineered sharp instruments; care in the use of sharp instruments; the use of appropriate gloves for surgical, obstetric and dental procedures and phlebot-omy; and the use of suitable impermeable gowns. Additionally the safe disposal of sharp instruments in point-of-use well-designed strong containers that are not overfilled and attention to safe systems of work, especially during the performance of exposure prone procedures (EPPs). Risks to patients from infected healthcare workers can occur in the course of performing EPPs but these are minimised by preplacement screening and immunisation processes. EPPs have been defined as 'those where there is a risk that injury to the healthcare worker may result in the exposure of the patient's open tissue to the blood of the worker'.

Hepatitis B

Causative organism: hepatitis B virus

Hepatitis B virus is a hepadnavirus with a small genome of partially double-stranded circular DNA. The surface protein hepatitis B surface antigen (HBsAg) is important in attachment to the host cell membrane. The genome has pre-S1, pre-S2 and S regions for manufacturing surface envelope proteins. Hepatitis B prevalence is highest in the Western Pacific and African regions, where 6% of the adult population is infected. In areas of high endemicity, the transmission of hepatitis B most commonly occurs through 'vertical transmission' from mother to child at birth (perinatal transmission) or through 'horizontal transmission' (exposure to infected blood), especially from an infected child to an uninfected child during the first five years of life. Sexual transmission is also a route of sig-nificance. Recognising these early life risks, around 189 countries now provide the vaccine for infants on a national level. For healthcare workers the most common cause is from contact with infected blood and body fluids. Occupational groups at risk include nurses, doctors, phlebotomists, laboratory and research staff and other categories of healthcare workers.

Infection may lead to full recovery, a chronic carrier state or liver failure and death. Carrier status is indicated by the presence of antigens: HBsAg with or without e-antigen (HBeAg), the latter a marker of increased infectiousness. Those with HBeAg as well as high levels of HBsAg and hepatitis B viral load (HBV DNA) have an increased risk of chronic liver disease and hepatocellular carcinoma. HBe (and HBs) carriers are infectious carriers, and the majority of cases of hepatitis B transmitted from healthcare workers to patients have involved such carriers. There have been 40 clusters of transmission of hepatitis B to patients worldwide since 1970, with 400 patients affected. Guidance for healthcare workers in the UK requires that those testing positive for HBsAg should be tested for HBV DNA. If they have an HBV DNA level at or above 200 IU ml^{-1} they are not allowed to undertake EPPs or to do clinical work in renal units. Notwithstanding this, work while on HBV antiviral treatment is allowed subject to periodic monitoring. Those who have anti-HBs levels of less than 10 mIU ml^{-1} post vaccination are required to be shown to be non-infectious and tested annually for HBsAg. Core antibody (anti-HBc) is a marker in carriers and also those who are naturally immune. It indicates previous or current infection and does not appear as a result of vaccination that uses recombinant HBsAg subunits.

Hepatitis B immunoglobulins have been administered to prevent infection soon after a needlestick injury or substantial contact with blood from a known hepatitis B carrier or case for non-immune exposed workers. Advice on administration of a booster dose of vaccine for responders varies by jurisdiction but is currently recommended in the UK for exposure from an HBsAg-positive source. Treatment of chronic infection consists of nucleoside analogues and/or pegylated interferon, which may result in seroconversion to anti-HBe and loss of HBsAg with or without seroconversion to anti-HBs.

The protection of individuals at risk can be achieved by vaccination (hepatitis B immunisation), which consequently also prevents hepatocellular carcinoma arising from hepatitis B infection. A full course of vaccination consists of three intramuscular (deltoid) injections of 0.5 ml of vaccine, with one month between the first and second doses and five months between the second and third doses. An accelerated course can be given with an initial dose, then a second dose one month later, a third dose after a further month and a fourth dose at one year after starting. Checking for seroconversion is recommended two months after the third dose. A booster dose is suggested after five years for healthcare workers in some jurisdictions such as the UK. Poor antibody response requires a second course of vaccine. The response rate is around 95% – some individuals do not produce antibodies in spite of several doses of vaccine. Carrier state, previous cleared infection, increasing age, chronic kidney disease, diabetes, immunosuppressant disease or medication can affect response. Counselling and advice are necessary before checking for antigen status to determine if non-response is due to carrier state. Implications for continuing or changing occupation or job activities in a known carrier should be considered by clinicians, nurses or occupational health staff providing advice to the individual.

Hepatitis C

Causative organism: hepatitis C virus
This bloodborne virus has features similar to hepatitis B. Infection can progress often asymptomatically to chronic liver disease with an increased risk of hepatocellular carcinoma. Hepatitis C virus (HCV) is an RNA virus in the Flaviviridae

family and it does not have the benefit of an available vaccine to prevent infection. Laboratory confirmation of the presence of hepatitis C viral RNA indicates infection. Healthcare workers who are HCV RNA positive should be restricted from performing EPPs. UK guidance advises that those who have been treated with direct-acting antiviral (DAA) therapy and who remain HCV RNA negative for at least three months after cessation of treatment should be permitted to return to performing EPPs at that time. As a further check, they should be shown still to be HCV RNA negative three months after. The US Centers for Disease Control and Prevention (CDC) reports the risk of percutaneous exposure to anti-HCV-positive blood or body fluids for infection to be 0.2%, and 0% for mucocutaneous exposure. While there is no post-exposure prophylaxis (PEP) follow-up testing is recommended at three to six weeks and again at four to six months post exposure. New infections can be identified and treated early with DAA since a sustained virological response greater than 90% is reported. People living with HCV should receive hepatitis A and B vaccine if they are not otherwise immune or infected.

Other hepatitis viruses

Hepatitis A virus (HAV) and hepatitis D virus (HDV or delta agent) are both capable of causing liver disease. Hepatitis A is transmitted through the faecal–oral route and a vaccine is available for conferring protection. The only healthcare occupational groups reported to be at increased risk are international travellers to high-risk countries such as humanitarian relief and overseas refugee workers, and people working with hepatitis A-infected primates. Laboratory workers working with the organism are suggested to be at risk in UK and Canadian guidance. The CDC does not consider staff of institutional care settings to be at risk whereas UK and Canadian guidance does, although it is agreed that routine immunisation of healthcare workers is not indicated. Hepatitis D is a 'satellite virus', meaning that it is replication deficient without the presence of HBV. Therefore, immunisation against HBV also protects against HDV, and is important for people living with HIV and HCV.

Human immunodeficiency virus

Causative organism: human immunodeficiency virus
HIV is an RNA virus belonging to the genus *Lentivirus* within the family of Retroviridae. It was first identified in the early 1980s, and it has been recognised that there are two viruses – HIV 1 and HIV 2 – both of which originally had zoonotic origin in the 1930s to 1940s. Since then several subtypes have been described. HIV 2 is mainly restricted to West Africa, with HIV 1 being responsible for around 37 million prevalent infections. UNAIDS (the Joint United Nations Programme on HIV and AIDS) estimated that, in 2019, of all people with HIV worldwide:

- 81% knew their HIV status
- 82% who knew their status were accessing anti-retroviral therapy
- 88% accessing anti-retroviral therapy were virally suppressed.

The infection is acquired through vertical transmission, unprotected sex, sharing needles and occupationally from needlestick injuries or possibly splashes involving samples of infected blood.

The acute seroconversion illness of HIV infection can be flu-like, sometimes with an erythematous maculopapular rash. These features may not be present or not recognised as they are non-specific. Generalised lymphadenopathy may be another presentation of HIV infection. Untreated the condition may otherwise be latent for perhaps as long as 10 years. As the CD4+ T-cell count eventually drops the risk of infection increases such that a CD4+ cell count of less than 200 cells mm^{-3} is a defining feature of the acquired immune deficiency syndrome (AIDS), as is the presence of a defining illness with recurrent, severe opportunistic infections such as the fungal *Pneumocystis jirovecii* pneumonia – the particular opportunistic organisms to some extent reflect their geographical spread. The risk of reactivation of latent *Mycobacterium tuberculosis* or active disease from new infection is increased at all stages but rises as CD4+ falls. There is also an increased risk of Burkitt's type lymphoma, immunoblastic lymphoma and primary brain lymphoma, which are increasing as a proportion of AIDS-defining conditions. Anti-retroviral therapy aims to suppress viral loads to low (<200 copies/ml) or undetectable (<20–75 copies/ml, depending on the assay used) levels. With early treatment and adherence, the life expectancy of a person living with HIV with no co-infection is similar to that of an uninfected person.

Although there are public concerns about the transmission of HIV from an infected healthcare worker to patients, the number of instances of transmission in this direction documented in the worldwide literature is very limited. The first case was that of an HIV-positive dentist in Florida infecting several of his patients, and the second case was that of an orthopaedic surgeon in France transmitting the infection to a patient during surgery. A third case occurred in 2006 in Spain, when HIV was transmitted from an obstetrician to a patient during a caesarean section. There is a further case of transmission to a patient on the basis of genetic similarity of the virus from a French nurse but the mode of transmission was never established.

CDC reports that, during 1985–2013, there were 58 confirmed and 150 possible cases of occupationally acquired HIV infection among healthcare workers. There has been only one documented case since 1997 in the UK of HIV seroconversion in a healthcare worker after occupational exposure. Splashes with body fluid are considered by CDC to present a 'near-zero' risk of transmission even if blood-stained, and contact of these body fluids with intact skin or mucous membranes is 'extremely low risk' while percutaneous exposure presents less than 1% risk of transmission. The estimated risk is 0.23% for becoming infected from a needlestick involving HIV-infected blood at work.

In the event of such an exposure PEP is available and should be administered as soon as possible post exposure. A full course of PEP consists of three (or more) newer anti-retroviral agents for four weeks for all occupational exposures to HIV. Medications included in an HIV PEP regimen should be selected to optimise side effect and toxicity profiles and a convenient dosing schedule along with an anti-emetic and antispasmodic medication supply to encourage completion of the PEP regimen. Testing of the source patient is helpful but should not cause delay in deciding to initiate and/or continue PEP. If the source patient is determined to be HIV negative, PEP should be discontinued and no follow-up HIV testing for the exposed provider is indicated. Follow-up and counselling of the healthcare worker is important to help manage the associated anxiety as well as for further care. Serological follow-up is also important with a baseline blood sample prior to PEP. This sample is tested for creatinine (and estimated glomerular filtration rate), alanine transaminase, HIV 1 antigen/antibody, hepatitis B serology if not protectively immunised, and hepatitis C. A pregnancy test should be done for all women of childbearing potential considering PEP. Further serology at six weeks and finally at four months post exposure with fourth-generation HIV antigen/antibody combination immunoassays follows according to CDC. UK guidance suggests that, for the majority of patients, a single fourth-generation HIV test performed 45 days after completion of PEP, or after exposure if PEP was not given, is enough to detect or exclude infection. In the meantime, although anxiety provoking, the healthcare worker is advised to use precautions to avoid possible secondary transmission, e.g. barrier contraception and avoiding blood or tissue donations, pregnancy and if possible, breastfeeding. There is no need to refrain from healthcare work while awaiting final serology for any consideration of possible transmission risk for patients given the remote likelihood of infection.

Tuberculosis

Causative organism: Mycobacterium tuberculosis

Among infectious diseases tuberculosis (TB) remains 'the captain of all these men of death', with 3836 people dying daily from TB in 2019. The rate of deaths was reducing at 1.6% per year but it is anticipated to increase following the global pandemic of SARS-CoV-2 owing to reduced case finding. Infection with TB leads to early primary disease in 5% of people without treatment. Reactivation of latent TB occurs in a further 5% of infected people in the absence of treatment. With intact cell-mediated immunity 90% of infected people live with latent TB. TB is recognised as being primarily transmitted by inhalation of aerosols (droplet nuclei). Reinfection can occur and is more likely in the 18 months before cell-mediated immunity fully develops. Disease progression after 18–24 months from initial infection is usually considered to be a reactivation.

Pulmonary TB manifests as persistent chronic cough of at least two to three weeks' duration, unless the person is HIV infected; a shorter duration of cough may occur in these cases, with fever and night sweats. As the condition progresses weight loss, anorexia, haemoptysis and chest pain may present. Extrapulmonary TB can also affect the bones, meninges and other parts of the body.

For the diagnosis of latent TB both the tuberculosis skin test (TST) and interferon-gamma release assay (IGRA) indicate a cellular immune response to *M. tuberculosis*. IGRA is more specific than TST when *Bacillus* Calmette–Guérin

(BCG) vaccination has been given. The implication of testing for latent TB is that further advice and treatment will be offered if it is present.

The risk of transmission of TB to healthcare workers is dependent on the patient source characteristics and the care activities (Box 4.1). Patient factors with higher risk include whether TB is pulmonary or laryngeal disease, acid-fast bacteria (AFB) smear-positive respiratory secretions, the presence of a cough, HIV infection and atypical manifestations of disease. A delayed patient diagnosis is also an exposure risk factor and occurs in around 50% of hospitalised patients. It has been shown that an average of 24 healthcare workers are exposed for each delayed diagnosis of TB.

The controls that should be in place include environmental (engineering) controls such as ventilation specifications for clinical areas and negative-pressure rooms and the use of upper room ultraviolet germicidal irradiation (UVGI) and high-efficiency particulate air (HEPA) filters. Administrative

---

Box 4.1 Risk Categories for Activities Performed by Healthcare Workers

- **High-risk activities**
  - Cough-inducing procedures (such as sputum induction)
  - Autopsy
  - Morbid anatomy and pathology examination
  - Bronchoscopy
  - Mycobacteriology laboratory procedures, especially handling cultures of *Mycobacterium tuberculosis*
- **Intermediate-risk activities**
  - Work requiring regular direct patient contact on units (such as emergency departments) where patients with respiratory tuberculosis (TB) disease may be present
  - Work in paediatric units where patients with TB may be admitted
  - Cleaning of rooms of patients with respiratory TB disease
- **Low-risk activities**
  - Work requiring minimal patient contact (such as clerical, reception and administration)
  - Work on units where patients with respiratory TB disease are unlikely to be present

(*Source:* Modified from Canadian Tuberculosis Standards, 7e. Public Health Agency of Canada, 2014.)

controls include organisational policies that separate suspect TB health facility attendees from unnecessary contact with others, reduce the time from arrival to diagnosis and placement of suspected or known cases in an airborne infection isolation room (AIIR). There would also be policies and practices for occupational health programmes to protect vulnerable healthcare workers, e.g. those who are immune compromised, and to allow early identification of occupational infection, with access to treatment, paid sick leave and workers' compensation. The latter would include reminders of the symptoms of TB and the need for prompt reporting of symptoms, with annual reminders for staff who have potential exposure. Contact tracing procedures would also be expected to be in place. Training is an important component of administrative policies. Personal protection controls would ensure the fit-testing and availability of respiratory protection before the need arises, e.g. face-fitted N95 or higher class filtering face piece respirators or powered air-purifying respirators for high-risk procedures.

There is also a concern regarding TB-infected healthcare personnel transmitting the infection to their patients. In the UK new healthcare workers are asked about a personal or family history of TB and to answer screening questions for symptoms and signs of TB. Documentary evidence of TB skin (or IGRA) testing within the past five years is checked and/or a BCG scar check by an occupational health professional since this vaccination continues to be recommended for healthcare workers in the UK. In countries where BCG is not routinely advised for healthcare workers the TST conversion rate from regular surveillance testing has been used as an index of healthcare-associated transmission. Current CDC guidance is that annual or other routine interval TB testing of healthcare personnel is not recommended unless there is a known exposure or ongoing transmission. This is because of known limitations to the IGRA and TST for serial testing. CDC allows either IGRA or TST to be used for healthcare worker screening whereas Canadian guidance recommends TST if serial testing is planned. In any case the results of both TST and IGRA should be interpreted with other relevant clinical information, such as age, BCG status, history of contact with active TB and factors that increase the risk of progression to active disease. Healthcare workers who report being, or are found to be, HIV positive during employment should have medical and occupational assessments of TB risk, and may need to modify their work to reduce exposure as a 'disability adjustment' to support them in mitigation of the risk.

Meticillin-resistant *Staphylococcus aureus*

This is a commensal present on the skin and in the nose and throat of about 1% of the general population, and does not usually pose a risk to healthy individuals. However, in immunocompromised or debilitated patients, and those with open surgical or traumatic wounds, the organism can cause an infection which is difficult to treat. In non-outbreak situations the prevalence of meticillin-resistant *Staphylococcus aureus* (MRSA) colonisation in healthcare workers has varied between 0.2% and 15%. Studies have shown that healthcare workers are rarely the source of an outbreak although screening in the outbreak situation will identify colonised staff. Inspection and swabbing of healthcare workers' hands may be the most useful action in an outbreak situation since damaged skin or nails is more likely to be associated with colonisation. There is no clear utility in routine screening of healthcare workers. Since MRSA is most frequently transmitted by direct skin-to-skin contact or fomites workers with MRSA infections should not be routinely excluded from work. It is reasonable to exclude such workers from activities where skin-to-skin contact with the affected skin area is likely to occur until their infections are healed. Additionally, consideration for exclusion should be given for exudative lesions and wounds that are draining and cannot be properly covered and contained with a clean, dry bandage or for those who cannot maintain good hygiene practices. Occupations affected apart from healthcare workers include prison staff and childcare, veterinary and other animal workers. In the case of the latter groups both companion animal- and livestock-associated MRSA are recognised.

Norovirus

This is also known as Norwalk virus (after an outbreak in Norwalk, Ohio) and winter vomiting disease, among others. Human noroviruses belong to the family Caliciviridae and are single-stranded RNA non-enveloped viruses, about 38 nm in diameter. Some resistance to infection is thought to be present in populations who only express the Lewis A (LeA) or LeX antigen (non-secretors). Antigenic drift of the virus means that the circulating dominant variants change every two to three years, allowing for reinfection of people immune to previous viruses.

Norovirus causes acute gastroenteritis, accounting for around 18% of cases worldwide and affecting approximately 685 million people annually. The clinical features are nausea, diarrhoea, vomiting, abdominal cramps, low-grade fever, chills, headache and malaise. The average incubation period is 33 hours. The illness is of a short duration, averaging 36–48 hours with a maximum of around five days, and recovery being usually complete. Diagnosis of outbreaks is often clinical, based on symptoms: vomiting in more than 50% of affected persons in the outbreak; the incubation period; duration of illness; and lack of identification of a bacterial pathogen in culture of stool since enzyme immunoassays are not sensitive and polymerase chain reaction (PCR) is not always specific, may not be locally available and is relatively costly.

Viral shedding in faeces lasts for between 18 hours and up to eight weeks post exposure whether symptomatically infected or not. Vomiting events may widely contaminate surfaces and present the possibility of aerosolisation and inhalation. Norovirus is environmentally persistent, lasting with infectious potential up to two weeks on surfaces and two months in water. The infection is highly contagious, with transmission mainly by the faecal–oral route. The impact of this infection is that, in settings such as hospitals, closure of wards may be necessary to contain the infection, and there may also be reduced staffing levels because of sickness absence and gastrointestinal illness precautions. Outbreaks of infection commonly occur in nursing homes, hospital wards, daycare centres, schools, cruise ships and restaurants, affecting workers and clients. Control is by attention to routine hygiene practices and infection control precautions.

4.3 Vector-borne infections

Malaria

Causative organism: Plasmodium falciparum and other species

This is an infection transmitted by female *Anopheles* sp. mosquitoes and is endemic in tropical and subtropical areas, such as parts of Africa and Asia. There are five species of protozoan parasites that cause malaria: *Plasmodium falciparum*, *Plasmodium vivax*, *Plasmodium malariae*, *Plasmodium ovale* and *Plasmodium knowlesi*. Following an infective bite the incubation period varies from 7 to 30 days. The appearance of symptoms can be longer if chemoprophylaxis has been taken. The organism enters red blood cells and causes haemolysis and anaemia. The presenting symptoms are 'flu-like', with fever, chills, sweats, headaches, nausea and vomiting, body aches and malaise. It also affects liver cells and the spleen, leading to hepatosplenomegaly. With infection by *P. falciparum*, cerebral malaria can result in delirium, coma and death. The presence of sickle-cell trait confers some protection against *falciparum* malaria.

Expatriate workers are a group identified as being at particular risk of malaria owing to lapses in the use of chemoprophylaxis. Occupational groups at risk include forestry workers, agricultural advisers, mine workers, military personnel and business travellers. Special consideration is required for those who may be at increased risk for severe malaria, e.g. pregnancy, those who have undergone splenectomy and those in immune-compromised states.

Provision of appropriate antimalarial chemoprophylaxis requires evaluation of the worker's exact travel itinerary to determine their malaria risk profile. Knowledge of the timing, type of travel and destination(s) is needed together with a discussion of the pros and cons of the available regimens so as to choose an option that is likely to have good adherence. The region(s) visited will determine whether the malaria encountered is likely to be chloroquine sensitive; resistant; or chloroquine and mefloquine resistant. Drug prophylaxis is not 100% effective, and all febrile illnesses occurring within a year of return from an endemic area should be investigated, with malaria being a possible diagnosis.

Occupational health departments should be aware of up-to-date national prophylaxis guidance, the possible side effects and contraindications to the use of such medication; for example, mefloquine should not be used in the first trimester of pregnancy and pilots are not permitted to use this medication, and proguanil may affect the efficacy of coumarin anticoagulants.

Education should be given on mosquito bite precautions, including that they bite day and night: use of long pants and tucked-in, long-sleeved shirts with closed-toe shoes or boots and a hat; light-coloured, loose clothes made of tightly woven materials such as nylon or polyester and permethrin-treated clothing; and approved insect repellent use. The use of long-lasting insecticidal (bed) nets is an evidence-based measure. Awareness of counterfeit drugs and the subsequent malaria susceptibility is also important. The provision of rapid diagnostic tests (RDTs) and standby emergency treatment (SBET) is advisable for those working in remote areas where diagnostic and treatment facilities may not be available within 24 hours. Adequate information and training on usage is required and it is not a substitute for antimalarial chemoprophylaxis. In some circumstances if malaria infection is acquired in the course of work and travel to an endemic area then workers' compensation may be available.

Lyme disease

Causative organism: Borrelia burgdorferi

This is a tick-borne disease that has deer and rodents as a reservoir and can be transmitted to humans. The bite of an infected tick of the genus *Ixodes* can transmit the spirochaete *B. burgdorferi*. The responsible species of tick varies geographically, with *Ixodes scapularis* being most common in eastern and midwestern USA and south-eastern and south central Canada; *Ixodes pacificus* in western USA and Canada; *Ixodes ricinus* in Europe; and *Ixodes persulcatus* in Asia. Occupational groups generally considered at risk are farmers, forestry workers, veterinary surgeons, military recruits and other outdoor workers.

There is often a small red bump at the site of a tick bite or after removal that resolves over a few days. A rash may subsequently manifest after 3–30 days with redness centred on the site of the bite which slowly increases and sometimes clears centrally, giving the classic 'bull's eye pattern' of erythema chronicum migrans. The rash may be accompanied by flu-like symptoms. Other disease presentations may occur if early infection is not treated; these include neurological symptoms, such as headaches, neck stiffness and facial nerve palsy, or cardiac complications caused by a carditis. The latter is more often asymptomatic with first-degree heart block found on electrocardiogram. Late disease may present with monoarticular arthritis, often affecting a knee joint.

Diagnostic testing is with a screening serology test such as immunofluorescence assay or enzyme-linked immunosorbent assay (ELISA) followed by Western blot for indeterminate or positive results. Antibody tests require at least two weeks to become positive. Treatment is with doxycycline at all stages of the infection for 14 days. Amoxicillin, azithromycin and cefuroxime are alternatives. For Lyme encephalitis or carditis intravenous ceftriaxone is used. Prevention is by education of workers about risks, tick avoidance measures, insecticide-treated clothing and insect repellent usage, performing tick checks following possible exposure, and showering or bathing within two hours of possible exposure.

4.4 Zoonotic infections

Anthrax

Causative organism: Bacillus anthracis

According to the World Health Organization there are small foci of animal disease in Canada and the USA, certain countries of Central and South America and Central Asia, several sub-Saharan African countries and western China. Sporadic cases and outbreaks continue to occur elsewhere. Historically, this Gram-positive, spore-forming bacillus was responsible for 'wool-sorter's disease', in which spores of the organism present in animal hides, hair, bone, fur, wool or horns were inhaled, causing pneumonic anthrax. More than 95% of human cases are cutaneous disease, when skin contact with spores leads to the formation of a characteristic ulcerative lesion, termed an 'eschar'. The eschar appears as a pustule with a ring of blisters and marked oedema. The incubation period ranges from a few hours to three weeks. For inhalational anthrax the median incubation period is four days but may be up to 11 days. Symptoms include fatigue, headache, nausea or vomiting, cough, dyspnoea and confusion. This may progress to severe respiratory distress and cyanosis, with meningitis occurring in about 50% of cases. Septicaemia may occur with any type of anthrax following lymphatogenous spread. Diagnosis can be confirmed on microscopy with or without direct fluorescent antibody stains. Bacterial growth on culture or PCR can be used to identify the toxin and capsule genes. Antibiotic treatment of anthrax depends on the presenting features and may require the administration of multiple antibiotics. Treatment with antitoxin is recommended in systemic disease. There are specific recommendations for PEP following aerosolized *B. anthracis* spores, e.g. bioterrorism. Anthrax immunisation is available for workers at risk, such as certain laboratory workers, some veterinary surgeons and workers handling animals or animal products likely to be contaminated, as well as for those in the military. The incidence of occupationally acquired anthrax has been reduced through animal vaccination and the treatment of animal hides and horns at the country of origin before they are exported for further processing.

Occupations at risk of anthrax are those that bring workers into contact with animals and their hides – cases have been reported in animal breeders, slaughterhouse workers, trappers and hunters, fur industry workers, tanning and leather industry workers, veterinary surgeons, and wildlife, agricultural and laboratory workers. More recently episodic cases have arisen in several countries of traditional drum-makers, who scrape hides, leading to cutaneous, inhalational and gastrointestinal anthrax. Outbreaks also occurred in postal workers in the USA in 2001 as a result of bioterrorism, with seven inhalational and three cutaneous anthrax cases.

Brucellosis

Causative organism: Brucella sp.

Brucella organisms have a worldwide distribution, especially in Mediterranean countries, Africa, the Middle East, India, Central Asia, Mexico and Central and

South America. Cattle are a common source of this zoonotic infection (*Brucella abortus*), although *Brucella melitensis* is the most prevalent cause of human brucellosis. The host range includes cattle, swine, goats, sheep, deer, caribou, elk, dogs and coyotes. Transmission occurs through direct contact with non-intact skin (abrasions) and mucous membranes; inhalation is also possible. Sources of infection include infected tissues, blood and body fluids such as urine and vaginal discharge and aborted fetuses; contact in abattoirs; and the ingestion of raw milk or cheese from infected animals. Infection can also be laboratory-acquired. The incubation period is variable: 5–60 days, but may be longer; patients present with intermittent fever, headache, weakness, profuse sweating and arthralgia. Because of a tendency for the fever to rise in the afternoon and subside at night it has been known as 'undulant fever'. Other features may include sacroiliitis and spondylitis, aseptic meningitis, endocarditis and hepatic abscess. Mild lymphadenopathy and hepatosplenomegaly occur in 20–25% of cases; other findings relate to specific organ involvement. Diagnosis is confirmed by isolation of organisms from blood, bone marrow or other body fluids or tissues. Serology and PCR can also be used. Treatment requires combination antibiotics – often doxycycline and an aminoglycoside – and continued treatment for six weeks. PEP for laboratory workers may require three weeks of doxycycline. Prevention measures involve appropriate hygiene measures in agricultural work and meat-processing as well as pasteurisation of milk and infection elimination strategies among animals.

Leptospirosis

Causative organism: Leptospira interrogans
Leptospirosis is a zoonotic disease caused by a spirochaete with many serovars. The more common are Hardjo, Icterohaemorrhagiae (rats), Canicola (dogs), Autumnalis, Hebdomadis, Australis and Pomona (swine and cattle). Transmission is by contact of skin or mucous membranes with contaminated water, soil or vegetation; coming into direct contact with urine or tissues of infected animals; inhalation of aerosolised contaminated fluids; and ingestion of contaminated foods. The incubation period is around 10 days. Occupations at risk include rice, sugar cane and rubber plantation workers; dairy and pig farmers; veterinary surgeons; abattoir workers; pest control (rodent) workers; sewage and canal workers; and military recruits. Many infections result in subclinical infection, but around 10% of symptomatic infections progress to severe illness with jaundice. The most common cause of death with leptospirosis is severe pulmonary haemorrhagic syndrome (SPHS), with a fatality rate of 50%. In other cases renal failure can cause death without dialysis support. The infection is described as biphasic, with antibiotic treatment most effective in early disease and of questionable benefit in late disease; however, the biphasic pattern is often not seen. Typical presentation includes fever, rigours, intense myalgia, headache, nausea, vomiting, diarrhoea and cough. Conjunctival suffusion, lymphadenopathy, hepatosplenomegaly and skin lesions may be found on examination. Patients may then recover within a week, followed by an aseptic meningitis, possibly Weil's disease, SPHS or a late-onset uveitis.

Because of the non-specific symptoms most cases are undiagnosed. As described above, early treatment is useful as it may avoid late complications. Laboratory testing is difficult as it still relies on the microscopic agglutination test or an ELISA, while culture requires specialised media and a high index of clinical suspicion during early disease but also takes some weeks. Treatment is with doxycycline for one week in early disease; in late disease intravenous penicillin may be useful. Other treatment is supportive, with mechanical ventilation or renal dialysis being required. Prevention is by use of appropriate clothing, hygiene measures such as handwashing and covering cuts with waterproof dressings; in some circumstances the use of a short course of prophylactic doxycycline may be appropriate, e.g. in military personnel and some agricultural workers.

4.5 Food- and waterborne infections

These include cholera, shigellosis, typhoid and paratyphoid fever and *Escherichia coli* infection. Occupational health practitioners may be involved in dealing with such infections: (i) if they occur in a food handler and (ii) when employees have to travel abroad during the course of their work.

The US Food and Drug Administration (FDA) identifies six highly infective pathogens that can easily be transmitted by food handlers and cause severe illness. The FDA calls these the 'big 6' and they include norovirus, HAV, *Salmonella* Typhi, *Shigella* spp., Shiga toxin-producing *E. coli* (STEC) and non-typhoidal *Salmonella*. Food handlers may both transmit and be carriers of infection while either symptomatic or asymptomatic. Where a food handler reports diarrhoea and vomiting there should be a restriction on their return to food handling for 48 hours following the cessation of symptoms. When a food handler is diagnosed as having enteric fever (includes typhoid and paratyphoid), six consecutive negative stool samples, each obtained one week apart commencing three weeks after completion of treatment, are recommended before return to work. Shigellosis with *Shigella dysenteriae, Shigella flexneri* or *Shigella boydii* requires two negative faecal specimens taken at intervals of not less than 48 hours. If the infection involves STEC or verocytotoxin-producing *E. coli* (VTEC), of which the most common strain is *E. coli* 0157:H7, two consecutive negative stool samples taken at least 48 hours apart are required. Non-typhoidal *Salmonella* requires exclusion for 48 hours following cessation of gastrointestinal symptoms. Jurisdictional guidelines may vary and should be checked. Prior to return to work food handlers should be reminded of the necessity for good hygiene practices.

For travellers abroad, immunisations for foodborne infections can be arranged based on an awareness of outbreaks of diarrhoeal diseases in the countries to which they travel. Typhoid vaccine may be administered parenterally (heat--killed organism or phenol-preserved antigen) or orally (live, attenuated vaccine) for travel to areas with a recognised risk of exposure to *Salmonella* Typhi. For cholera, the vaccine available is less than 60% effective.

Hepatitis A as described in Section 4.2 ('Other hepatitis viruses').

There is no effective vaccine against *E. coli* or shigellosis. Travellers abroad should exercise food and water precautions, including ice. Readers are referred to other texts regarding the management of travellers' diarrhoea.

4.6 Silicotuberculosis

The inhalation of extraneous substances may cause direct damage to the lung architecture, leading to a predisposition for infection. Among other effects the inhalation of cigarette smoke is known to impair mucociliary clearance by paralysis of cilia, and promoting a change in the nature of the respiratory epithelium. The excessive inhalation of so-called nuisance dusts can also overwhelm these clearance mechanisms. There is also the example of pneumococcal pneumonia and increased occurrence in welders, probably because of the effects of inhaled iron and other metal fumes. An association that has long been recognised is that between silicosis and TB, with most studies being conducted in mining populations. For workers who have an established diagnosis of silicosis the relative risk is about 3.0 for the development of pulmonary TB. There is also a nearly four times greater risk of extrapulmonary TB, with pleural TB being the most common site. Both more intense exposures to silica and an increased severity of silicosis are associated with pulmonary TB. Silica exposure without silicosis may also be associated with pulmonary TB. Silica particles are phagocytosed by macrophages, causing inflammasome activation with autophagy and the release of intracellular silica, leading to an inflammatory cycle. When present there is a concomitant increase in intracellular replication of *M. tuberculosis*, which is also released from macrophages. However the interaction between silica and *M. tuberculosis* remains incompletely understood. It is known from genotyping studies that TB infections are passed between mineworkers. The risk of the development of both silicosis and pulmonary TB continues following the cessation of exposure to silica. Extending the treatment of pulmonary TB by two months in this situation may improve cure rates and reduce relapse, but further research is needed to confirm this suggestion. As mentioned previously HIV infection is significantly associated with TB and there is a combined effect with silica exposure and silicosis. Therefore, the population rates of TB and of HIV infection both influence the likelihood of silicotuberculosis.

Further Reading

Boggild, A., Brophy, J., Charlebois, P. et al. (n.d.) *Canadian recommendations for the prevention and treatment of malaria. An Advisory Committee Statement (ACS) from the Committee to Advise on Tropical Medicine and Travel (CATMAT) Public Health Agency of Canada.* https://www.canada.ca/en/public-health/services/catmat/canadian-recommendations-prevention-treatment-malaria.html (accessed 8 March 2021).

Centers for Disease Control and Prevention (2020). *CDC Yellow Book: Health Information for International Travel.* https://wwwnc.cdc.gov/travel/page/yellowbook-home (accessed 15 March 2021).

Centers for Disease Control and Prevention (2021). *TB Screening and Testing of Health Care Personnel.* https://www.cdc.gov/tb/topic/testing/healthcareworkers.htm (accessed 6 March 2021).

Centers for Disease Control and Prevention (2021). *Malaria.* https://www.cdc.gov/parasites/malaria/index.html (accessed 8 March 2021).

Chiodini, P.L., Patel, D., and Whitty, C.J.M. (2019). *Guidelines for Malaria Prevention in Travellers from the United Kingdom, 2019.* London: Public Health England.

Cresswell F and the British Association for Sexual Health and HIV/British HIV Association Guideline Writing Group (2021). *UK Guideline for the use of HIV Post-Exposure Prophylaxis 2021.* https://www.bhiva.org/file/6074031a87755/PEPSE-guidelines.pdf (accessed 6 March 2021).

Moorman, A.C., de Perio, M.A., Goldschmidt, R. et al. (2020). Testing and clinical management of health care personnel potentially exposed to hepatitis C virus — CDC Guidance, United States, 2020. *MMWR Recommendations and Reports* 69 (RR-6): 1–8. https://doi.org/10.15585/mmwr.rr6906a1.

National Institute for Health and Care Excellence (2016). *Tuberculosis. NICE guideline NG33.* Last updated: 12 September 2019. www.nice.org.uk/guidance/ng33 (accessed 6 March 2021).

Public Health Agency of Canada (2014). *Canadian Tuberculosis Standards*, 7e. Ottawa: Public Health Agency of Canada. https://www.canada.ca/content/dam/phac-aspc/migration/phac-aspc/tbpc-latb/pubs/tb-canada-7/assets/pdf/tb-standards-tb-normes-ch4-eng.pdf (accessed 6 March 2021).

Public Health Agency of Canada (2021). *Pathogen Safety Data Sheets.* https://www.canada.ca/en/public--health/services/laboratory-biosafety-biosecurity/pathogen-safety-data-sheets-risk-assessment.html (accessed 8 March 2021).

Public Health England (2020). *Integrated Guidance on Health Clearance of Healthcare Workers and the Management of Healthcare Workers Living with Bloodborne Viruses (Hepatitis B, Hepatitis C and HIV). Guidance from the UK Advisory Panel for Healthcare Workers Infected with Bloodborne Viruses (UKAP).* London: Public Health England.

CHAPTER 5

Clinical Evaluations

5.1 Pre-placement

Pre-placement, sometimes termed pre-employment, assessment is a function carried out by almost all occupational health services. Preferably, the assessment should be undertaken following a job offer (pre-placement); in many jurisdictions, to do otherwise may be a prima facie case of discrimination on the grounds of disability if the job is withdrawn. But in parts of the world the reality is that workers have to pass a medical assessment to be employed (thus a pre-employment). The main purpose is to ensure that if the person has a pre-existing illness, disability or susceptibility that may make the performance of the proposed job difficult or unsafe for the individual, co-workers or third parties, e.g. visitors or customers, it is considered and mitigated as far as is reasonable. Pre-existing disorders present before commencing work can add to the liability of the employer in the event of future claims for work-related disease, e.g. hearing loss. The assessment is also used to see to what extent the workplace and the job can be adapted to meet the needs of the worker with a disability, and it provides baseline data for future assessments. However, these aims are sometimes complemented by other aims, which attempt to make full use of the presence of the new employee at the occupational health department. Thus, the pre-placement examination may be used to introduce the facilities of the service to the new starter, to bring the worker's immunisations up to date and to reinforce advice on health promotion. If the worker meets the criteria for employment, they will usually also meet the health criteria for joining the company's pension scheme where one is available. Generally, it is now accepted that pre-placement

Pocket Consultant: Occupational Health, Sixth Edition. Kerry Gardiner, David Rees, Anil Adisesh, David Zalk, and Malcolm Harrington.
© 2022 John Wiley & Sons Ltd. Published 2022 by John Wiley & Sons Ltd.

assessments are poor at identifying adequately work applicants who may in time need frequent absences from work or who may become disabled from chronic medical conditions, such as poor mental health. So, directing the pre-placement evaluations to these objectives is discouraged.

The implementation of legislation on disability discrimination in many countries has led to a review of the basis for pre-employment examinations. Such examinations of prospective candidates or those on an interview shortlist would be better replaced by pre-placement assessment of the candidate selected after interview where they are still permissible. This is in any case more cost-effective, as it avoids the performance of several assessments for the eventual selection of one individual. Importantly, in some jurisdictions excluding a prospective employee from employment must be evidence-based; the risks associated with the person's medical condition and the nature of the work must be explicit. Rejecting human immunodeficiency virus (HIV)-positive applicants merely because of their infection unrelated to the job requirements is an example. Partly for this reason, the content of the pre-employment examination should be informed by an occupational risk exposure profile (OREP), which is an account of the hazards associated with the specific occupation, so that work restriction or exclusion is linked to job exposures. Such measures may be termed 'bona fide' job requirements, that is, they are demonstrably justifiable.

Employing a person with existing health conditions should take account of the possible expertise and contribution of the individual to the job, rather than just the apparent cost implications of the conditions alone. An individual with a chronic ailment that is well controlled by regular treatment may indeed contribute more to a job than an equivalent 'healthy' individual with less experience or poor motivation. Such decisions are not medical judgements and generally the foreseeability of the effects of a medical condition may be limited to a few years.

Pre-placement assessments vary in content and length, depending on the aims. Some are directly to obtain information that is essential to ensure no contraindication between the person's health status and the proposed job. Others may include opportunistic general health and lifestyle matters on a voluntary basis so that individual health promotion can be facilitated. Questions and examinations unrelated to the aims of the pre-placement assessment should not be asked at the same time to avoid discrimination, or the perception of it. The trend in pre-placement questionnaires is towards fewer questions that are more focused.

Medical confidentiality requirements mean that prospective employers are generally not informed of the details of applicants' conditions; rather, only their employability and any work restrictions necessitated by their health.

5.2 Fitness for work

Fitness for work is a complex topic that is generally covered poorly in undergraduate training of physicians and other practitioners who may become part of the occupational health team. Work has many benefits: financial, of course, but also psychological and physical health ones. Legislation on employment equity, disability discrimination prevention and related matters governs many aspects of fitness to work. Also, retaining skilled and experienced workers, older people among them, in the workforce is advantageous for the economy. For these and other reasons enabling people to continue working is important and unnecessary declarations of unfitness to work are to be avoided. Return to work as soon as is manageable, even in a reduced or modified role, is encouraged because the longer the absence the less likely a successful return to employment. Some countries, notably the UK, have active rehabilitation and return to work programmes.

Impairment is a change in the normal structure or function – say limited movement of a knee joint – that can cause a disability (the resulting loss of ability to do something like climbing stairs or kicking a ball), but will only be a participation restriction at work if it results in the inability to fulfil a work role: lifts (elevators) may make climbing stairs unnecessary and few of us need to kick a ball at work. Consequently, activity limitations may confer no participation restrictions for a particular job and a functional assessment weighed against the requirements of the actual work tasks of the individual in the usual job or in a modified role need to be considered in fitness for work assessments.

Exploring alternative or modified work tasks or work processes (work accommodation) is a core and sometimes statutory aspect of retaining people at work. There are many ways to accommodate workers with impairments. Short duration, troublesome tasks that exacerbate asthma – cleaning tasks for instance – can be allocated to co-workers; the physical work environment can be modified for wheelchairs and flexible working hours or more frequent rest periods introduced.

Essentially, fitness to work evaluations are a weighing-up of the functional capacity of a person against the requirements of the job. Doctors without knowledge of the job requirements should be wary of making precise judgements about fitness to work in a particular job. In this situation, it is preferable to describe the impairment and disability caused by it and leave the fitness to work decision to the occupational health service, assuming there is one. Functional capacity assessments can be comprehensive and include general health, ability to travel to and from work, manual skills, vision, mental state, capacity to communicate, alertness, risk to others in doing the work and many other domains. Prognosis and possible optimalisation of treatment of medical conditions are also considerations. The job needs should inform the domains to be evaluated. Detailing the requirements of the job may also be complex and extend well beyond physical demands; suitability for shift work and interfacing with customers are two examples among many. Occupational therapists are a major resource in assessing functional capacity and suitability for aspects of work, but they are in short supply in most low- and middle-income countries. The utility of functional capacity assessments to predict a sustained return to work is limited compared with that for the short term. Authors of fitness to work reports should be cautious about making far-reaching statements about fitness to work outside of the job in question such as 'unfit for work in the open labour market' unless objective evidence to support this is at hand.

Occupational health services can play a role in maintaining fitness for work through activities to prevent deterioration of health by deleterious life-style factors such as smoking, poor diet, lack of exercise and alcohol consumption.

Post-sickness absence review

Some occupational health departments review workers who return after a period of sickness absence. The reason for the review is to ensure that the person has no residual effects from the cause of the sickness absence that may affect the return to work. Although hospital physicians and general practitioners (family physicians) often indicate the duration of absence required and the fitness for return to work, this may be performed without a full appreciation of the job duties or work environment. Hence, occupational health staff can consider these factors in conjunction with those providing clinical care. Close liaison between occupational health services and physicians responsible for treatment facilitates successful return to work after sickness.

Sickness absence or absence attributed to sickness often includes absence for social, family and personal reasons other than illness. Sympathetic review and assistance by occupational health staff may reduce the likelihood of recurrence of absence for these reasons. Sickness absence policies often make the distinction between frequent, short-term absences and long-term spells of absence (e.g. more than four weeks of continuous absence). Long-term absence results from chronic ailments, acute conditions requiring a waiting period for surgery, incomplete recovery from illness or post-surgical complications or recuperation.

Frequent, short-term absences are often difficult to manage. This is especially so if the stated causes for these absences vary, suggesting that there may be factors other than a chronic underlying illness. These could include work-related factors, such as job dissatisfaction; individuals who are prone to frequent, short-term infections; non-work factors, such as illness in a family member; or drug and alcohol problems. However, there may be relevant organisational policies to support workers with these issues which may reduce absences.

Retirement on grounds of ill health

One of the functions of occupational health services is to assess workers wishing to retire from their jobs on health grounds. These include workers with chronic illnesses or incomplete recovery from treatment, where the continuing safe and efficient performance of their work is in doubt. Pension entitlements may be brought forward for those who are successful. The replacement of an experienced worker who retires early could be a problem for the organisation. The occupational health staff also have to consider whether the individual is capable of doing other jobs in spite of the illness. If so, redeployment of the worker to a different job within the company is a suitable alternative.

5.3 Taking an occupational history

This is a full description of the individual's previous jobs and occupational exposures, usually from the time of leaving school to date. It is a crucial part of any medical examination and, indeed, every medical student and occupational health student should be taught to take an occupational history. If the occupational history is incomplete or not taken, an important aspect of a patient's history will be omitted. This could lead to an error in diagnosis or a delay in diagnosis and management. In some circumstances, an *exposure* history rather than an occupation history is appropriate. This is especially so if the occupational history does not explain the clinical features. In asbestos-mining areas asbestos-related diseases may be due to casual childhood employment, environmental exposure or contamination of homes by asbestos mine employees. Mercury is widely used to extract gold in artisanal and illicit gold mining; poisoning may occur in miners but also in those in proximity to the extraction site. It is not unusual for artisans to work additionally to their formal employment during 'leisure time' and hobbies may contribute to occupational exposure, pottery for example. Hobbies may entirely explain some diseases: the amateur boat builder may become sensitised to isocyanates; or the bird fancier may develop extrinsic allergic alveolitis.

Table 5.1 shows a format for obtaining a full occupational history. The information can be provided by the worker filling in the table or, more usually, by a healthcare worker interview. For the former method it is often necessary for the information to be supplemented by direct questioning so that key facts are ascertained. Information about past occupations can be as relevant as that about the present job. Previous occupations may be the cause of the patient's current health problems, particularly for diseases of long latent period, such as cancer or asbestosis. For these cases, a detailed past history is vital.

Some stated occupations, such as 'civil servant', 'operator' or 'retired', need further clarification, as these vague terms do not give much indication of occupational exposures.

The occupational history should contain information on the following items for each job:

- job title
- description of tasks/duties within the job title
- employer and nature of the company/industry
- duration of employment in each job
- hours of work, including overtime and shift work
- exposure to occupational hazards
- provision and use of personal protective equipment
- sickness absence, especially for work-related ill health or injury.

TABLE 5.1

Format for obtaining full occupational history.

Workplace (employer's name and location)	Dates worked from	Dates worked to	Full/part time	Describe type of industry	Describe job title and duties	Known health hazards in workplace (dusts, solvents, etc.)	Usual frequency of exposure to the hazards[a]	Types of protective equipment used	Were you ever off work for a work-related health problem or injury?

[a] Ascertain whether exposure is daily for most of the shift, infrequent during the shift, once per week, once per month etc.

5.4 Health or medical surveillance

The term 'health or medical surveillance' has been used for the scheduled periodic medical/physiological assessment of exposed workers, with a view to protecting workers and preventing occupationally related diseases. Surveillance in public health is the collection of information, usually on a disease, for the purposes of interventions to reduce its occurrence or impact. This should be true of surveillance in occupational health as well. Deviations from health or disease detected by medical assessments of workers should result in a review of workplace exposures and improved control if necessary. Examinations only directed to an individual's condition without intention to address the cause is better termed screening. Screening may be useful: medical conditions unrelated to work may necessitate work accommodation or treatment and the workplace is a useful site for public health programmes such as HIV detection and prevention, but in the main medical data collected on workers should be linked to exposure data to inform improvements in exposure control or the placement of employees in more suitable jobs. For example, audiometry that identifies accelerated decline in hearing, even if clinically unimportant, should lead to the evaluation of workplace noise control.

Periodic health surveillance is most useful and cost-effective when it is targeted to detect specific deviations from health associated with actual work exposures experienced by the employee. Non-specific medical evaluations and multiple tests often result in false positives, i.e. tests that are outside the normal reference range but inconsequential to health or abnormal but unrelated to work. False positives are problematic in occupational health because they require further evaluations of the employee, sometimes invasive or costly ones, and the question of who pays for them may be contentious. Focused testing using the minimum number of necessary investigations should be the aim. Health surveillance should also be subject to cost–benefit analysis. It may be more beneficial to health to use the money that would have been spent on medical evaluations on exposure control, making medical investigations unnecessary or less frequently required.

In some situations, scheduled periodic evaluations should be complemented by encouraging workers to present to the occupational health department in between them. This is particularly true for acute conditions that can manifest over a short time, such as metal poisoning, work-related asthma, dermatitis, tuberculosis and other occupational infections.

Medical surveillance is required by law for some groups of workers exposed to specific hazards in the workplace. This activity, when carried out by occupational health departments, requires that the medical or physiological assessments are valid and that information is sought on the nature and extent of occupational exposures. The legal requirements vary between countries; some examples are included below.

- Periodic audiometry as part of the assessment of noise-exposed workers is common worldwide. A decline in a worker's hearing should prompt evaluation of noise control, consideration of improvement in hearing protectors, workers' compensation if appropriate and possible relocation of the affected employee, bearing in mind that introducing a replacement worker into excessive noise may be illegal and is certainly a questionable practice.

- Commonly, examinations of workers exposed to ionising radiation, asbestos, silica, tuberculosis in health workers, metal (lead, mercury, manganese, arsenic), welding fume and coal mine dust are mandatory or necessary.
- Examination of the hands and nose in workers exposed to chromic acid mist and other hexavalent chromium compounds. The rationale for periodic assessment is the early detection of 'chrome ulcers' on the skin of the hands and nasal septal ulceration or perforation, all recognised pathological effects from such exposure. Nasal examination requires experience in detecting such pathology with the aid of a nasal speculum. As for detecting skin ulceration, more frequent self-examination by individual workers with referral to occupational health is better than less frequent skin examinations of all exposed workers by occupational health staff.
- Exposure to respiratory sensitisers. The periodic review of symptoms, with lung function assessment, is recommended for workers exposed to isocyanates, platinum salts, laboratory animal dander, glutaraldehyde and other recognised respiratory sensitisers. The symptom enquiry includes wheeze, breathlessness, chest tightness and nocturnal cough. The lung function tests include spirometry and peak flow determinations. The effectiveness of occasional lung function testing in detecting asthma is questionable. Spirometry can detect obstruction of the airways during an asthma attack, but could well be normal in between attacks in someone with asthma. This limitation illustrates the need for access to occupational health services between scheduled evaluations when symptoms occur.

There are other periodic medical assessments that do not fit with the description of health surveillance provided earlier. These are medical examinations of special groups, where their state of health may affect the safety of the public. Two examples follow.

- *Professional drivers.* Those who drive passenger-carrying vehicles or large goods vehicles are required to have periodic medical assessments to ensure that they have not developed a disease or disability that might affect their fitness to drive and pose a danger to the public. Conditions generally specified that will bar such drivers include uncontrolled epilepsy, severe mental health conditions and liability to sudden attacks of severe giddiness or syncope (fainting spells). Further detailed advice is available in the UK Driver and Vehicle Licensing Agency's guide on the fitness to drive (https://www.gov.uk/guidance/assessing-fitness-to-drive-a-guide-for-medical-professionals).
- *Food handlers.* The medical surveillance of this group of staff is intended primarily to protect the products from contamination by infected material (see Section 4.5).

Exit medicals are undertaken close to when employees leave the enterprise; the last periodic medical may serve as the exit medical. However, if a disease could have arisen between the time of the last period medical and the worker's departure date from the enterprise, using the last period medical would be inappropriate. The exit medical should describe occupational exposures as well as health at the time, especially causally related to the job's hazards. One setting in which the exit medical is useful is when a worker is likely to move to a workplace with the same or similar exposures: noise is a good example; audiometry results and noise levels and duration are very helpful for the next employer's occupational health service. Results from the exit medical can, with the worker's consent, be used for pre-placement medical purposes by the next employer for workers who move frequently among employers – artisans who do temporary work at many enterprises are among them. The absence of exposure-related deviations from health at exit does not protect the employer from liability for long-latency disease that can arise post exposure, for instance cancer and pneumoconioses. But the absence of conditions that present during exposure, such as noise-induced hearing loss, does provide protection.

5.5 Medical records

Many jurisdictions have regulations stipulating that occupational medical records must be kept for lengthy periods, even 40 years or more. If a company closes, it may be mandatory to transfer the records to a state or other facility. Workers should also have the right of access to their own records. Additionally, records need to be kept safely so that they are unavailable to individuals without good reasons to access them. In the main, access is restricted to the occupational health service and staff of occupational health enforcement agencies. Because individual informed consent would usually be necessary to use these records for research, it is useful to obtain this consent at the pre-placement examination or soon after. It is advisable to get approval for the consent process from an ethics committee or institutional review board.

Records on individual workers that are maintained by occupational health services include the following.

- Pre-placement questionnaires and examinations.
- Occupational history information, including data on previous occupations, present job and change in job within the same organisation.
- Visits to the occupational health service, including the reasons for and outcomes of the visits. This includes periodic attendance for periodic medical assessments, health surveillance for exposure to specific agents, emergency first aid treatment for accidents and injury, visits for advice and counselling and, in some cases, visits for the treatment of minor ailments.
- Results of physiological tests, e.g. lung function tests, audiometry or vision screening.
- Results of other laboratory investigations, e.g. antigen status and antibody levels for specific infections, biological monitoring and biological effect monitoring results and blood and urine test results.

- Occupational/industrial hygiene data. These are often kept by the occupational/industrial hygiene or safety department, separately from the medical records. However, if there is to be regular evaluation of occupational exposure and effect, it would be sensible for the two data sets to be brought together and compared by the relevant specialties.
- Immunisation records, including vaccination for travel and for specific protection against occupational infections in health workers.
- Communications and reports from family physicians, hospital medics, physiotherapists and other healthcare practitioners providing treatment for the worker.
- Consent forms, including those for access to medical reports and those allowing disclosure of certain information to management.
- Data on smoking history or alcohol consumption and current medications.

Some occupational health services still maintain the above range of medical records in files and paper format. They can be filed in alphabetical order, by work department or by work or personal identification number. Increasingly, computer systems are being used for the storage of medical records. Commercial software systems are now available for such tasks as tracking immunisation status, automatic printing of reminder letters and aggregating and summarising data for groups of workers. The potential for using data kept in this format for epidemiological studies is good; however, the usefulness of the data is only as good as the completeness, consistency and accuracy of recording. There are differences, even for recording data on diagnosis. Hence, low back pain could be recorded as sciatica, lumbago, myositis or backache. Attempts have been made to develop uniform recording systems for occupational health data, with varying success. Where computer systems are used to store and retrieve occupational health records, the security of the system must be ensured. In addition to physical safeguards, such as locks and keeping the system in a locked secure room, computer software is also available to provide password protection, anti-virus mechanisms and a system audit trail and to limit the number of individuals who have access to and who can modify some or all of the records. There should also be provisions for the back-up storage of data in the event of disaster or system failure. Advances in computerisation have meant the availability of equipment, such as scanners and storage systems, that can facilitate the safekeeping and processing of large amounts of data. Where data about individuals are stored on a computer, there are legal provisions in many countries, such as the UK's General Data Protection Regulation (UK GDPR), to safeguard the accuracy and availability of that data. Paper copies or originals of some historical documents, especially those that have medicolegal implications, should still be kept.

Further Reading

Hobson, J. and Smedley, J. (2019). *Fitness for Work: the Medical Aspects*, 6e. Oxford, UK: Oxford University Press.

CHAPTER 6

Occupational Toxicology

6.1 General principles of toxicology

Toxicology is the study of substances that can have adverse health effects on living organisms, especially in relatively small doses. All substances are capable of causing harm; it is the dose that determines the likelihood of ill-health effects (paraphrasing Paracelsus). Other determinants include the physical and chemical form of the agent, the route of administration and the susceptibility of the individual. The subject area is of relevance to occupational health professionals as they have a major interest in controlling exposure and preventing ill health from exposure to toxic substances encountered in work situations. Some areas of specialisation in toxicology are forensic toxicology, clinical toxicology, regulatory toxicology, behavioural toxicology, and occupational and environmental toxicology.

Hazard and risk

The terms 'hazard' and 'risk' are often confused and used interchangeably. A clear distinction should be made between the two. 'Hazard' refers to the potential to cause harm, whereas 'risk' refers to the likelihood of harm occurring and also takes into account the severity of the effect.

Pocket Consultant: Occupational Health, Sixth Edition. Kerry Gardiner, David Rees, Anil Adisesh, David Zalk, and Malcolm Harrington.
© 2022 John Wiley & Sons Ltd. Published 2022 by John Wiley & Sons Ltd.

A good substance to exemplify the difference is asbestos. It is a recognised hazard, causing harm to the respiratory system (among other target organs). However, the risk of these effects occurring depends on the nature and extent (duration and concentration) of exposure. If asbestos is present within sealed insulating material, then the risk to health of those who work in the building is very small; however, if workers attempted to undertake maintenance work on the asbestos (thereby breaking the 'seal') then this would liberate substantial quantities of asbestos fibres into the local atmosphere, which would be inhaled, thereby posing an appreciable risk. The hazard in these two situations is the same, but the risk is hugely different.

Differences in toxicity due to different forms of chemicals

Physical form

Lead ingots do not pose a risk to health from skin absorption or inhalation. However, if the ingots are heated above the melting point of lead (>330 °C), the lead will vaporise, oxidise and condense, creating lead oxide fumes – and it is this form of lead that, when inhaled and absorbed, causes systemic (whole body) toxicity.

Spillages of salts of mercury in powder form underneath floorboards may not pose as much of a risk to health as spillages of mercury metal – as the metal is liquid and volatile. It vapourises easily at room temperature to produce mercury in a form that can be inhaled to cause mercury poisoning.

The solubility of chemicals in water can determine their bioavailability and rate of clearance. Compounds that are poorly soluble can persist at the site of entry into the body and may exert long-term pathological effects. This may be the reason why less soluble forms of nickel salts, such as sulphides and oxides of nickel, are respiratory carcinogens, with less evidence for a similar effect from the more soluble forms.

Chemical form

Cyanide is highly toxic to biological enzyme systems, yet hydrocyanic acid (HCN) and sodium cyanide (NaCN) have differing degrees of lethality. HCN is a gas and NaCN is a white crystalline powder, which when dissolved in water or acids, for example gastric hydrochloric acid, releases HCN. Thiocyanate (SCN^-) contains sulphur linked to the cyanide radical, yet it is relatively non-toxic compared with hydrogen cyanide. Indeed, the rationale behind the administration of sodium thiosulphate in cases of cyanide poisoning is to convert the cyanide to thiocyanate, so that the latter can be safely excreted via the urine.

Organic and inorganic forms

Organic and inorganic compounds of the same metal may have different toxic properties. Inorganic lead poisoning causes colic, constipation, malaise, anaemia and encephalopathy, whereas the predominant clinical features of poisoning by organic lead compounds, such as tetraethyl lead (TEL), are those of a toxic organic psychosis – mainly psychiatric symptoms. Also, blood lead levels form a good indicator of excessive absorption of inorganic lead, whereas for organic lead urinary lead levels are a better marker for biological monitoring (see Section 12.6).

Inhalation of inorganic tin, such as tin oxide, leads to a characteristic chest radiograph with no functional changes. The condition, referred to as stannosis, is relatively benign, despite the gross radiological picture. Similar effects are seen with the inhalation of barium sulphate dust – causing baritosis – and iron oxide particles – causing siderosis. However, the inhalation of fumes of organic tin compounds, such as tributyl tin, causes irritant effects to the respiratory tract. Other organic tin compounds, such as triethyl tin, have been described as causing cerebral oedema, and triphenyl tin acetate causes hepatic damage.

Valency states

Compounds of metals with different valency states may differ in their toxic and biological properties. For example, chromium compounds may have a valency of 0–6. Chromium metal (valency 0) is relatively inert. Trivalent chromium compounds are an essential dietary requirement, Cr(III) having a role in glucose metabolism. Some hexavalent compounds, for example calcium chromate, are pulmonary carcinogens, whereas trivalent compounds are not.

Extent of halogenation

Polychlorinated biphenyls (PCBs) can exist as many different isomers. The extent of chlorination of the biphenyl component affects the properties of the PCB, such as the electrical and thermal resistance. The site and extent of chlorination also affects the toxicity. This is also true of polybrominated biphenyls, where the extent of bromination determines the physical and toxicological properties.

The substitution of all four hydrogen atoms on the methane molecule produces carbon tetrachloride, with well-recognised hepatotoxic properties. If only three hydrogen atoms on methane are replaced by chlorine, chloroform gas is formed. This has anaesthetic properties and is also hepatotoxic. With only two hydrogen atoms replaced by chlorine, methylene chloride is produced. This agent is used as a paint stripper and causes an increase in carboxyhaemoglobin when absorbed. Neither carbon tetrachloride nor chloroform has this property.

Similarly, by substituting all four hydrogen atoms on ethylene with chlorine, tetrachloroethylene (perchloroethylene) is produced. This is the most common solvent used for dry-cleaning clothes. Substituting three hydrogen atoms results in trichloroethylene, used widely as a degreasing agent. When only one hydrogen atom is replaced by chlorine, monochloroethylene (vinyl chloride) is produced. Trichloroethylene and perchloroethylene are hepatotoxic and liquid at room temperature. Vinyl chloride is gaseous, has anaesthetic properties and is the only chlorinated ethylene compound known to cause angiosarcoma of the liver (in rodents and humans).

Exposure, absorption and metabolism

The main routes of entry for toxic substances into the body are:

- Inhalation – for gases, vapours, dusts, fumes and other aerosols (e.g. mists).
- Skin absorption – especially for fat-soluble substances. An 'Sk' notation in the UK's Health and Safety Executive's document on Workplace Exposure Limits (EH40/2005 – updated annually) indicates those chemicals that can be absorbed through the skin. The American Conference of Governmental Industrial Hygienists, Inc. (ACGIH) publication on threshold limit values (TLVs) also provides a 'Skin' notation against those chemicals where skin and mucosal absorption can lead to systemic effects.
- Ingestion – rarer for occupational agents but can result from the consumption of food and drink at process areas in workplaces. Inhaled particles trapped on the mucociliary escalator may also be coughed up and then ingested before being cleared via the gastrointestinal tract.
- Inoculation – this is often viewed in the context of exposure to biological rather than chemical hazards, for example needlestick injuries as a means of occupational transmission of bloodborne infections such as hepatitis B. However, in the administration of medications using hypodermic needles by healthcare workers, vets and farmers, inoculation incidents have resulted in cases of severe local tissue damage and systemic effects. Also, injection guns used in engineering processes have caused oil-based products to be accidentally injected into fascial spaces in the hands, resulting in tissue necrosis.

Toxic agents may have a local effect at the site of entry or may be distributed via the blood to have effects on other target organs, for example liver, lungs, central and peripheral nervous system, bone marrow and kidneys.

- Local effects – include skin and mucous membrane irritation, for example to the eyes, nose, throat and lower respiratory tract. The potential for skin contact with chemicals used in the workplace is considerable, and hence contact dermatitis is a common occupational disease. The respiratory tract is the obvious site for effects from inhaled toxic substances. Whether the upper or lower respiratory tract or other target organs are affected by inhaled toxins depends on the speed and efficiency of pulmonary clearance, on the solubility of the chemical and potentially on the aerodynamic diameter of the particle to which the substance is absorbed or adsorbed.
- Systemic effects – can be caused by the chemical itself or by metabolites usually produced on passage through the liver. Metabolites excreted via the urine can affect the bladder whereas those excreted through the bile can affect the lower gastrointestinal tract. Fat-soluble toxic agents are distributed to organs with a high lipid content, for example beneath the skin; around the liver and kidneys; to the bone marrow; and to the brain and spinal cord. Adipose tissue acts as a depot for the storage and slow release of these fat-soluble agents. Therefore, some of these agents, for example organic solvents, have a prolonged effect and an extended half-life.

Detoxification

Several enzymatic reactions are responsible for the detoxification of absorbed chemicals. These include enzymes that are part of the cytochrome P450 mixed function oxidase system in the liver microsomes. Other enzymes are dehydrogenases and reductases. The metabolic processes involve phase I reactions, such as oxidation, reduction and hydrolysis, and phase II reactions, such as conjugation with glucuronic acid. The conversion of bilirubin into bilirubin glucuronide is an example of a phase II reaction. This is part of the normal body mechanism for dealing with bilirubin produced by the breakdown of haemoglobin at the end of the 120-day lifespan of red blood cells. Bilirubin is fat soluble, but on glucuronidation it is converted to a water-soluble form, which is then easily excreted via the bile.

The purpose of detoxification is to produce a less toxic metabolite that can then be excreted. However, the process is imperfect, and at times a more toxic compound or one with carcinogenic or mutagenic properties is produced. Pro-carcinogens, for example polycyclic aromatic hydrocarbons (PAHs), are chemicals that do not exert a carcinogenic effect directly, but on metabolism the ultimate or proximate carcinogen is produced. This is believed to be the mechanism by which the urinary bladder becomes the site for malignant change from exposure to PAHs and to β-naphthylamine. PAHs are absorbed via the lungs, where they are transported to the liver. The metabolites produced are excreted via the kidneys and, for the period of contact with the bladder before the urine is voided, the metabolites exert a carcinogenic effect on the bladder epithelium.

Excretion

Occupational agents that are systemically absorbed are excreted as the parent chemical compounds or after conversion to other metabolites. The main routes of excretion are:

- via the urine, e.g. aluminium and cobalt
- through the bile, e.g. silver and copper
- in the breath, e.g. organic solvents, such as ethanol, toluene and trichloroethylene.

Ingested compounds that are poorly absorbed via the gastrointestinal tract are excreted in the faeces.

Small amounts of absorbed compounds may also be excreted in sweat, milk, tears and saliva. They may also be found in keratinous tissues of hair and nails. There is a time delay between the systemic absorption of a chemical and its excretion. The clearance of perchloroethylene, for example, occurs in several phases: a rapid phase within hours and a slow phase over several days or weeks. This information is important for biological monitoring (see Section 12.6) and the interpretation of the results.

Variability of response to toxic agents

Not everyone reacts equally to a given dose of a toxic material. The factors that contribute to individual variability include:

- age
- sex

- size
- ethnic group
- genetic make-up – including inherited differences in speed of metabolism of absorbed chemicals, for example slow and fast acetylators of certain drugs; another example is individuals with glucose 6-phosphate deficiency, who can have haemolytic episodes on exposure to fava beans or naphthalene
- immune status
- atopy – defined as a propensity to produce immunoglobulin E (IgE) antibodies in response to exposure to common environmental allergens; it manifests as an individual or family history of asthma, eczema or hay fever, with increased serum IgE and/or positive skin-prick tests to recognised allergens
- nutritional state
- co-existing disease (and its treatment)
- concomitant exposure to other synergistic or antagonistic chemicals (including prescribed medications, e.g. barbiturates, steroids and alcohol)
- previous exposure to the toxic agent; the administration of halothane has caused toxic hepatitis in some individuals who have had previous exposure to this anaesthetic agent; in addition, previous exposure to allergens may cause sensitisation, so that subsequent exposure to smaller doses can result in severe effects.

Classification of toxic substances

There is no single suitable classification of toxic substances. Various authorities use systems based on physical, chemical, physiological or biological properties or some combination of these. Classification of toxic chemicals based on physical properties can have categories as solids, liquids, semi-solids and gases or vapours. A chemical classification can subdivide chemicals into elements and compounds, with compounds being further categorised as organic or inorganic and halogenated or non-halogenated. Organic compounds can be aromatic (ring structures based on the presence of one or more benzene rings) or aliphatic (primarily straight-chained formulae). A physiological/biological classification includes categories as irritants, sensitisers, carcinogens, etc.

LD_{50}

Acute toxicity looks at lethal effects following oral, dermal or inhalation exposure. One index of acute toxicity in animal studies is the LD_{50}. This is the dose of a test chemical that causes death in 50% of exposed laboratory animals. There is a variation in LD_{50} results depending on the test animal species used, and also on the route of exposure. Hence, LD_{50} data should specify these parameters and standardise against the mass of the organism (rat/mouse/etc.) to enable comparison with humans. Similarly, LC_{50} is the concentration of the agent that causes death in 50% of animals. There are five categories of severity for LD_{50} and LC_{50}, where category 1 requires the least amount of exposure to be

TABLE 6.1

Categories of LD_{50} and LC_{50}.

Method of administration	Category				
	1	2	3	4	5
Oral: LD_{50} measured in mg/kg of bodyweight	5	50	300	2000	5000
Dermal: LD_{50} measured in mg/kg of bodyweight	50	200	1000	2000	5000
Gas inhalation: LC_{50} measured in ppmv	100	500	2500	20000	–
Vapour inhalation: LC_{50} measured in mg/l	0.5	2.0	10	20	–
Dust and mist inhalation: LC_{50} measured in mg/l	0.05	0.5	1.0	5.0	–

LC_{50}, the concentration of a test chemical that causes death in 50% of exposed laboratory animals; LD_{50}, the dose of a test chemical that causes death in 50% of exposed laboratory animals; ppmv, parts per million volume.

lethal and category 5 requires the most exposure to be lethal. Table 6.1 shows the upper limits for each category.

NOAEL
A different approach from the toxicity rating of chemicals is the determination of the NOAEL (no observable adverse effect level). This is the maximum dose that produces no observable adverse effects in a group of test animals or epidemiological studies of exposed humans. The NOAEL is sometimes used in setting occupational exposure standards, adding an appropriate safety factor to produce a standard that protects the majority of exposed workers. The safety factor used seems arbitrary and may differ depending on the anticipated adverse effects from excessive exposure, or even from one expert committee to another.

Problems with LD_{50} and NOAEL
The above grading systems do not take into account slow or delayed death. The extrapolation of such ranges of toxicity from different animal species to humans must also be exercised with caution, especially when varying results are obtained between different species of test animal. It is important to be aware of the limitations of LD_{50} values. Unfortunately, health and safety standards are sometimes based on such values and the justification for their use in workplace control criteria is weak. There continues to be an urgent need for the development of methods other than animal testing to determine the toxicity of chemicals to humans.

GHS hazard statements

These risk phrases are used internationally, not just in Europe, and there is an ongoing effort towards complete international harmonisation using the *Globally Harmonized System of Classification and Labelling of Chemicals* (GHS) – an internationally agreed standard managed by the United Nations (UN) that was set up to replace the assortment of hazardous material classification and labelling schemes previously used around the world. Core elements of the GHS include standardised hazard testing criteria, universal warning pictograms and harmonised safety data sheets that provide users of dangerous goods with a host of information. The system acts as a complement to the UN numbered system of regulated hazardous material transport. Implementation is managed through the UN Secretariat. Although adoption has taken time, the system has been enacted to significant extents in most major countries of the world. This includes the European Union (EU), which has implemented the UN's GHS into EU law as the CLP Regulation, and the USA's Occupational Safety and Health Administration standards.

Hazard statements are part of the GHS, forming standardised phrases for chemical substance hazards and mixtures that are intended to be translated internationally. Formerly known as risk or R-phrases, hazard statements serve the same purpose and are a key element for container labelling under GHS along with product identification, hazard pictograms, signals words (Danger or Warning where necessary), precautionary statements for handling to minimise user risks and the supplier's identity. Hazard statements each have a three-digit code and are grouped together by physical, health and environmental hazards so the numbers do not flow consecutively within each category. Although there are some country-specific hazard statements, below is a complete list of hazard statements that should appear on labels and safety data sheets used around the world.

Physical hazards
- H200   Unstable explosive
- H201   Explosive, mass explosion hazard
- H202   Explosive, severe projection hazard
- H203   Explosive; fire, blast or projection hazard
- H204   Fire or projection hazard
- H205   May mass explode in fire
- H206   Fire, blast or projection hazard: increased risk of explosion if desensitising agent is reduced
- H207   Fire or projection hazard: increased risk of explosion if desensitising agent is reduced
- H208   Fire hazard: increased risk of explosion if desensitising agent is reduced
- H220   Extremely flammable gas
- H221   Flammable gas
- H222   Extremely flammable aerosol
- H223   Flammable aerosol

- H224   Extremely flammable liquid and vapour
- H225   Highly flammable liquid and vapour
- H226   Flammable liquid and vapour
- H227   Combustible liquid
- H228   Flammable solid
- H229   Pressurised container: may burst if heated
- H230   May react explosively even in the absence of air
- H231   May react explosively even in the absence of air at elevated pressure and/or temperature
- H232   May ignite spontaneously if exposed to air
- H240   Heating may cause an explosion
- H241   Heating may cause a fire or explosion
- H242   Heating may cause a fire
- H250   Catches fire spontaneously if exposed to air
- H251   Self-heating: may catch fire
- H252   Self-heating in large quantities: may catch fire
- H260   In contact with water releases flammable gases which may ignite spontaneously
- H261   In contact with water releases flammable gas
- H270   May cause or intensify fire: oxidiser
- H271   May cause fire or explosion: strong oxidiser
- H272   May intensify fire: oxidiser
- H280   Contains gas under pressure: may explode if heated
- H281   Contains refrigerated gas: may cause cryogenic burns or injury
- H290   May be corrosive to metals

Health hazards
- H300   Fatal if swallowed
- H301   Toxic if swallowed
- H302   Harmful if swallowed
- H303   May be harmful if swallowed
- H304   May be fatal if swallowed and enters airways
- H305   May be harmful if swallowed and enters airways
- H310   Fatal in contact with skin
- H311   Toxic in contact with skin
- H312   Harmful in contact with skin
- H313   May be harmful in contact with skin
- H314   Causes severe skin burns and eye damage
- H315   Causes skin irritation
- H316   Causes mild skin irritation
- H317   May cause an allergic skin reaction
- H318   Causes serious eye damage
- H319   Causes serious eye irritation
- H320   Causes eye irritation
- H330   Fatal if inhaled
- H331   Toxic if inhaled

- H332   Harmful if inhaled
- H333   May be harmful if inhaled
- H334   May cause allergy or asthma symptoms or breathing difficulties if inhaled
- H335   May cause respiratory irritation
- H336   May cause drowsiness or dizziness
- H340   May cause genetic defects
- H341   Suspected of causing genetic defects
- H350   May cause cancer
- H351   Suspected of causing cancer
- H360   May damage fertility or the unborn child
- H361   Suspected of damaging fertility or the unborn child
- H361d   Suspected of damaging the unborn child
- H361D   May damage the unborn child
- H361f   Suspected of damaging fertility
- H361F   May damage fertility
- H362   May cause harm to breastfed children
- H370   Causes damage to organs
- H371   May cause damage to organs
- H372   Causes damage to organs through prolonged or repeated exposure
- H373   May cause damage to organs through prolonged or repeated exposure
- H300 + H310   Fatal if swallowed or in contact with skin
- H300 + H330   Fatal if swallowed or if inhaled
- H310 + H330   Fatal in contact with skin or if inhaled
- H300 + H310 + H330   Fatal if swallowed, in contact with skin or if inhaled
- H301 + H311   Toxic if swallowed or in contact with skin
- H301 + H331   Toxic if swallowed or if inhaled
- H311 + H331   Toxic in contact with skin or if inhaled
- H301 + H311 + H331   Toxic if swallowed, in contact with skin or if inhaled
- H302 + H312   Harmful if swallowed or in contact with skin
- H302 + H332   Harmful if swallowed or if inhaled
- H312_H332   Harmful in contact with skin or if inhaled
- H302 + H312 + H332   Harmful if swallowed, in contact with skin or if inhaled
- H303 + H313   May be harmful if swallowed or in contact with skin
- H303 + H333   May be harmful if swallowed or if inhaled
- H313 + H333   May be harmful in contact with skin or if inhaled
- H303 + H313 + H333   May be harmful if swallowed, in contact with skin or if inhaled
- H315 + H320   Causes skin and eye irritation

Environmental hazards
- H400   Very toxic to aquatic life
- H401   Toxic to aquatic life

- H402   Harmful to aquatic life
- H410   Very toxic to aquatic life with long-lasting effects
- H411   Toxic to aquatic life with long-lasting effects
- H412   Harmful to aquatic life with long-lasting effects
- H413   May cause long-lasting harmful effects to aquatic life
- H420   Harms public health and the environment by destroying ozone in the upper atmosphere
- H433   Harmful to terrestrial vertebrates

The GHS classification criteria related to health are given below (there are also classifications for physical hazards, environmental hazards and a classification for mixtures).

- *Acute toxicity* includes five GHS categories from which the appropriate elements relevant to transport, consumer, worker and environmental protection can be selected. Substances are assigned to one of the five toxicity categories on the basis of LD_{50} (usually oral, dermal) or LC_{50} (inhalation).
- *Skin corrosion* means the production of irreversible damage to the skin following the application of a test substance for up to four hours. Substances and mixtures in this hazard class are assigned to a single harmonised corrosion category.
- *Skin irritation* means the production of reversible damage to the skin following the application of a test substance for up to four hours. Substances and mixtures in this hazard class are assigned to a single irritant category. For those authorities, such as pesticide regulators, wanting more than one designation for skin irritation, an additional mild irritant category is provided.
- *Serious eye damage* means the production of tissue damage in the eye, or serious physical decay of vision, following application of a test substance to the front surface of the eye, which is not fully reversible within 21 days of application. Substances and mixtures in this hazard class are assigned to a single harmonised category.
- *Eye irritation* means changes in the eye following the application of a test substance to the front surface of the eye, which are fully reversible within 21 days of application. Substances and mixtures in this hazard class are assigned to a single harmonised hazard category. For authorities, such as pesticide regulators, wanting more than one designation for eye irritation, one of two subcategories can be selected, depending on whether the effects are reversible in 21 or 7 days.
- *Respiratory sensitiser* means a substance that induces hypersensitivity of the airways following inhalation of the substance. Substances and mixtures in this hazard class are assigned to one hazard category.
- *Skin sensitiser* means a substance that will induce an allergic response following skin contact. The definition for 'skin sensitiser' is equivalent to 'contact sensitiser'. Substances and mixtures in this hazard class are assigned to one hazard category.
- *Germ cell mutagenicity* means an agent giving rise to an increased occurrence of mutations in populations of cells and/or organisms. Substances and

mixtures in this hazard class are assigned to one of two hazard categories. Category 1 has two subcategories.

- *Carcinogenicity* means a chemical substance or a mixture of chemical substances that induce cancer or increase its incidence. Substances and mixtures in this hazard class are assigned to one of two hazard categories. Category 1 has two subcategories.
- *Reproductive toxicity* includes adverse effects on sexual function and fertility in adult males and females, as well as developmental toxicity in offspring. Substances and mixtures with reproductive and/or developmental effects are assigned to one of two hazard categories, 'known or presumed' and 'suspected'. Category 1 has two subcategories for reproductive and developmental effects. Materials that cause concern for the health of breastfed children have a separate category: effects on or via lactation.
- *Specific target organ toxicity* category distinguishes between single and repeated exposure for target organ effects. All significant health effects not otherwise specifically included in the GHS that can impair function, both reversible and irreversible, immediate and/or delayed, are included in the non-lethal target organ/systemic toxicity class. Narcotic effects and respiratory tract irritation are considered to be target organ systemic effects following a single exposure. Substances and mixtures of the single-exposure target organ toxicity hazard class are assigned to one of three hazard categories. Substances and mixtures of the repeated exposure target organ toxicity hazard class are assigned to one of two hazard categories.
- *Aspiration hazard* includes severe acute effects such as chemical pneumonia, varying degrees of pulmonary injury or death following aspiration. Aspiration is the entry of a liquid or solid directly through the oral or nasal cavity, or indirectly from vomiting, into the trachea and lower respiratory system.

Threshold for toxic effect

For toxic chemicals, there is a threshold dose below which there is no observed effect (the NOAEL). Above this threshold, the higher the dose the greater the effect, and/or the greater the number of individuals affected. However, this threshold varies between species, and also within the same species depending on factors such as age, state of health and diet. For some carcinogenic compounds, for example genotoxic carcinogens, there may be no threshold. Each exposure, regardless of magnitude, adds to the risk of an effect. Hence, there is a need to keep exposures as low as feasible for carcinogens. For allergens, the threshold for sensitisation may be relatively high, but, once sensitised, the individual can react to minute amounts of the causative agent.

Short-term tests for carcinogenicity

The basis of some short-term tests for carcinogenicity lies in the demonstration that chemical agents have mutagenic properties. The possibility of carcinogenesis is inferred from showing mutagenesis. The development of short-term tests arose because of several factors. These included the costs of performing animal tests and the time period required before results were obtained. Short-term tests can produce results within several days, whereas animal tests may take several months or years to complete. With the numbers of new chemicals being introduced, there were also insufficient facilities for carrying out animal tests on all new chemicals. Another factor was the interest in developing alternative test systems that do not require animal experiments. Toxicologists explored the development of short-term screening tests, using mainly bacterial systems or cell lines. Many such tests have been produced, with varying degrees of success and predictive value. The variety of tests include the Ames test; sister chromatid exchange (SCE); the dominant lethal test; the micronucleus test; the Styles cell transformation test; and the detection of adducts. Details of three of these tests are described below.

Ames test

One variant of this test relies on the use of histidine-dependent *Salmonella typhimurium* on culture plates. The test material is added, and the number of colonies of the bacteria that can grow in the absence of histidine indicates the extent of reverse mutation of the bacteria. A proportion of the bacteria undergo reverse mutation, so that the bacteria can survive in the absence of the amino acid histidine. The extent of reverse mutation is compared between plates with the test material and control plates without. A significant difference in the number of colonies in the test versus control plates indicates mutagenicity, and therefore inferred carcinogenicity of the test material.

As described, the test is quite good at detecting direct carcinogens, such as alkylating agents. However, for indirect carcinogens, such as aromatic amines and PAHs, an additional step is required to convert the indirect carcinogen to the ultimate carcinogen before it can cause any mutagenic effect. This step is the addition of liver homogenate from rats or mice, termed the S9 mix, to the test system. The S9 mix refers to the centrifugation of minced liver at $9000\,\text{rev}\,\text{min}^{-1}$. The rationale behind the use of liver homogenate is to supply sufficient enzymes to effect the transformation of pro-carcinogen to ultimate carcinogen. An additional procedure that can be included is the parenteral administration of phenobarbitone or Aroclor 1254 to the rodents before harvesting the liver for the preparation of the S9 mix. Phenobarbitone or Aroclor enhances the production of liver enzymes, and can increase the enzyme content in the S9 mix. Other variants of the Ames test use strains of *Escherichia coli* instead of *S. typhimurium*.

SCE

This test is used to detect genetic damage by chemicals. The reasoning behind this approach is that chemicals that can cause deoxyribonucleic acid (DNA) damage are likely to possess carcinogenic activity. Cellular genetic material is examined during mitosis after the addition of the test chemical. DNA damage results in the exchange of material between pairs of chromatids at this stage of cell division. The difference in the extent of DNA exchange between cells exposed to the test chemical and those exposed to a control compound indicates whether the test material is carcinogenic.

Detection of adducts

Carcinogens can react with sites on the purine or pyrimidine bases of cellular DNA to produce adducts. These adducts can be detected in urine samples or in haemoglobin or white blood cells. The basis for detecting the presence of such adducts is that they indicate an effect from exposure to a carcinogen and, in theory, this might be of use in a screening programme. However, there are many unanswered questions, such as the specificity and sensitivity of these adducts as an indicator of carcinogen exposure, their persistence, their variability in biological samples, dietary and non-occupational factors that may contribute to adduct formation and the within- and between-laboratory variability in the detection of adducts. Hence, DNA adducts are interesting research tools, but they currently have little applied value in occupational health practice.

6.2 Metals, metalloids and transition metals

Aluminium (Al)

Occurrence. Metalliferous ores, mainly as alumina, bauxite (Al_2O_3).

Properties. Light, white metal.

Uses. Alloys; engine and aircraft components; window frames; and food containers. Oxides used as abrasives. Insoluble salts, such as hydroxide, used in antacid preparations.

Metabolism. Ingested aluminium salts are poorly absorbed from the gastrointestinal tract. Can interfere with phosphate absorption. Excreted in the faeces. Once absorbed, aluminium is largely excreted in the urine. Lung retention is also possible.

Health effects. Acute: massive oral doses cause gastrointestinal irritation, but whether long-term sequelae, such as encephalopathy, can occur is disputed (some of those affected by the Camelford water supply incident in the UK continued to complain of a range of symptoms decades after the event). Chronic: Shaver's disease (a form of pulmonary fibrosis) was described in 1947 in workers who inhaled aluminium fumes in the manufacture of alumina abrasives, but this effect has not been described in subsequent studies. Workers in the aluminium smelting and refining industries can develop 'pot room asthma' and have an increased risk of bladder cancer. However, none of these effects is considered to be due directly to aluminium or aluminium salts. Fluorosis used to occur in such workers and those in neighbouring areas from fluoride ore smelting. The putative association between aluminium absorption and Alzheimer's disease is unresolved, but support for the hypothesis has waned.

Biological monitoring. Not widely done but there is a German Biological Exposure Index of $50\,\mu g\,g^{-1}$ creatinine based on a NOAEL for the occurrence of subtle neurotoxic effects. The body burden of aluminium appears to be little affected by non-dietary intake.

Measurement. Sampled onto cellulose ester membrane filters using SIMPEDS/ Higgins and Dewell cyclones at 2.21min^{-1} for respirable dust and the Institute of Occupational Medicine (IOM)/seven-hole UK Atomic Energy Authority (UKAEA) head for total inhalable dust. If necessary, acid (HNO_3) digestion and atomic absorption spectrophotometry (US National Institute for Occupational Safety and Health [NIOSH] 7013).

Workplace exposure limits. Aluminium alkyl compounds UK Health and Safety Executive (HSE) workplace exposure limit (WEL) – eight-hour time-weighted average (TWA), 2mg m^{-3}.

Aluminium metal, HSE WEL: eight-hour TWA, total inhalable – 10mg m^{-3}; respirable dust – 4mg m^{-3}.

Aluminium oxides, HSE WEL: eight-hour TWA, total inhalable – 10mg m^{-3}; respirable dust – 4mg m^{-3}.

Aluminium salts (soluble), HSE WEL: eight-hour TWA, total inhalable – 2mg m^{-3}.

Antimony (Sb)

Occurrence. Metalliferous ores, usually as sulphide (Sb_2S_3).

Properties. Silvery-white, soft metal with properties very similar to arsenic. Stibine (SbH_3) is a gas formed from antimony on reaction with nascent hydrogen.

Uses. Alloys, notably in lead-acid batteries; flame retardants; electronics; paint pigment; rubber compounding.

Metabolism. Few severe poisonings – probably similar to arsenic.

Health effects. Vomiting and eye, skin and mucous membrane irritation, which may be severe. Characteristic skin changes occur; known as antimony dermatosis. A benign pneumoconiosis has been described. Stibine is a haemolytic agent. Cardiac arrhythmias and mild jaundice have been reported.

Health surveillance. Safe Work Australia recommends physical examination, noting any skin changes or lesions, and standardised lung function questionnaire and spirometry.

Measurement. Antimony and compounds (particulate): sampled onto cellulose acetate filter (pore size, $0.8 \mu m$) at an air flow rate of around 21min^{-1} for subsequent analysis for Sb using atomic absorption spectrophotometry.

Workplace exposure limits. Antimony and compounds, except stibine (as Sb), HSE WEL: eight-hour TWA, 0.5mg m^{-3}.

Arsenic (As)

Occurrence. Widely dispersed in nature, usually in association with metalliferous ore, for example arsenopyrite (FeAsS). It is therefore a by-product of both ferrous and non-ferrous smelting, mainly as the trioxide (As_2O_3). Major public health issue in several countries owing to contaminated drinking water. Rice is an important source of inorganic As in the diet, and seafood and seaweed of organic arsenic.

Properties. A steel-grey brittle metal. Compounds of arsenic include As_2O_3, a crystalline solid, trivalent and pentavalent forms and arsine (AsH_3) gas.

Uses. Alloys; insecticides; fungicides; rodenticides; pigments; and decoloriser in glass and paper making.

Metabolism. Normal body constituent because of wide dispersion in nature. Stored in keratin. Excretion of inorganic arsenic is mainly in the urine as As(III), As(V) and the major metabolites monomethylarsonic acid (MMA) and dimethylarsinic acid (DMA).

Health effects. Acute: severe respiratory irritation, headache, abdominal pain, diarrhoea, and vomiting → shock. Skin irritation and allergy are possible. See also arsine (see Section 6.2). Chronic: gastrointestinal symptoms occasionally, peripheral neuropathy – mainly sensory – keratoses and dermatitis, melanosis of face and trunk, with or without areas of 'raindrop' depigmentation. Equivocal evidence of liver damage – vascular or parenchymal in type. Carcinogenic changes in skin, lungs and bladder (International Agency for Research on Cancer [IARC] group 1). Organic As is much less toxic than inorganic As and health effects are not a concern.

Health surveillance and biological monitoring. Periodic review of skin, respiratory and other symptoms. Inorganic arsenic and its metabolites in urine are widely used for measuring uptake. Many jurisdictions have a urinary standard for inorganic As and DMA and MMA of $35\,\mu g\,g^{-1}$ of creatinine. If total urinary As is measured, concentrations may be elevated owing to dietary organic As (arsenobetaine) unless dietary restrictions precede urine collection. Arsenic levels in hair and nails are less reliable.

Measurement. Arsenic and compounds (particulate): sampled onto a treated cellulose ester filter (pore size, $0.8\,\mu m$) at an air flow rate of around $21\,min^{-1}$ for subsequent analysis for arsenic using atomic absorption spectrophotometry.

Workplace exposure limits. Arsenic and compounds, except arsine (as As), HSE WEL: eight-hour TWA, $0.1\,mg\,m^{-3}$ (carcinogen notation).

Beryllium (Be)

Occurrence. Mainly as beryllium aluminium cyclosilicate ($3BeO.Al_2O_3.6SiO_2$) and bertrandite ($Be_4Si_2O_7(OH)_2$).

Properties. A very light, hard, non-corrosive, grey metal.

Uses. Alloys; electronics; nuclear reactors and weapons; aerospace; and ceramics.

Metabolism. Absorption is poor from the gut, but good from the lungs. Protein bound with liver, spleen and skeleton deposition. Urinary excretion variable.

Health effects. Acute: chemical pneumonitis, cough, chest pain, dyspnoea and pneumonia. Conjunctivitis, rhinitis and pharyngitis. Skin irritant and sensitiser. Chronic: sarcoid-like granulomata – mainly in the lungs, but occasionally subcutaneous. The lung lesions can lead to progressive interstitial fibrosis with hilar lymphadenopathy resulting in cor pulmonale. Beryllium is probably a lung carcinogen. Chest radiography in severe cases shows widespread nodules, $1–5\,\mu m$ in size, which may coalesce.

Health surveillance. Beryllium lymphocyte proliferation tests are used to monitor sensitisation. Respiratory symptoms and spirometry, and chest radiography if indicated.

Measurement. Sampled onto cellulose acetate filter (pore size, 0.8 μm) at an air flow rate of around 1 l min^{-1} for subsequent analysis after treatment for Be using atomic absorption spectrophotometry (30 minutes at 0.025 mg m^{-3}).

Workplace exposure limits. Beryllium and beryllium compounds (as Be), HSE WEL: eight-hour TWA, 0.002 mg m^{-3} (carcinogen notation).

Cadmium (Cd)

Occurrence. Cadmium sulphide (CdS), usually in association with zinc ore.

Properties. Soft, ductile, silvery-white metal, which is corrosion resistant and electropositive.

Uses. Alloys; alkaline storage batteries; electroplating; pigments; and nuclear reactors (neutron absorber).

Metabolism. Mainly absorbed through inhalation. Bound to plasma globulin, with accumulation in the kidney and lesser amounts in the liver. Urinary excretion is slow (hence the long half-life of Cd) unless there is renal damage.

Health effects. Cadmium fumes can cause a severe chemical pneumonitis that can lead to pulmonary oedema and death, importantly after a latent period. (Welding Cd alloys can generate high levels of fumes.) Mucous membrane irritation may also occur. Chronic: non-specific features include gastrointestinal disturbance, yellow rings on the teeth and anosmia. The main target organs are, however, the lungs and kidneys. Emphysema can be severe and is usually focal (α_1-antitrypsin may have a role in the pathogenesis of emphysema in cadmium-exposed workers). Nephrotoxicity is usually manifested as tubular damage with proteinuria (especially β_2-microglobulins), glycosuria and amino aciduria. Hypertension has been implicated as a sequelae of chronic cadmium exposure. Lung carcinoma is thought by many to follow chronic exposure (IARC group 1), but the case for prostate and renal cancers is weaker. Bone damage has been reported following environmental exposure (itai-itai disease is an oft-cited example) but less so in workers.

Health surveillance and biological monitoring. Lung function tests, urinalysis for low-molecular-weight proteins as markers of tubular injury – β_2-microglobulins not uncommonly. Cadmium in urine is indicative of body burden and to some extent recent exposure, but is a poor estimate of effect. Renal cortical cadmium levels are more reliable, but difficult to measure (neutron activation analysis).

Measurement. Sampled onto cellulose acetate filter (pore size, 0.8 μm) at an air flow rate of 2 l min^{-1} for subsequent analysis after treatment for cadmium using atomic absorption spectrophotometry (UK Methods for the Determination of Hazardous Substances [MDHS] 10/2 and 11).

Workplace exposure limits. Cadmium and cadmium compounds, except cadmium oxide fume, cadmium sulphide and cadmium sulphide pigments (as Cd), HSE WEL: eight-hour TWA, 0.025 mg m^{-3} (carcinogen notification [cadmium metal, cadmium chloride, fluoride and sulphate]).

Cadmium oxide fume (as Cd), HSE WEL: eight-hour TWA, 0.025 mg m^{-3}; 15-minute short-term exposure limit (STEL), 0.05 mg m^{-3} (carcinogen notification).

Cadmium sulphide and cadmium sulphide pigments (respirable dust (as Cd)), HSE WEL: eight-hour TWA, 0.03 mg m^{-3} (carcinogen notification – cadmium sulphide).

Chromium (Cr)

Occurrence. Chromite ore (FeO.Cr$_2$O$_3$).

Properties. Hard, corrosion-resistant, grey metal. Several valency states including divalent, trivalent and hexavalent.

Uses. Stainless steel and other alloys; electroplating; pigments; and leather tanning.

Metabolism. Essential trace element. Better absorption for hexavalent than trivalent forms. Hexavalent forms enter cells and are reduced intracellularly to trivalent chromium. Excretion mainly in the urine in trivalent form.

Health effects. Mainly due to hexavalent chromium compounds. Hexavalent salts are irritant and corrosive, causing chronic skin, nasal (chrome ulcers) and respiratory tract irritation. Chrome compounds are sensitisers and may cause dermatitis (e.g. cement dermatitis – chrome content in cement is being reduced in several regions) and asthma. Chromate ore workers have an increased incidence of lung carcinoma, thought to be due to the slightly soluble hexavalent chromium compounds of strontium, calcium and zinc. Chromium platers, exposed to chromic acid mist, have also been reported to have an excess of lung cancer (IARC group 1).

Health surveillance and biological monitoring. Examination of the skin and nasal septum. Respiratory symptoms and lung function tests as indicated. End-of-shift urinary chromium.

Measurement. Chromium, chromates, soluble chromic and chromous salts: sampled onto cellulose acetate filter (pore size, 0.8 µm) at an air flow rate of around 1.5 l min^{-1} for subsequent analysis for Cr using atomic absorption spectrophotometry. Chromic acid and chromates: sampled onto polyvinyl chloride (PVC) filter (pore size, 5 µm) at an air flow rate of around 1 l min^{-1} for subsequent colorimetric analysis.

Workplace exposure limits. Chromium metal, Cr(II) and Cr(III) compounds as Cr, HSE WEL: eight-hour TWA, 0.5 mg m^{-3}. Cr(VI) compounds as Cr, HSE WEL: eight-hour TWA, 0.01 and 0.025 mg m^{-3} (if process generated) (carcinogen, sensitiser and biological monitoring guidance value notification).

Lead (Pb)

Occurrence. Mainly as the sulphide (PbS), in association with other metallic sulphates.

Properties. Soft, bluish-grey metal. Heavy, malleable and ductile. Inorganic and organic compounds.

Uses. Pipes; sheet metal; foil; ammunition; pigments; solders; lead batteries (manufacture and recycling); and anti-knock additive to petrol (organic compound only), although a rare use nowadays.

Metabolism. Poorly absorbed through the gut (10%), but dependent on the calcium and iron content of the diet. Pulmonary absorption more effective. Transported in form bound to red cell membrane and stored mainly in bone. Excretion mainly urinary.

Health effects. Inorganic. Acute: non-specific with lassitude, abdominal cramps and constipation, myalgia and anorexia. Chronic: peripheral motor neuropathy (especially wrist drop, although this is rarely seen nowadays) and anaemia are the main late manifestations. Disturbances of haem synthesis and a slowing of motor nerve conduction times can be detected soon after excessive absorption has commenced. Renal damage and encephalopathy are rare and usually confined to children. Reproductive effects occur in women (serious prenatal outcomes, among others) and men. Organic, differs from inorganic in being primarily associated with psychiatric manifestations, such as insomnia, hyperexcitability and even mania.

Biological monitoring. Blood lead. UK suspension level: 60 µg per 100 ml for men and 30 µg per 100 ml for women; many jurisdictions have lower levels. For instance the American College of Occupational and Environmental Medicine advises removal of women trying to become pregnant if they continue to have lead exposures causing a blood lead >5 µg per 100 ml. Zinc protoporphyrin infrequently used. (For organic lead absorption, urinary lead estimation is more useful.)

Occupational hygiene measurement. Inorganic lead: sampled onto cellulose acetate filter (pore size, 0.8 µm) in a single-hole holder at an air flow rate of around 11 min^{-1} for subsequent analysis after treatment for Pb using atomic absorption spectrophotometry. Note that filters should be partially covered, as with UKAEA-type holders. Organic lead: sampled through a charcoal tube at an air flow rate of 1000 ml min^{-1} for subsequent analysis of Pb using atomic absorption spectrophotometry.

'Lead in air standard' (The Control of Lead at Work Regulations 1998). Lead other than alkyls, eight-hour TWA, 0.15 mg m^{-3}. Lead alkyls, eight-hour TWA, 0.10 mg m^{-3}.

Manganese (Mn)

Occurrence. Widely occurring as MnO_2, $MnSiO_3$.

Properties. Reddish-grey, hard metal. Decomposes in water.

Uses. Alloys; dry-cell batteries; potassium permanganate; glass and ceramics; matches; anti-knock agent in gasoline; fungicides.

Metabolism. Essential trace element. Poorly absorbed from the gut, somewhat better from the lungs. Accumulates in the kidney, liver, bone, and brain (basal ganglia). Excretion largely through the gut. Transport in body is intracellular. Excess Mn activates superoxide dismutase, leading to reactive oxygen species in mitochondria; it may also have a pro-inflammatory effect in the brain.

Health effects. Acute: manganese oxide fume is a respiratory and mucous membrane irritant and may cause metal fume fever. Chronic: slow onset (one to two years) with headache, asthenia, poor sleep and disturbed mental state. Neurological signs are primarily of the basal ganglia and symmetrical with the globus pallidus most affected → parkinsonism, 'manganism'. Suggestive evidence that Mn is associated with increased incidence of idiopathic Parkinson's disease.

Health surveillance and biological monitoring. Assessment of central nervous system (CNS) symptoms and signs, especially the extrapyramidal system. Blood Mn levels are poorly correlated with air concentrations in individuals.

Measurement. Sampled onto cellulose acetate filter (pore size, $0.8 \mu m$) at an air flow rate of $1.5 l \, min^{-1}$ for subsequent analysis for Mn using atomic absorption spectrophotometry (NIOSH 7300).

Workplace exposure limits. Manganese and its inorganic compounds (as Mn), HSE WEL: inhalable fraction: eight-hour TWA, $0.2 \, mg \, m^{-3}$ and respirable fraction eight-hour TWA, $0.05 \, mg \, m^{-3}$.

Mercury (Hg)

Occurrence. Mainly as sulphide ore (HgS), rarely as liquid metal.

Properties. Liquid at normal temperature and pressure. Therefore has a measurable vapour pressure. Mixes in a unique fashion with other metals (amalgams).

Uses. Scientific instruments; amalgams; dental amalgam (fillings); 'silvering'; solders; pharmaceuticals; paints; seed dressings (organic compounds only); and explosives. Major modern concern is extensive use of mercury in artisanal and illegal gold mining; affecting the workers, surrounding communities and the environment. The Minamata Convention on Mercury (2013) is a multicountry agreement to reduce mercury use.

Metabolism. Metallic (elemental) mercury rapidly absorbed by inhalation and poorly absorbed from the gut. Salts quickly absorbed by all routes. Inorganic salts more readily absorbed through the gut and excreted by kidneys than organic compounds. Organics (methyl mercury mainly) have a predilection for the CNS.

Health effects. Inorganic. Acute: rare in industry. Febrile illness with pneumonitis. If severe, can cause oliguric renal failure. Chronic: slow onset with peculiar neuropsychiatric disorder (erethism) with features of anxiety, neurosis, timidity and paranoia. Accompanied by gingivitis, excessive salivation, intention tremor, jerky micrographia and scanning speech. Upper motor neuron lesions and visual field constriction more commonly associated with organic mercurialism. Anterior capsule of the lens of the eye may be discoloured. Nephrotic syndrome.

Biological monitoring. Mercury in urine (preferably 24-hour specimen) for longer term exposure or blood for acute exposure. The UK biological monitoring guidance value is $20 \, \mu mol \, mol^{-1}$ creatinine for urinary mercury. This is equivalent to $35 \, \mu g \, g^{-1}$ creatine, a common limit value. Dietary intake of fish and shellfish can increase levels and should be noted.

Measurement. Mercury vapour: measured with a direct-reading instrument using ultraviolet light (interfered with by the presence of oil mist vapour). Organic compounds: sampled through adsorbent tube (Hopcalite) at an air flow rate of $50 \, ml \, min^{-1}$ for subsequent analysis for Hg using atomic absorption spectrophotometry (MDHS 16). By diffusive sample (see MDHS 58).

Workplace exposure limits. Mercury and divalent inorganic compounds including mercuric oxide and mercuric chloride (measured as mercury), HSE WEL: eight-hour TWA, $0.02 \, mg \, m^{-3}$.

Nickel (Ni)

Occurrence. Sulphide ore extracted by separation or Mond process (unique reaction of nickel with carbon monoxide to produce nickel carbonyl $Ni(CO)_4$).

Properties. Hard, ductile, magnetic, silvery-white metal. Low corrosion.

Uses. Alloys (especially with steel); electroplating; oil catalyst; coins; ceramics; and batteries.

Metabolism. Many compounds, soluble and insoluble. Poor absorption of insoluble compounds, wide bodily distribution, especially the brain and lungs. Rapid excretion in the urine and faeces.

Health effects. Allergic contact dermatitis common (occupational and non-occupational, e.g. jewellery) and asthma. Nickel carbonyl inhalation can cause pneumonitis. Chronic: chronic rhinitis and sinusitis, carcinoma of the nose and nasal sinuses associated with exposure to Ni, although exact aetiological agent is uncertain – nickel oxides and sulphides or even nickel arsenide.

Health surveillance and biological monitoring. Respiratory and skin symptoms followed by appropriate investigations. Skin patch tests to diagnose nickel skin sensitisation. Urinary nickel concentrations sampled end of shift, end of the working week. Results are influenced by the solubility of the Ni compound.

Measurement. Sampled onto cellulose acetate filter (pore size, 0.8 μm) at an air flow rate of around 2 l min^{-1} for subsequent analysis for Ni using atomic absorption spectrophotometry (MDHS 42/2).

Workplace exposure limits. Nickel and its inorganic compounds (except nickel tetracarbonyl): water-soluble nickel compounds (as Ni) nickel, HSE WEL: eight-hour TWA, 0.1 mg m^{-3} and water-insoluble nickel compounds (as Ni), HSE WEL: eight-hour TWA, 0.5 mg m^{-3} (skin and carcinogen [nickel oxides and sulphides] and sensitiser [nickel sulphate] notification).

Phosphorus (P)

Occurrence. Wide, usually as phosphates of calcium.

Properties. Three allotropic forms – white (or yellow), which spontaneously ignites, and red and black, the most toxic. Can form the gaseous hydride phosphine (PH_3), as well as organic compounds.

Uses. Agriculture; baking powder; detergents; explosives; paper; and printing. Phosphoric acid has several applications, among them as an anti-rust agent.

Metabolism. Rapid absorption by ingestion or inhalation.

Health effects. Acute: phosphorus oxides cause severe pneumonitis. White phosphorus can cause severe burns and liver damage. Chronic: 'phossy jaw' – now virtually unknown. A severe, painful necrotic disease of the bone – usually the mandible; notably a related condition – bisphosphonate-related osteonecrosis of the jaw – occasionally occurs with use of these drugs.

Health surveillance. Dental surveillance (state of teeth) with further specialist investigation if indicated.

Measurement. Phosphoric acid: sampled onto solid sorbent tube (Tenax) for subsequent analysis using a gas chromatography flame ionisation detector (NIOSH 7905). Phosphoric acid: sampled onto solid sorbent tube (washed silica gel) for subsequent analysis using ion chromatography (NIOSH 7903). Phosphorus compounds: bubbled into distilled water for subsequent colorimetric analysis (NIOSH 6402).

Workplace exposure limits. Phosphorus pentachloride, HSE WEL: eight-hour TWA, 0.1 ppm and 0.87 mg m^{-3}; 15-minute STEL, 0.2 ppm and 2 mg m^{-3}.
Phosphorus trichloride, HSE WEL: eight-hour TWA, 0.2 ppm and 1.1 mg m^{-3}; 15-minute STEL, 0.5 ppm and 2.9 mg m^{-3}.
Phosphorus (yellow), HSE WEL: eight-hour TWA, 0.1 mg m^{-3}; 15-minute STEL, 0.3 mg m^{-3}.
Phosphoryl trichloride, HSE WEL: eight-hour TWA, 0.2 ppm and 1.3 mg m^{-3}; 15-minute STEL, 0.6 ppm and 3.8 mg m^{-3}.

Platinum (Pt)
Occurrence. Alluvial deposits and ores such as cooperite and braggite.
Properties. Soft, ductile, malleable, non-corrosive, white metal.
Uses. Electrical contacts; catalysts (including automotive); alloys; jewellery; photography; and anti-cancer drugs. Other platinum group metals such as palladium are replacing platinum to some extent, e.g. in catalysts.
Metabolism. Excretion in the urine. However, soluble platinum compounds may bind to protein, and binding to DNA is a feature of drugs like cisplatin and carboplatin.
Health effects. Acute: nasal irritation. Chronic: platinum asthma (not due to the metal, especially after exposure to chloroplatinic acid or one of its salts). Dry, scaly skin irritant or allergic dermatitis. Cisplatin (IARC group 2A, probably carcinogenic to humans).
Health surveillance. Platinum salt skin prick tests. Respiratory and skin symptoms. Pulmonary function tests. Pre-placement atopy testing was done but is now discouraged.
Biological monitoring. Platinum in urine, samples collected end of shift, end of the working week.
Measurement. Sampled onto cellulose acetate filter (pore size, 0.8 μm) at an air flow rate of around 2 l min^{-1} for subsequent analysis using atomic absorption spectrophotometry.
Workplace exposure limits. Platinum compounds, soluble (except certain halogeno-Pt compounds) (as Pt), HSE WEL: eight-hour TWA, 0.002 mg m^{-3}.
Platinum metal, HSE WEL: eight-hour TWA, 5 mg m^{-3}.

Thallium (Tl)
Occurrence. As a complex with copper, silver and selenium, $(TlCuAg)_2Se$.
Properties. Soft, malleable, silvery-grey metal. Soluble in acids. Oxidises in air.
Uses. Rodenticide; insecticide; electronics; optical equipment; alloys; fireworks; dyes.
Metabolism. Readily absorbed by all routes. The similar ionic radius and electrical charge to potassium (K^+) means it interferes with ion transport channels. Excretion is slow with a biological half-life up to 30 days; poisoning is cumulative.
Health effects. Acute: vomiting, diarrhoea, abdominal pain and anxiety state. Acute ascending polyneuritis. Chronic: anorexia, polyneuritis, alopecia, albuminuria and ocular lesions. Mees' lines on the nails.

Health surveillance. Medical surveillance of peripheral nervous system and CNS. Hair loss has been described with thallium over-exposure.

Biological monitoring. Thallium in urine, samples collected end of shift, end of the working week.

Measurement. Sampled onto cellulose acetate filter (pore size, 0.8 µm) at an air flow rate of around 2 l min^{-1} for subsequent analysis using atomic absorption spectrophotometry (NIOSH 7300).

Workplace exposure limits. Thallium, soluble compounds (as TI), HSE WEL: eight-hour TWA, 0.1 mg m^{-3} (skin notation).

Vanadium (V)

Occurrence. Carnotite, patronite and vanadinite with most vanadium recovered from impurities in magnetite. Also a by-product of oil-burning furnaces when vanadium pentoxide is deposited in the flues.

Properties. Grey-white lustrous powder.

Uses. Alloys with steel increase the hardness and malleability of products. Catalyst; insecticide; and dyes.

Metabolism. Inhalation is the main route of entry. Rapid renal excretion.

Health effects. Acute: respiratory symptoms; severe pneumonitis (usually due to exposure to flue dust) with mucous membrane irritation and gastrointestinal disturbances. Chronic: chronic bronchitis; asthma; eczematous skin lesions; a fine tremor of extremities; and greenish discoloration of tongue.

Biological monitoring. Urinary vanadium for exposure to vanadium pentoxide end of shift, end of the working week sample.

Measurement. Vanadium oxides sampled onto a PVC filter in a Higgins and Dewell cyclone for subsequent analysis using X-ray powder diffraction.

Workplace exposure limits. Vanadium pentoxide, HSE WEL: eight-hour TWA, 0.05 mg m^{-3}.

Zinc (Zn)

Occurrence. As sulphide or carbonate.

Properties. High corrosion resistance. Poor conductor.

Uses. Galvanising; alloys, e.g. brass (5–40% Zn); dyes; and electroplating.

Metabolism. Essential trace element, for example carbonic anhydrase is a zinc-containing enzyme. Also thought to be an important factor in wound healing. Poorly absorbed. Faecal excretion.

Health effects. Acute: metal fume fever. Can occur with fume of other metals, but zinc is the most common agent. Symptoms resemble influenza and commence within 12 hours of exposure. Recovery is rapid with no sequelae. Zinc chloride is a skin and lung irritant.

Health surveillance. Review of symptoms and pulmonary function tests where indicated.

Measurement. Zinc fume: sampled onto cellulose acetate filter (pore size, 0.8 µm) at an air flow rate of around 2 l min^{-1} for subsequent analysis using atomic absorption spectrophotometry. Zinc distearate: sampled onto a weighed glass fibre filter for gravimetric analysis.

Workplace exposure limits. Zinc chloride fume, HSE WEL: eight-hour TWA, $1\,mg\,m^{-3}$; 15-minute STEL, $2\,mg\,m^{-3}$.

Zinc distearate, HSE WEL: inhalable dust, eight-hour TWA, $10\,mg\,m^{-3}$; 15-minute STEL, $20\,mg\,m^{-3}$; respirable dust, eight-hour TWA, $4\,mg\,m^{-3}$.

6.3 Organic chemicals

In general, organic chemicals are carbon-containing compounds. Carbon has a valency of four and a unique ability to form chain or ring structures. Aliphatic compounds are hydrocarbons with a chain structure, for example *n*-hexane. Aromatic compounds have ring structures based on benzene.

e.g. Aliphatic compound = *n*-hexane.

e.g. Aromatic compound = benzene

Aromatic compounds are rings:

e.g. benzene

(abbreviated)

These two groups have differing properties, depending not only on their configuration but also on the elements attached to the 'unoccupied' valency arms.

Organic compounds that are important for industrial processes are frequently hydrocarbons (methane and benzene) or hydrocarbons with some hydrogen atoms replaced by halogens, such as chlorine. The chlorinated hydrocarbons are fat-soluble and are often non-flammable, non-combustible and non-explosive.

As a *general* rule, increasing the chlorination of aliphatic hydrocarbons leads to increasing toxicity, whereas the reverse is true of aromatic hydrocarbons. Many chlorinated hydrocarbons are hepatotoxic.

Aromatic organic compounds

Aniline

NH₂

Properties. Colourless, oily liquid with a fish-like odour. Molecular weight (MW), 93.13.

Uses. Dyes; herbicides; explosives; pharmaceuticals; and rubber processing.

Metabolism. Skin and lung absorption. Converts haemoglobin (where iron is in ferrous state) to methaemoglobin (where iron is in ferric form), with a resulting diminution of the oxygen-carrying capacity of the blood. This is the basis for methylene blue in the treatment of, for example, congenital and idiopathic methaemoglobinaemia as it reduces methaemoglobin to haemoglobin.

Health effects. Acute: mild skin irritant. Moderate exposure may only cause mild cyanosis. Severe poisoning results in anoxia and death. Effects may be delayed for a few hours after exposure. Haemolysis is associated with Heinz bodies from oxidative stress.

Biological monitoring. Urine analysis of post-shift total aniline; aminophenol can also be measured, however medications such as paracetamol (acetaminophen) can interfere. Methaemoglobin levels are used for acute intoxication.

Measurement. Sampled onto a silica gel tube at an air flow rate of $200\,\text{ml}\,\text{min}^{-1}$ for subsequent analysis using gas chromatography (NIOSH 2002). Colorimetric detector tubes are also available.

Workplace exposure limits. HSE WEL: eight-hour TWA, 1 ppm and $4\,\text{mg}\,\text{m}^{-3}$ (skin notation).

Benzene

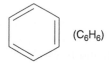 (C₆H₆)

Occurrence. By-product of petroleum and coke-oven industries.

Properties. Colourless, flammable liquid. The fat solvent par excellence. MW, 78.11.

Uses. The initial compound is used in the production of numerous organic aromatics, including styrene, phenol and cyclohexane, as well as many plastics, paints, glues, dyes and pharmaceuticals.

Metabolism. Lung and skin absorption with ready transportation and uptake by fatty tissue, e.g. brain and bone marrow. Excretion occurs through the lungs, particularly at higher exposures; at lower concentrations, excretion is predominantly in the urine as conjugated phenols (catechol and hydroquinone). Minor metabolites are *t,t*-muconic acid and S-phenylmercapturic acid (SPMA).

Health effects. Chronic: bone marrow depression with a delayed effect, in some cases of many years. The early symptoms and signs are vague, but, later, tiredness and spontaneous bleeding may occur as anaemia, pancytopenia and/or thrombocytopenia become more severe. Aplastic anaemia, acute myeloblastic leukaemia and acute erythroleukaemia are the most feared effects of chronic exposure.

Health surveillance. Baseline and periodic – usually annual – complete blood counts are generally advised to detect early haemopoietic effects. Biological monitoring uses post-shift urinary SPMA levels, which increase approximately linearly with airborne benzene concentrations between 0 and 80 ppm. Urinary *t,t*-muconic acid in urine is not useful for monitoring low-level (<1 ppm) airborne benzene exposure owing to dietary sources of production.

Measurement. Sampled onto a charcoal tube at an air flow rate of $200\,ml\,min^{-1}$ for subsequent analysis using gas chromatography (MDHS 17). Colorimetric detector tubes are also available.

Workplace exposure limits. HSE WEL: eight-hour TWA, 1 ppm and $3.25\,mg\,m^{-3}$ (carcinogen and skin notation).

Dinitrophenol

Properties. Explosive, yellow, crystalline solid. MW, 184.11.

Uses. Explosives, dyes, timber preservative, insecticides.

Metabolism. Absorbed through the gastrointestinal tract, skin and respiratory tract. Effects enhanced by heat and alcohol. Excretion is slow, urine becomes orange and skin is turned yellow. Dinitrophenol and its homologue dinitro-orthocresol interfere with temperature regulation by the uncoupling of oxidative phosphorylation. This leads to an increase in metabolic rate.

Health effects. Acute: sudden onset of chest pain and dyspnoea with or without hyperpyrexia, profuse sweating and thirst, leading to shock and cardiovascular collapse in acute poisoning. Methaemoglobinaemia may be present. Chronic: similar to acute effects with or without liver tenderness and jaundice. Cataract formation. Dinitrophenol has been widely available and used for weight loss, especially in 'bodybuilding'.

Biological monitoring. Urine analysis for dinitrophenol or its metabolite 2-amino-4-nitrophenol has limited use.

Isocyanates

(Toluene diisocyanate
two isomers)

(e.g. toluene diisocyanate (TDI)
Properties. Colourless liquid. MW, 174.16.
Uses. Polyurethane production varying from flexible form (TDI) to rigid types (diphenylmethane diisocyanate; MDI); spray paints; and adhesives. Methyl isocyanate an intermediate for carbamate pesticides.
Metabolism. Exposure is through the respiratory tract and skin. There is haptenisation by binding to albumin and other proteins. Metabolism leads to urinary excretion as the corresponding diamine conjugate, e.g. TDI as toluene diamine.
Health effects. Acute: respiratory irritation in all exposed at high concentrations, and development of pulmonary sensitisation and occupational asthma in some individuals. Methyl isocyanate, an aliphatic compound responsible for the Bhopal incident, causes pulmonary oedema and other irritant effects. Chronic: hypersensitivity pneumonitis, chronic obstructive pulmonary disease, allergic contact dermatitis.
Health surveillance. Periodic review of respiratory symptoms with a validated questionnaire. Biological monitoring for the urinary diamines with urine samples collected post shift or post exposure for intermittent usage.
Measurement. Air is drawn through an impregnated tape. The resulting stain is examined photometrically. Proprietary instruments available. A colorimetric detection tube for TDI is available. Alternatively, a measured volume of sample air is drawn through a glass impinger (bubbler) containing 1-(2-methoxyphenyl)-piperazine for subsequent analysis using high-pressure liquid chromatography (MDHS 25). In another method, a measured volume of sample air is drawn through a glass impinger containing dimethylformamide and dilute hydrochloric acid for subsequent colorimetric analysis (MDHS 49).
Workplace exposure limits. HSE WEL: isocyanates, all (as –NCO) except methyl isocyanate: eight-hour TWA, $0.02\,\mathrm{mg\,m^{-3}}$; 15-minute STEL, $0.07\,\mathrm{mg\,m^{-3}}$.

Chlorinated naphthalenes

$$C_{10}H_{(8-n)}Cl_{n}$$

Properties. A group of compounds with varying degrees of chlorination. The higher the chlorine content, the higher the melting point.

Uses. Wire insulation and flame resistance in condensers.

Metabolism. Inhalation of fumes, accidental ingestion and possible percutaneous absorption of liquids. Activation of the aryl hydrocarbon receptor, leading to expression of cytochrome CYP1A1 in skin. There is also a concentration of dioxins in the skin compartment relative to the blood.

Health effects. Acute: little effect. Chronic: two distinct effects: (i) chloracne from systemic and possibly skin absorption of halogenated hydrocarbons (see also Section 3.4, 'Skin'); (ii) transient hepatotoxicity.

Health surveillance. Reporting of skin symptoms by those exposed and skin examination. Liver function tests where liver damage is suspected.

Organophosphates

Organophosphates (OPs) are a group of carbon-based compounds with phosphorus in the general chemical formula. They are used as pesticides, for example in sheep dip to control sheep scab and other parasites. Examples include malathion, parathion, dichlorvos and triorthocresylphosphate (TOCP). Parathion is an aromatic compound, but malathion and TOCP are aliphatic. Unfortunately, deliberate ingestion of OP pesticides remains common in some low- and middle-income countries, accounting for one in seven suicides globally. Instances of Novichok OP agent poisoning have been well publicised in recent years.

Parathion

$$(C_2H_5O)_2 - \overset{\displaystyle\|}{\underset{\displaystyle S}{P}} - O - \!\!\!\bigcirc\!\!\!- NO_2$$

Metabolism and toxicity. OPs that are absorbed systemically by inhalation, through the skin and by ingestion inactivate acetylcholinesterase at synapses in the nervous system by phosphorylation of the enzyme. Percutaneous absorption is likely to be a major route. This inactivation of the cholinesterase allows prolonged action of acetylcholine released at synapses and nerve endings. Effects of OP poisoning are therefore those of excessive cholinergic activity. Red cell and plasma cholinesterase is also inhibited but the temporal effects may differ from those on the nervous system. Low red cell or plasma cholinesterase is consistent with OP exposure but a baseline level is required for biological effect monitoring, to show a fall. OPs are metabolised to dialkyl phosphates, which are then excreted in the urine and can also be used for biological exposure monitoring.

Health effects. Acute: cholinergic effects, such as chest tightness, wheezing, slurred speech, blurred vision, sweating, salivation, abdominal cramps, diarrhoea and vomiting. Chronic: neuropsychiatric effects following chronic exposures with learning and memory difficulties and weakness are reported. Some

OPs, such as TOCP, can cause a delayed, sometimes irreversible, peripheral neuropathy owing to their effect on neuropathy target esterase.

Biological monitoring. Plasma or red cell cholinesterase levels can be determined. Plasma cholinesterase measures pseudo-cholinesterase (butyrylcholinesterase) activity. Red blood cell cholinesterase is preferred for biological monitoring as it determines true acetylcholinesterase levels. Red cell cholinesterase should not fall by more than 30% of an individual's baseline level as this indicates substantial exposure. Some laboratories will have levels of precision that mean smaller differences are of significance. Biological monitoring programmes: for example in pesticide applicators baseline levels should be determined when there has been a 60-day exposure-free period, ideally with two samples a few days apart and a post-application determination of cholinesterase activity. Note: some persons have genetically low plasma cholinesterase. Urinary dialkyl phosphate levels can be used post shift and pre-shift the next day as indicators of the extent of exposure.

Measurement. Sampled onto a solid sorbent tube for subsequent analysis using gas chromatography–flame photometric detector (NIOSH 5600).

Workplace exposure limits. Malathion: HSE WEL: eight-hour TWA, $10\,\mathrm{mg\,m^{-3}}$ (skin notation).

Phenol

OH

Properties. Colourless crystals. Also known as carbolic acid in solution; was used by Lister in his historic carbolic disinfectant sprays. MW, 94.11.

Uses. Insecticides; disinfectants; pharmaceuticals; perfumes; and explosives.

Metabolism. Readily absorbed by all routes; sulphate and glucuronide conjugates excreted in the urine. Higher exposures lead to oxidation to quinones and excreted in the urine; homogentisic acid can be formed, causing ochronosis.

Health effects. Acute: powerful skin corrosive, exacerbated by local anaesthetic properties. Headache, dizziness, weakness, dysrhythmia, convulsions. Chronic: chronic dermatitis from low concentrations following repeated skin contact, severe scarring from phenol splashes. Renal failure. Weight loss, gastrointestinal disturbances.

Biological monitoring. Following systemic absorption – total phenol in the urine at the end of the shift from hydrolysis of conjugates.

Measurement. Air is drawn through a 0.1N solution of sodium hydroxide in a bubbler at an air flow rate of $1000\,\mathrm{ml\,min^{-1}}$; the acidified solution is analysed using a gas chromatograph. Colorimetric detection tubes are also available.

Workplace exposure limits. HSE WEL: eight-hour TWA, 2 ppm and $7.8\,\mathrm{mg\,m^{-3}}$; 15-minute STEL, 4 ppm and $16\,\mathrm{mg\,m^{-3}}$ (skin notation).

Styrene (vinyl benzene)

Properties. Colourless liquid. MW, 104.15.

Uses. Solvent for synthetic rubber; chemical intermediate; manufacture of polymerised synthetics; and glass-reinforced plastics (in boat building). Also ingredient in acrylonitrile–butadiene–styrene co-polymer.

Metabolism. Absorbed through the lungs and skin, enhanced by respiratory exertion. Rapidly metabolised to mandelic acid and, to a lesser extent, phenyl-glyoxylic acid and excreted in the urine.

Health effects. Acute: acute mucous membrane irritation. Drowsiness, diminished cognitive and perceptual skills. Chronic: fissured dermatitis, colour vision disturbance (blue/yellow) and other features of CNS depression. Styrene is probably carcinogenic to humans (IARC group 2A).

Biological monitoring. Urinary mandelic acid and phenylglyoxylic acid concentrations together or mandelic acid alone in end-of-shift samples. Alcohol intake during the exposure period inhibits mandelic acid excretion.

Measurement. Sampled onto a charcoal tube at an air flow rate of $200\,ml\,min^{-1}$ for subsequent analysis using gas chromatography (MDHS 44).

Workplace exposure limits. HSE WEL: eight-hour TWA, $430\,mg\,m^{-3}$ and 100 ppm; 15-minute STEL, $1080\,mg\,m^{-3}$ and 250 ppm.

Toluene (methyl benzene)

Properties. Colourless liquid. MW, 92.14.

Uses. Benzene manufacture; paint solvent; component of petrol.

Metabolism. Rapidly absorbed through the lungs and skin, and excreted as hippuric acid with about 1% as o-cresol in the urine.

Health effects. Acute: narcotic. Conjunctival irritation. Cardiac dysrhythmias (has caused deaths in 'glue-sniffers'). Chronic: irritant dermatitis, chronic toxic encephalopathy, possible ototoxicity.

Biological monitoring. Urinary *o*-cresol or toluene at end of shift. Blood or breath toluene can also be measured. Alcohol intake causes high blood toluene.

Measurement. Sampled onto a charcoal tube at an air flow rate of $1000\,ml\,min^{-1}$ for subsequent analysis using gas chromatography. Colorimetric detection tubes are also available.

Workplace exposure limits. HSE WEL: eight-hour TWA, $191\,mg\,m^{-3}$ and 50 ppm; 15-minute STEL, $384\,mg\,m^{-3}$ and 100 ppm (skin notation).

Xylene

3 isomers:
ortho-   meta-   para-

Properties. Colourless liquid. MW, 106.17. Three isomers (ortho, meta and para).

Uses. Solvent; chemical intermediate.

Metabolism. Rapidly absorbed from the lungs; skin absorption, metabolised and excreted in the urine as methyl hippuric acid.

Health effects. Acute: mucous membrane irritation. Narcotic. Chronic: irritant dermatitis, possible chronic toxic encephalopathy, possible ototoxicity.

Biological monitoring. Urinary methyl hippuric acid, interference by alcohol and aspirin. Blood and breath xylene.

Measurement. Sampled onto a charcoal tube at an air flow rate of $1l\,min^{-1}$ for subsequent analysis using gas chromatography (NIOSH 1501).

Workplace exposure limits. HSE WEL: eight-hour TWA, $220\,mg\,m^{-3}$ and 50 ppm; 15-minute STEL, $441\,mg\,m^{-3}$ and 100 ppm (skin notation and biological monitoring guidance value).

Aliphatic organic compounds

Acrylonitrile

Properties. Explosive, flammable liquid. Readily polymerised. MW, 53.06.

Uses. Manufacture of synthetic rubber, acrylic resins and fibres.

Metabolism. Skin and lung absorption. Toxicity due to the release of cyanide radical (CN^-), being a cyanogen. Excreted as thiocyanate in urine.

Health effects. Acute: vapour is severe eye and respiratory irritant and skin vesicant on contact. Headache, weakness, dizziness → asphyxia and death. Similar to cyanide poisoning but slower onset. Chronic: skin sensitiser, anaemia with erythropenia and leucopenia. Possibly carcinogenic to humans (IARC group 2B).

Biological monitoring. N-(2-Cyanoethyl)valine in blood is specific to acrylonitrile, SCN and (CN) blood levels; can all be used as biomarkers for the assessment of acrylonitrile exposure and toxicity.

Measurement. Sampled onto a charcoal tube at an air flow rate of $200\,ml\,min^{-1}$ for subsequent gas chromatographic analysis. Colorimetric detector tubes are also available (MDHS 1).

Workplace exposure limits. HSE WEL: eight-hour TWA, $4.4\,mg\,m^{-3}$ and 2 ppm (skin and carcinogen notation).

Carbon disulphide

Properties. Colourless liquid. MW, 76.16.

Uses. Solvent for fats, sulphur, rubber oils. Preparation of viscose rayon.

Metabolism. Absorbed through the lungs and skin. Slow metabolism and excretion with main concentration build-up in the brain.

Health effects. Acute: severe eye, skin and mucous membrane irritant. Dizziness, headaches, psychosis, drowsiness. Chronic: four distinct syndromes:

1. Parkinsonian-like clinical features due to damage to the corpus striatum and globus pallidus
2. peripheral neuropathy affecting motor and sensory nerves as well as ocular nerves
3. psychotic conditions (rarely seen nowadays, but lesser neuropsychiatric states are still described)
4. cardiovascular disease – possibly due to increased blood cholesterol and β-lipoprotein, leading to ischaemic heart disease and increased intima–media thickness as well as peripheral vascular damage.

Biological monitoring. 2-Thiothiazolidine-4-carboxylic acid (TTCA) in urine at the end of shift, noting that dithiocarbamate pesticides and rubber accelerators, such as thiuram and disulfiram (Antabuse), as well as dietary cabbage consumption can give rise to urinary TTCA.

Measurement. Sampled onto a charcoal tube at an air flow rate of $200\,ml\,min^{-1}$ for subsequent analysis using gas chromatography. Colorimetric detection tubes are also available.

Workplace exposure limits. HSE WEL: eight-hour TWA, $15\,\mathrm{mg\,m^{-3}}$ and $5\,\mathrm{ppm}$ (skin notation).

Carbon tetrachloride

$$
\begin{array}{c}
\mathrm{Cl} \\
| \\
\mathrm{Cl-C-Cl} \\
| \\
\mathrm{Cl}
\end{array}
$$

Properties. Colourless, non-flammable liquid with a sweet but unpleasant smell. Combustion yields phosgene gas. MW, 153.82.
Uses. Many former uses are now restricted and it is used as a feedstock chemical. Solvent; degreaser; manufacture of refrigerants such as Freon; in fire extinguishers; adhesives; paints; and coatings.
Metabolism. Absorbed through the lungs, skin and gut and stored in fatty tissues. Excreted unchanged through the lungs, although some is metabolised and excreted in the urine.
Health effects. Acute: nausea, vomiting, drowsiness, dizziness, eye and skin irritation. Chronic: dry, scaly dermatitis. Centrilobular necrosis with or without fatty degeneration of the liver. Acute oliguric renal failure. There is a synergistic effect if there is concomitant exposure to alcohol.
Biological monitoring. Blood concentration is of limited value.
Measurement. Sampled onto a charcoal tube at an air flow rate of $1000\,\mathrm{ml\,min^{-1}}$ for subsequent analysis using gas chromatography. Colorimetric detection tubes are also available.
Workplace exposure limits. HSE WEL: eight-hour TWA, $6.4\,\mathrm{mg\,m^{-3}}$ and $1\,\mathrm{ppm}$; 15-minute STEL, $5\,\mathrm{ppm}$, $32\,\mathrm{mg\,m^{-3}}$ (skin notation).

Chloroform

$$
\begin{array}{c}
\mathrm{H} \\
| \\
\mathrm{Cl-C-Cl} \\
| \\
\mathrm{Cl}
\end{array}
$$

Properties. Clear, colourless, non-flammable liquid with characteristic odour. MW, 119.38.
Uses. Fat solvent, manufacture of fluorocarbons, plastics. Abandoned as an anaesthetic agent due to its hepatotoxicity.
Metabolism. Absorbed through the lungs and skin. Stored in fatty tissue and slowly excreted through the lungs and, to a lesser extent, the kidneys.
Health effects. Acute: eye, skin and respiratory irritant. Potent anaesthetic, dysrhythmia. Chronic: liver enlargement and damage potentiated by alcohol use. Renal failure. Chronic dry, scaly dermatitis.
Biological monitoring. Blood concentration is of limited value. *Measurement*. Sampled onto a charcoal tube at an air flow rate of $1000\,\mathrm{ml\,min^{-1}}$ for subsequent analysis using gas chromatography.

Workplace exposure limits. HSE WEL: eight-hour TWA, $9.9\,mg\,m^{-3}$ and $2\,ppm$ (skin notation).

Ethylene oxide

$$HC_2 \overset{\diagdown}{\underset{O}{\diagup}} CH_2$$

Properties. Colourless, flammable gas (odour detection, 500 ppm). Heavier than air.
Uses. Chemical intermediate in the production of ethylene glycol and polyester fibres with dichlorodifluoromethane (to lower the risk of explosion and fire). It is used as a general purpose gaseous sterilising agent, particularly in hospitals.
Metabolism. Inhaled as a gaseous agent and skin absorption can also occur; the liquid form may cause skin blistering. Soluble in water; it is a highly reactive epoxide and an alkylating agent. Converted to ethylene glycol and thiodiacetic acid.
Health effects. Acute: narcotic properties with CNS depression. In high concentrations (several hundred parts per million), it can cause nausea, vomiting, headache and mucous membrane and eye irritation. Chronic: probably capable of causing peripheral neuropathy and encephalopathy. Sensitising agent causing anaphylaxis, urticaria and asthma. Considered carcinogenic to humans (IARC group 1) owing to association with lymphatic and haematopoietic cancers.
Biological monitoring. Urinary thioether excretion and blood ethylene glycol have been used for research purposes.
Measurement. Sampled onto a charcoal tube with an optimum volume of just less than $5\,l$ ($10\,ml\,min^{-1}$ for eight hours; maximum, $200\,ml\,min^{-1}$). Desorbed with CS_2 for subsequent analysis using gas chromatography.
Workplace exposure limits. HSE WEL: eight-hour TWA, $1.8\,mg\,m^{-3}$ and $1\,ppm$ (skin and carcinogen notation).

Formaldehyde

$$H-\overset{\overset{\textstyle O}{\|}}{C}-H$$

Properties. Colourless gas with a pungent odour. Commonly used as an aqueous solution (formalin) of 34–38% formaldehyde. MW, 30.03.
Uses. Plastics and resin manufacture; preservative; intermediate in chemical manufacture; embalming and healthcare use. Used also in textile industry as a crease-resistant agent, and with urea or phenol as a binding agent.
Metabolism. Mainly by inhalation. Metabolised in the liver and excreted in the urine and exhaled air. Converted to formate in many tissues on direct contact, including red blood cells.
Health effects. Acute: severe mucous membrane and skin irritation. Brown discolorations of the skin and the nails. Chronic: allergen for skin; although not

generally considered a respiratory sensitiser, it is a respiratory tract irritant. Formaldehyde causes cancer of the nasopharynx and leukaemia in animal studies and is associated in human studies; it is therefore considered to be carcinogenic to humans (IARC group 1).

Biological monitoring. None in common use. Formate in urine is not useful because of its variability.

Measurement. Air is bubbled through a 0.5% solution of 3-methyl-2-benzothiazolone hydrazone in a bubbler at a flow rate of 1 l min^{-1}. The resulting solution is analysed by colorimetric means. Colorimetric detector tubes are also available (MDHS 19).

Workplace exposure limits. HSE WEL: eight-hour TWA and 15-minute STEL, 2.5 mg m^{-3} and 2 ppm (carcinogen notation).

Ketones and ethers

Ketones   and   Ethers

Uses. Solvents.

Examples of ketones: dimethylketone (acetone), methylethylketone (MEK), methyl-*n*-butylketone (MnBK) and methylisobutylketone (MiBK).

Example of ethers: diethylether, diisopropyl ether.

Metabolism. Typically by inhalation; also by skin contact. MnBK is biotransformed to 2,5-hexanedione.

Health effects. Acute: upper respiratory tract irritants. Cause dermatitis. Chronic: narcotic. MnBK can cause peripheral neuropathy. Neurotoxic effects potentiated by concomitant exposure to MEK and/or MiBK. Bis(chloromethyl)ether is a strong alkylating agent and a potent lung carcinogen.

Biological monitoring. Non-specific. Exceptions: MEK, MiBK and 2,5-hexanedione (for MnBK) in end-of-shift urine.

Measurement. Ethers and ketones are sampled by drawing air through a Tenax tube at a flow rate of 200 ml min^{-1} for subsequent analysis using gas chromatography.

Workplace exposure limits. Diethylether, HSE WEL: eight-hour TWA, 310 mg m^{-3} (100 ppm); 15-minute STEL, 620 mg m^{-3} and 200 ppm.

Methylethylketone (butan-2-one) (MEK), HSE WEL: eight-hour TWA, 600 mg m^{-3} and 200 ppm; 15-minute STEL, 899 mg m^{-3} and 300 ppm (skin notation and biological monitoring and guidance value).

Methylbutylketone (hexan-2-one) (MBK), HSE WEL: eight-hour TWA, 21 mg m^{-3} and 5 ppm (skin notation).

Methylisobutylketone (4-methylpentan-2-one) (MiBK), HSE WEL: eight-hour TWA, 208 mg m^{-3} and 50 ppm; 15-minute STEL, 416 mg m^{-3} and 100 ppm (skin notation and biological monitoring and guidance value).

Methyl alcohol (methanol)

```
      H
      |
H —— C —— OH
      |
      H
```

Properties. Colourless liquid which smells like ethanol. MW, 32.04.
Uses. Celluloid manufacture; paint remover; varnishes; antifreeze; cements; fuel additive.
Metabolism. Absorbed by all routes and slowly metabolised to formaldehyde and formic acid.
Health effects. Acute: headache, dizziness, dermatitis, conjunctivitis, CNS depression. Chronic: there is a symptom-free period for 12–24 hours, sometimes longer, after a significant acute exposure. This is followed by metabolic acidosis with varying optic nerve and retinal damage with blindness. Ingestion of 4–15 ml has been enough to cause blindness.
Biological monitoring. Urine methanol levels at end of the shift.
Measurement. Sampled onto a silica gel tube at an air flow rate of 50 ml min^{-1} for subsequent analysis using gas chromatography. A general alcohol detector tube is available.
Workplace exposure limits. HSE WEL: eight-hour TWA, 266 mg m^{-3} and 200 ppm; 15-minute STEL, 333 mg m^{-3} and 250 ppm (skin notation).

Methyl bromide (bromomethane)

```
      H
      |
H —— C —— Br
      |
      H
```

Properties. Colourless, odourless gas. MW, 94.94.
Uses. Fire extinguishers; refrigerant; insecticide; and fumigant.
Metabolism. Rapidly absorbed by inhalation, and toxic probably directly and through metabolites such as inorganic bromide.
Health effects. Acute: late onset, up to 48 hours delay, of acute respiratory tract irritation and pulmonary oedema. The gas can penetrate clothing and cause irritation or burns. Nausea, vomiting, headaches and convulsions may also occur. Chronic: recovery from the acute attack is usual, but prolonged exposure or delayed treatment can cause peripheral neuropathy, tremor, renal failure and chronic toxic encephalopathy.
Biological monitoring. Urine or blood can be used for analysis of inorganic bromide; the blood half-life is about 14 days, so sample timing is not important.
Measurement. Sampled onto two large charcoal tubes in series at an air flow rate of 1000 ml min^{-1} for subsequent analysis using gas chromatography. Colorimetric detection tubes are also available.

Workplace exposure limits. HSE WEL: eight-hour TWA, $20\,mg\,m^{-3}$ and $5\,ppm$; 15-minute STEL, $59\,mg\,m^{-3}$ and $15\,ppm$ (skin notation).

Methylene chloride (dichloromethane)

$$
\begin{array}{c}
\text{H} \\
| \\
\text{H} - \text{C} - \text{Cl} \\
| \\
\text{Cl}
\end{array}
$$

Properties. Non-flammable, colourless liquid. MW, 84.93.

Uses. Paint and varnish remover; insecticide; fumigant; solvent; and fire extinguisher.

Metabolism. Skin and lung absorption. Metabolism results in the production of carbon monoxide and an increase in carboxyhaemoglobin.

Health effects. Acute: skin and mucous membrane irritant. Acute intoxication with stupor, numbness and tingling of limbs following inhalation due to narcotic effect. Chronic: dry, scaly dermatitis. Can precipitate cardiac ischaemia owing to increase in carboxyhaemoglobin.

Biological monitoring. Carboxyhaemoglobin levels in blood and carbon monoxide in exhaled air. Smoking affects biological monitoring results. Methylene chloride itself can be measured in blood or exhaled breath but this is not the preferred method because of the short half-life (<1 hour). Urine levels reflect the average blood value between urine voiding.

Measurement. Sampled onto a charcoal tube at an air flow rate of $1000\,ml\,min^{-1}$ for subsequent analysis using gas chromatography. Colorimetric detection tubes are also available (NIOSH 1012).

Workplace exposure limits. HSE WEL: eight-hour TWA, $363\,mg\,m^{-3}$ and $100\,ppm$; 15-minute STEL, $706\,mg\,m^{-3}$ and $200\,ppm$ (skin notation and biological monitoring guidance value).

Tetrachloroethane

$$
\begin{array}{c}
\text{H} \quad\ \text{H} \\
| \qquad | \\
\text{Cl} - \text{C} - \text{C} - \text{Cl} \\
| \qquad | \\
\text{Cl} \quad\ \text{Cl}
\end{array}
$$

Properties. Heavy, non-flammable liquid with a phenolic odour. MW, 167.85.

Uses. Solvent; chemical intermediate.

Metabolism. Rapid absorption from the skin and lungs. Slowly metabolised and excreted in the urine. Main metabolites trichloroacetic acid (TCA) and oxalic acid.

Health effects. Acute: gastrointestinal and upper respiratory tract irritation. CNS depression. Chronic: hepatic: hepatomegaly and hepatic failure; neurological: polyneuropathy, particularly of the extremities; renal: albuminuria; dermatological: dry, scaly dermatitis.

Health surveillance and biological monitoring. Non-specific. Organ function tests may be of use.

Measurement. Sampled onto a charcoal tube at an air flow rate of $200\,ml\,min^{-1}$ for subsequent analysis using gas chromatography (NIOSH 1019).

Workplace exposure limits. ACGIH TLV: eight-hour TWA, $6.9\,mg\,m^{-3}$ and 1 ppm (skin notation).

Tetrachloroethylene (perchloroethylene)

$$
\begin{array}{ccc}
Cl & & Cl \\
\diagdown & & \diagup \\
& C = C & \\
\diagup & & \diagdown \\
Cl & & Cl
\end{array}
$$

Properties. Non-flammable liquid with characteristic ether-like odour. MW, 165.8.

Uses. Solvent in adhesives and sealants; degreaser; widely used as dry-cleaning agent; it was used as a fumigant.

Metabolism. Readily absorbed through the lungs and skin. Metabolised to TCA and excreted in small amounts in the urine, but mainly excreted unchanged in the breath. Slow elimination with blood levels detectable several days after a single exposure.

Health effects. Acute: powerful narcotic. Can cause mucous membrane and skin irritation as well as liver damage. Chronic: chronic toxic encephalopathy and liver damage, possible renal effects.

Biological monitoring. Urine TCA (end-of-working-week sample); however, this is a poor indicator. Blood or breath samples pre-shift at the end of a working week with analysis for perchloroethylene are preferred.

Measurement. Sampled onto a charcoal tube at an air flow rate of $1000\,ml\,min^{-1}$ for subsequent analysis using gas chromatography.

Workplace exposure limits. HSE WEL: eight-hour TWA, $138\,mg\,m^{-3}$ and 20 ppm; 15-minute STEL, $689\,mg\,m^{-3}$ and 40 ppm (skin notation).

1.1.1-Trichloroethane

$$
\begin{array}{ccc}
H & Cl & \\
| & | & \\
H - C - C - Cl & \\
| & | & \\
H & Cl &
\end{array}
$$

Properties. Non-flammable liquid, sweet, chloroform-like odour. MW, 133.4.

Uses. Chemical intermediate; solvent; and degreasing agent.

Metabolism. Readily absorbed through the lungs and easily absorbed through the skin. Metabolised to TCA and excreted in the urine. Mostly excreted unchanged in the breath.

Health effects. Acute: mucous membrane and skin irritant, narcotic, capable of sensitising the myocardium to adrenaline, thereby causing dysrhythmias. Chronic: dry, scaly dermatitis.

Biological monitoring. Urinary TCA collected end of shift, at the end of the working week. Blood or breath trichloroethane collected pre-shift at the end of the working week.

Measurement. Sampled onto a charcoal tube at an air flow rate of $1000\,ml\,min^{-1}$ for subsequent analysis using gas chromatography (NIOSH 1003).

Workplace exposure limits. HSE WEL: eight-hour TWA, $555\,mg\,m^{-3}$ and 100 ppm; 15-minute STEL, $1100\,mg\,m^{-3}$ and 200 ppm.

Trichloroethylene

Properties. Non-flammable liquid. MW, 133.41.

Uses. Degreasing agent; formerly an anaesthetic agent.

Metabolism. Readily absorbed through the lungs and, to a lesser extent, the skin. Metabolised to chloral hydrate and then to TCA or its glucuronide, and trichloroethanol excreted in the urine. Elimination of TCA takes longer than 24 hours, with a consequent increase during the working week.

Health effects. Acute: powerful narcotic, action exacerbated by ethanol. Consistent exposure to trichloroethylene and alcohol consumption responsible for 'degreaser's flush'. Mild respiratory and skin irritant. Cardiac dysrhythmias. Chronic: peripheral neuropathy has been reported. A known human carcinogen, with a well-established link to kidney cancer (IARC group 1). Limited evidence for associations with non-Hodgkin's lymphoma and liver cancer.

Biological monitoring. Urinary TCA collected end of shift, at the end of the working week.

Measurement. Sampled onto a charcoal tube at an air flow rate of $1000\,ml\,min^{-1}$ for subsequent analysis using gas chromatography.

Workplace exposure limits. HSE WEL: eight-hour TWA, $550\,mg\,m^{-3}$ and 100 ppm; 15-minute STEL, $820\,mg\,m^{-3}$ and 150 ppm (carcinogen and skin notation).

Vinyl chloride (monochloroethylene)

Properties. Flammable gas with pleasant odour. MW, 62.5.

Uses. Polymerised to plastics; solvent in rubber manufacture. Previously used as aerosol propellant and has anaesthetic properties.

Metabolism. Rapidly absorbed by inhalation and partially excreted by the same route. Rapid clearance from the blood through poorly understood metabolic pathways. Biotransformation to the reactive chloroethylene oxide in the liver may be important. It is possible that some of the health effects are related to the immune reaction to vinyl chloride–protein complexes, which are considered 'foreign'.

Health effects. Acute: narcotic. Chronic: fatigue, lassitude, abdominal pain. Raynaud's phenomenon, which can be severe. Acro-osteolysis of fingertips, leading to pseudo-clubbing and scleroderma-like changes. Angiosarcoma of the liver is rare, but invariably fatal. Occurred following high exposures in workers clearing vinyl chloride monomer polymerisation chambers.

Health surveillance. Many jurisdictions require a periodic clinical history; physical examination with or without liver function monitoring, which is not of much value for present exposure levels.

Measurement. Sampled onto two charcoal tubes in series at an air flow rate of 50 ml min^{-1} for subsequent analysis using gas chromatography (NIOSH 1007). Colorimetric detector tubes are also available.

Workplace exposure limits. HSE WEL: eight-hour TWA, 2.6 mg m^{-3}, 1 ppm (carcinogen notation).

Further Reading

Agency for Toxic Substances and Disease Registry (ATSDR) (2021). Toxicological Profiles. https://www.atsdr.cdc.gov/toxprofiledocs/index.html (accessed 5 September 2021).

GESTIS Substance Database (2018). Information system on hazardous substances of the German Social Accident Insurance. https://www.dguv.de/ifa/gestis/gestis-stoffdatenbank/index-2.jsp. Accessed 5th September 2021.

Safe Work Australia. Health Monitoring Guides (2020). Health monitoring when you work with hazardous chemicals - Guide for workers. https://www.safeworkaustralia.gov.au/sites/default/files/2020-10/Health%20Monitoring%20Guidance%20-%20Workers%20-%20Final.pdf. Accessed 5th September 2021.

CHAPTER 7

Occupational Cancer

7.1 Introduction

Volumes have been written on this subject, but space allows only the briefest survey here. A short historical account is followed by an annotated list of some of the characteristics of occupational cancer and by some lists indicating the probable and possible human carcinogens of occupational origin.

7.2 Historical perspective

The first recognised association between cancer and occupation was made in 1775 by Percival Pott, a surgeon at St Bartholomew's Hospital, London. He noted an

Pocket Consultant: Occupational Health, Sixth Edition. Kerry Gardiner, David Rees, Anil Adisesh, David Zalk, and Malcolm Harrington.
© 2022 John Wiley & Sons Ltd. Published 2022 by John Wiley & Sons Ltd.

increased incidence of scrotal cancer in chimney sweeps and, rejecting the venereal aetiology popular in his day, thought that the tumour was more likely to be due to soot. Further observations later linked other components of fossil fuel with skin cancer – notably of the scrotum – but it took many long and arduous laboratory experiments before the link was confirmed experimentally in the first quarter of the twentieth century. The compounds implicated were all polynuclear aromatic hydrocarbons, examples of which include the following:

Benzo(a)pyrene   Dibenz(a,b)anthracene

In 1895, Ludwig Rehn described bladder tumours in workers in the aniline dye industries. Subsequently, a range of aromatic amines have been noted to be bladder carcinogens. Examples include the following:

2-Naphthylamine   4-Aminobiphenyl

Benzidine   Methyene-bis-O-chloraniline

Despite the length of time that has elapsed since the discovery of these carcinogens, workers are still contracting tumours from these or similar agents, and will continue to do so. This is partly because of the legacy of a long latent period (sometimes exceeding 40 years) and partly because effective substitutes of such materials have not always been available; in some cases, such as benzene and vinyl chloride monomer, society has chosen to continue to use these agents – albeit more safely.

7.3 Theories of chemical carcinogenesis

Chemicals form the bulk of the occupationally related carcinogens, and it is important to distinguish between the different classes. In brief, two broad groups are postulated. Genotoxic carcinogens pose a clear qualitative hazard to health as they are capable of altering cellular genetic material, and thus should theoretically cause cancer after a single exposure. On the other hand, epigenetic carcinogens seem to be without direct effect on genetic material and require high or prolonged exposure for effect. The genotoxic carcinogens probably have no safe threshold; the epigenetic carcinogens may have.

A tentative classification, which seems reasonable in animal models, can be expressed as shown in Table 7.1.

7.4 Characteristics of occupational carcinogens

Tumours of occupational origin are usually indistinguishable, histopathologically and symptomatically, from non-occupational tumours. Nevertheless, there are some characteristics of note.

TABLE 7.1

Classification of chemical carcinogens.

Type	Mode of action	Example
Genotoxic		
Direct action	Interacts with DNA	Bis(chloromethyl)ether
Secondary action	Requires conversion to direct type	2-Naphthylamine
Inorganic	Affects DNA replication	Nickel salts
Epigenetic		
'Solid state'	Mesenchymal cell effects	Asbestos
Hormone	Endocrine effect ± promoter	Diethylstilboestrol
Immunosuppressor	Stimulates certain tumour growth	Azathioprine
Co-carcinogen	Enhances genotoxic types when given at same time	Ethanol
Promoter	Enhances genotoxic types when given subsequently	Bile acids

- They tend to occur earlier than 'spontaneous' tumours of the same site.
- Exposure to the putative agent is repeated, but not necessarily continuous.
- The latent period is 10–40 years for solid organ cancers but can be shorter for other malignancies, such as leukaemia.
- Rare tumours that occur more frequently than expected in a population of workers.
- Despite widely differing estimates of the proportion of all cancers caused by occupation, the true figure probably lies in the range of 3–8%. However, if one adds in the interaction of occupational exposures with other risk factors, for example asbestos and cigarette smoking, the range doubles to 5–15%. For some shop floor groups in some industries, and for some tumour sites, such as lung and bladder, the risks can rise to 20–40%. Multiple chemical exposures, which are the norm in modern industry, make it exceedingly difficult, however, to isolate particular individual chemicals as the guilty parties. The role of synergism is probably important, although still largely unquantified.

7.5 Known or suspected occupational carcinogens

The length of the list and its individual members vary according to which organisation has compiled it. Perhaps the most widely accepted list is that of the International Agency for Research on Cancer (IARC). Soon after the IARC was established in 1965, it started to receive frequent requests for advice on the carcinogenicity of chemicals, including requests for lists of established and suspected human carcinogens. In 1970, an IARC Advisory Committee on Environmental Carcinogenesis recommended 'that a compendium on carcinogenic chemicals be prepared by experts. The biological activity and evaluation of practical importance to public health should be referenced and documented'. The next year, the IARC Governing Council adopted a resolution that IARC should prepare 'monographs on the evaluation of carcinogenic risk of chemicals to man', which became the initial title of the series. In succeeding years, the scope of the programme broadened as monographs were developed for complex mixtures, occupational exposures, physical agents, biological organisms, pharmaceuticals and other exposures. In 1988 'of chemicals' was dropped from the title, and in 2019 'evaluation of carcinogenic risks' became 'identification of carcinogenic hazards', in line with the objective of the programme.

Evaluation and rationale

Consensus evaluations by a Working Group of the strength of the evidence of cancer in humans, the evidence of cancer in experimental animals and the mechanistic evidence are made using transparent criteria and defined descriptive terms. The Working Group then develops a consensus overall evaluation of the strength of the evidence of carcinogenicity for each agent under review.

This evaluation will utilise data from three sources with their respective outcomes.

1. Carcinogenicity in humans
   a. Sufficient evidence of carcinogenicity
   b. Limited evidence of carcinogenicity
   c. Inadequate evidence of carcinogenicity
   d. Evidence suggesting a lack of evidence of carcinogenicity

2. Carcinogenicity in experimental animals
   a. Sufficient evidence of carcinogenicity
   b. Limited evidence of carcinogenicity
   c. Inadequate evidence of carcinogenicity
   d. Evidence suggesting a lack of evidence of carcinogenicity

3. Mechanistic evidence
   a. Strong mechanistic evidence
   b. Limited mechanistic evidence
   c. Inadequate mechanistic evidence

Once the Working Group has considered all of the data then the substance/agent is classified into one of four categories:

1. the agent is carcinogenic to humans (group 1)
2. the agent is probably carcinogenic to humans (group 2A)
3. the agent is possibly carcinogenic to humans (group 2B)
4. the agent is not classifiable.

This list is also presented in Table 7.2.

In addition to (or in conjunction with) the IARC list of group 1 carcinogens there are studies that suggest links between certain tumours and certain industries or materials. Table 7.3 lists the occupations recognised as presenting a carcinogenic risk.

7.6 Work attribution of cancers

Level of probability to attribute cancer to work exposure

In many jurisdictions and for many purposes – workers' compensation among them – the test of whether a cancer is attributable to work is the balance of probability, meaning greater than 50% probability and thus a material contribution to causation. Accordingly, attribution can be positive even in the face of substantial uncertainty. The question of 'How can I *prove* a cancer is due to work?' therefore only arises in circumscribed situations: criminal negligence may be one, but even here the test is not certainty but rather beyond reasonable doubt. Some of the subjectivity in determining likely attribution can be ameliorated by applying an arithmetic test: if the workplace exposure circumstances of the afflicted

TABLE 7.2

Integration of streams of evidence in reaching overall classifications (the evidence in *bold italic* represents the basis of the overall evaluation).

Stream of evidence			Classification based on strength of evidence
Evidence of cancer in humans[a]	Evidence of cancer in experimental animals	Mechanistic evidence	
Sufficient	Not necessary	Not necessary	**Carcinogenic to humans (group 1)**
Limited or inadequate	*Sufficient*	*Strong (b)(1) (exposed humans)*	
Limited	*Sufficient*	Strong (b)(2–3), limited or inadequate	**Probably carcinogenic to humans (group 2A)**
Inadequate	*Sufficient*	*Strong (b)(2) (human cells or tissues)*	
Limited	Less than sufficient	*Strong (b)(1–3)*	
Limited or inadequate	Not necessary	*Strong (a) (mechanistic class)*	
Limited	Less than sufficient	Limited or inadequate	**Possibly carcinogenic to humans (group 2B)**
Inadequate	*Sufficient*	Strong (b)(3), limited or inadequate	
Inadequate	Less than sufficient	*Strong b(1–3)*	
Limited	*Sufficient*	*Strong (c) (does not operate in humans)[b]*	
Inadequate	*Sufficient*	*Strong (c) (does not operate in humans)[b]*	**Not classifiable as to its carcinogenicity to humans (group 3)**
All other situations not listed above			

[a] ***Human*** cancer(s) with highest evaluation.
[b] ***The*** strong evidence that the mechanism of carcinogenicity in experimental animals does not operate in humans must specifically be for the tumour sites supporting the classification of sufficient evidence in experimental animals.

TABLE 7.3

Occupations recognised as presenting a carcinogenic risk.

Industry	Occupation	Site of tumour	Likely carcinogen
Agriculture, forestry, fishing	Farmers, seamen, vineyard workers	Skin	Ultraviolet light
	Mining arseniferous ores	Lung, skin	Arsenical insecticides
	Mining iron ore	Lung, skin	Arsenic
	Mining tin	Lung	? Radon
	Mining asbestos	Lung, bone marrow	? Radon
	Mining uranium	Lung, pleura and peritoneum	Asbestos
		Lung	
Petroleum	Wax pressing	Scrotum	Polynuclear aromatics
Painting	Painting	Lung,? bladder	?
Metal	Aluminium production	Bladder,? lung	Polynuclear aromatics
	Copper smelting	Lung,? sinonasal	Arsenic
	Chromate production	Lung,? sinonasal	Chromium compounds
	Chromium plating	Lung	Chromium compounds
	Ferrochromium production	Lung	Chromium compounds
	Iron/steel production/ founding	Lung	Benzo(a)pyrene
	Nickel refining	Nasal sinuses, lung	Nickel compounds
	Pickling operations	Larynx, lung	Acid mists
Transport	Shipyards	Lung, pleura and peritoneum	Asbestos
Chemicals	BCME and CMME production	Lung	BCME, CMME
	Vinyl chloride production	Liver	VCM
	Isopropyl alcohol production (manufacture by strong acid method)	Paranasal sinuses	? Acid mists
	Chromate pigment production	Lung	Chromium compounds

(Continued)

TABLE 7.3 (Continued)

Industry	Occupation	Site of tumour	Likely carcinogen
	Dye manufacture and users	Bladder	Aromatic amines
	Auramine and poison gas manufacture	Lung	Mustard gas
	Production of inorganic acid mists (strong) containing sulphuric acid	Larynx, lung	Sulphuric acid
Rubber	Rubber manufacture	Lymphatic and haemopoietic systems, bladder	Benzene, aromatic amines
	Calendering, tyre curing and tyre building	Lymphatic and haemopoietic systems	Benzene
	Cable making, latex production	Bladder	Aromatic amines
Construction, maintenance	Installation of insulation, demolition	Lung, pleura and peritoneum	Asbestos
Leather	Boot and shoe making	Nose, bone marrow	Leather dust, benzene
Wood pulp and paper	Furniture making	Nasal sinuses	Wood dust
Electric/ electronics	Engineering	Bone marrow, brain	? Fluxes, ?? EMF
Healthcare industry	Pharmaceutical manufacturing		
	Pharmacies	Bone marrow	Cytotoxic drugs
	Nursing		
	Radiology	Bone marrow	Ionising radiation
	Caring for patients	Hepatoma	
		Kaposi's sarcoma	Hepatitis B and C
		Non-Hodgkin's lymphoma	HIV
	Sterilisation unit	Lymphatic and haemopoietic systems	Ethylene oxide

BCME, bis (chloromethyl) ether; CMME, chloromethyl methyl ether; EMF, electromagnetic field; HIV, human immunodeficiency virus; VCM, vinyl chloride monomer.

person have been shown to be associated with a relative effect estimate – hazard ratio, odds ratio, incidence rate ratio, for instance – for a tumour of around 2 or greater, then the balance of probability test of work attribution can be reasonably assumed to have been met. For the minority of agents – ionising radiation and asbestos are examples – the balance of probability determination is based on generally accepted dose–responses. Lung cancer risk from asbestos is approximately double that of an unexposed population after an exposure of 25 fibres per millilitre year (the equivalent of air concentrations of 5 fibres per millilitre for five years or 1 fibre per millilitre for 25 years, etc.) So, if the concentrations of asbestos over the exposure years can be estimated, the balance of probability threshold can be tested in a fairly standard manner. Unfortunately, in most settings attribution to work is more subjective, but there are approaches to attribution which result in a satisfactorily robust opinion for most circumstances. One such approach is outlined here.

An approach to determining the probability of a material workplace contribution

The initial step is to get confirmation of a specific malignancy, preferably from a histological report, because patient-derived information may be unintentionally unreliable: lung cancer on history may be secondary to colon or liver cancer, for instance. An exploration of exposures to workplace lung carcinogens would thus be unhelpful in this case.

Lifetime occupational exposure should then be obtained, by an occupational history usually, although objective measurements may be available; radiation dosimetry is one such exception. Some tumours are relatable to occupations and work processes rather than to identified individual carcinogens, so these work features should be part of the occupational history. Latency from first exposure to disease onset and frequency, duration and perceived intensity of exposure are also essential elements of the occupational history.

Whether there is an established association between the specific cancer and the exposure circumstances should then be sought. Some workplace exposures are commonplace, as are some tumours; spurious associations between them are accordingly inevitable. For this reason, it is inadvisable to search for individual studies on exposure–cancer associations; authoritative independent assessments are preferable, those of the IARC foremost among them. One advantage of the IARC system is that substances or settings classified as 1 or 2A are widely accepted as established human carcinogens for purposes of attribution. The IARC monographs typically provide the exposure settings connected to the increased cancer risk, latency, and the exact nature of the causative chemicals, for example, so the circumstances of the individual under investigation can be weighed against these. The monographs also summarise the magnitudes of the relative risks found in the studies that contributed to the carcinogenic classification, so circumstances producing relative risks of 2 or greater may be reported and are valuable, as exemplified by silica. Radiological silicosis has typically been found to increase lung cancer occurrence by twofold or greater, but not so silica without the pneumoconiosis. Accordingly, many jurisdictions restrict workers' compensation for silica-exposed workers with lung cancer to those with radiological disease.

Almost all cancers are associated with more than one risk, so even if an established workplace risk has been identified its contribution relative to others needs to be judged, a somewhat rough approximation in the main. This step necessitates identification of risk factors consistently and firmly established with the malignancy. Authoritative textbooks, IARC classifications, systematic reviews and meta-analyses should be used as tentative associations are not of interest. The contribution of non-workplace and workplace factors should then be estimated. Latency from first occupational exposure to cancer onset is a key consideration. This apportionment among risk factors may be relatively straightforward. According to the IARC renal cancer is associated with tobacco smoking, trichloroethylene, X-radiation and gamma-radiation. But associations with obesity and hypertension are also consistently reported in methodologically sound studies. A long-term smoker with chronic hypertension and only occasional recent use of trichloroethylene who develops renal cancer would struggle to meet the balance of probability test for a material occupational contribution. Many cases are, of course, more difficult. It is also important to bear in mind that risk factors may interact more than additively: workplace exposures may have made a material contribution even if another risk factor predominated; without the occupational exposure the risk may have been substantially lower.

A report with a conclusion about the probability of a material workplace contribution and the reasons for this decision is useful. An expression of uncertainty is often warranted, as is referral to a specialist in complex cases. A conclusion may be along the lines of: 'On the balance of probability wood dust was a major contributor to the employee's nasal cavity cancer because in similar exposure circumstances the IARC has determined that wood dust is an established human carcinogen (group 1). The employee has other risk factors for nasal cancer, but these are considered minor contributors because exposure to them was short-term and less than typically associated with nasal cavity cancer'.

7.7 Prevention

Workplace screening for occupational cancers

On the face of it, screening workers exposed to occupational carcinogens for early detection and initiation of treatment seems sensible, even ethically required. But this is only true if early detection and treatment result in longer survival, or at least a period of better quality of life, and if the positives of screening outweigh the negatives. Unfortunately, these conditions are rarely met.

It is true that studies have shown that early detection of some cancers by screening increases survival time from diagnosis to death, an ostensibly favourable outcome of the intervention. Regrettably, biases explain much of the apparently longer lives. One of these is lead time bias. Cancers detected pre-symptomatically by screening are usually at an early stage, and death from them typically occurs relatively long after diagnosis. On the other hand, without screening tumours are diagnosed when sufficiently advanced to be symptomatic, and even to have spread. Survival from diagnosis to death is shorter than for their screened counterparts. But both screened and unscreened may die at the same time; all screening achieved was to push back diagnosis, rather than push forward death. Even screening for malignant melanoma, a skin cancer associated with sun-exposed occupations, is not supported or refuted by current evidence from population studies (Johansson et al. 2019).

False positives – meaning positive tests of health effects unrelated to workplace factors or due to imperfect test performance – detected during workplace screening are problematic. And such false positives may be common, as exemplified by screening for lung cancer. The National Lung Screening Trial in the USA showed a 20% reduction in mortality from lung cancer in subjects screened with low-dose computed tomography (CT) compared with those who had standard chest radiographs (National Lung Screening Trial Research Team 2011). In all, about 25 000 CTs were done and 650 lung cancers diagnosed, but over 12 700 participants without the cancer required diagnostic follow-up because of CT abnormalities. Positive screening tests usually need confirmatory evaluation, sometimes with expensive and invasive investigations. Besides the issue of who pays for these investigations, questions about work attribution can be difficult to manage: it is reasonable for workers to conclude that, since screening was thought to be necessary, a cancer detected by it is work-related. Rejecting this notion, no matter how valid, may engender mistrust in management and the occupational health service.

The problems with screening for occupational cancers do not mean that the workplace is not a useful setting for public health authority-supported cancer screening programmes as part of comprehensive worker health programmes.

Before instituting screening for occupational cancers some questions should be satisfactorily answered:

- Is there clear benefit from early detection of the cancer?
- Is the screening test acceptable to workers and without undue harm (anxiety included)?
- How common will false positives be, and will they be manageable?
- Will positive screening tests require invasive or expensive confirmatory investigations, and who will pay for them?
- Would the money be better spent on controlling exposures?

In conclusion, currently few if any occupational cancer screening programmes can be justified, especially in resource-constrained settings. But new evidence along with technological advances may change this; keeping up with the literature is thus advisable.

Further Reading

Johansson, M., Brodersen, J., Gøtzsche, P.C., and Jørgensen, K.J. (2019). Screening for reducing morbidity and mortality in malignant melanoma. *Cochrane Database of Systematic Reviews* 6: CD012352. https://doi.org/10.1002/14651858.CD012352.pub2.

Loomis, D., Guha, N., Hall, A.L., and Straif, K. (2018). Identifying occupational carcinogens: an update from the IARC monographs. *Occupational and Environmental Medicine* 75: 593–603. https://doi.org/10.1136/oemed-2017-104944.

The National Lung Screening Trial Research Team (2011). Reduced lung-cancer mortality with low-dose computed tomographic screening. *The New England Journal of Medicine* 365: 395–409. https://doi.org/10.1056/NEJMoa1102873.TABLE 3.8

CHAPTER 8

Occupational Hygiene – Gases, Vapours, Dusts and Fibres

8.1 Introduction

This chapter aims to provide an abridged account of the sources/uses, health effects and measurement requirements for a number of chemical substances presenting as gases, vapours, dusts or fibres. It complements the material in Chapter 6.

In terms of the types of activity that generate the majority of exposures in the working environment (gases/vapours and dusts/fibres), the following is a short list of periodic and/or continuous processes.

Exposure generation

1. 'Material handling' that generates dust/fibres, gases or vapours:
    - debagging
    - pouring of liquids

Pocket Consultant: Occupational Health, Sixth Edition. Kerry Gardiner, David Rees, Anil Adisesh, David Zalk, and Malcolm Harrington.
© 2022 John Wiley & Sons Ltd. Published 2022 by John Wiley & Sons Ltd.

- transfer of material from one container to another
- transfer of material from one mode of transport to another
- blending
- stirring or agitating
- screening or sieving
- crushing or grinding
- emptying
- recharging
- sampling.
2. Processes causing emission of (mainly) vapours, but also particles:
   - stirring and agitating
   - surface coating
   - drying
   - spraying
   - dipping
   - curing
   - baking
   - welding
   - sampling.
3. Processes producing mainly dust, but also some fume or gas:
   - machining
   - drilling
   - planing
   - sanding
   - milling
   - cutting
   - sawing
   - dismantling
   - demolition.

Fugitive emissions (in terms of random/unexpected releases) produce gases, liquids and vapours, and occur as a result of leaks from:

- fractured or corroded pipes, vessels and containers
- poorly made joints or the breakdown of seals on joints
- along the shafts of valves
- along the shafts of pumps
- spills and collisions.

Workplace exposure limits

Heading into 2020, the Health and Safety Executive (HSE) in the UK updated document Environmental Hygiene 40 (EH40), which contains occupational exposure limits (OELs) for use with the Control of Substances Hazardous to Health (COSHH) Regulations 2002. Under the COSHH regulations, there were two types of OELs for hazardous substances: occupational exposure standards

(OESs) and maximum exposure limits (MELs). However, as a result of concerns expressed by the Health and Safety Commission's Advisory Committee on Toxic Substances (ACTS) about how well employers and other stakeholders understood OELs, and about how widely these were being used in industry, this system of two distinct standards has been discontinued in favour of a single type of OEL, which is known as the workplace exposure limit or WEL. Hence, the Control of Substances Hazardous to Health (Amendment) Regulations 2004 removed the OESs and MELs and replaced them with WELs in conjunction with eight principles of good practice for control. In addition, some former OESs have been removed and not converted to WELs because of doubts that the original limits were not soundly based.

WELs are concentrations of hazardous substances in the air, averaged over a specified period of time referred to as a time-weighted average (TWA). Two time periods are used: long-term (eight hours) and short-term (15 minutes). Short-term exposure limits (STELs) are set to help prevent effects, such as eye irritation, that may occur following exposure for a few minutes.

Setting exposure limits

HSE has established WELs to prevent excessive exposure to specified hazardous substances by containing exposure below a set limit. A WEL is the maximum concentration of an airborne substance averaged over a reference period, to which employees may be exposed by inhalation.

Derivation of WELs

The first stage in the derivation of the WEL involves an assessment of the toxicology of the substance concerned. The purpose of this assessment is to identify the potential for a substance to produce adverse human health effects and to understand the exposure–response relationships for these effects. In the context of setting OELs, there are certain key reference points on the exposure–response curve. These are the 'no observed adverse effect level' (NOAEL) and the 'lowest observed adverse effect level' (LOAEL) (see Section 6.1). The concept of NOAEL/ LOAEL is generally agreed to have practical relevance in the OEL context only for those substances or toxicological mechanisms that have a 'threshold' of effect. For example, eye irritation caused by an acid vapour will only occur above a certain threshold exposure concentration, and thus the concept of a NOAEL will apply. In contrast, for substances such as DNA-reactive chemicals that cause cancer by a genotoxic mechanism, although in theory a threshold may exist (because of biochemical defence and repair mechanisms), currently available techniques do not allow the reliable identification of a clear threshold or NOAEL. (The NOAEL is the highest point on the exposure–response curve at which no adverse health effects are observed; the LOAEL is the lowest point on the exposure–response curve at which adverse health effects are observed. See Chapter 6.)

If a NOAEL (or LOAEL) can be identified, then this value is taken as a starting point for estimating the highest level of occupational exposure at which no adverse health effects would be expected to occur in workers or their progeny following exposure over a working lifetime. Given that, in many cases, NOAELs/LOAELs are obtained from studies in animals, numerical 'uncertainty factors' (safety factors) are usually applied in order to arrive at this estimated desired level of exposure. These factors are applied to take account of toxicological uncertainties such as possible species differences in response, and also to take account of human variability in responsiveness.

Having determined the highest level of occupational exposure at which no adverse health effects would be predicted to occur, the next stage is to determine whether this level of exposure is currently being achieved in the workplace. If not, then consideration would be given to the potential for improving existing standards of control such that this level of exposure could be reasonably achieved. If ACTS considers this level of exposure is reasonably practicable, then the WEL will be proposed at this level.

This route to deriving the WEL will result in a limit set at a level at which no adverse health effects would be expected to occur in workers or their progeny, based on the known and/or predicted effects of the substance, and would also be reasonably practicable for industry to achieve.

There are some categories of substance for which this route to deriving a WEL, based on the concept of a NOAEL/LOAEL, will not be possible:

A. Genotoxic carcinogens: for such substances, there are no currently available techniques by which it is generally accepted that a NOAEL can be reliably identified; hence an approach based on a NOAEL cannot be applied.

B. Asthmagens: although the concept of a NOAEL may be valid, the quality of the available data means that it is generally not possible to identify a threshold level of occupational exposure below which there would be no risk of developing the disease.

C. Mixtures of variable composition such as metalworking fluids (MWFs): the variable composition means that MWFs pose a variable hazard. A defined position on the likely human health effects and the identification of a single NOAEL value is not possible.

D. Any other substance for which the balance of doubt and uncertainty about likely health effects is such that a NOAEL or threshold for effect cannot be confidently identified or predicted. This is more likely to apply to substances with inadequate toxicity data sets. Expert judgement on a case-by-case basis will be needed to determine whether a particular data set is adequate to predict health effects confidently.

E. For some substances, a NOAEL/LOAEL may be identifiable from which it is possible to estimate a level of exposure at which no adverse human health effects would be predicted to occur. However, after due consideration of the costs and efficacy of available control solutions, ACTS may consider that it would not be reasonably practicable to control below this desired level of exposure across all industry sectors.

For substances belonging in one of the above categories A–E, the WEL would be derived by identifying a level of exposure that would represent a standard of control commensurate with good occupational/industrial hygiene practice. In determining this level, the severity of the likely health effects and the cost and efficacy of control solutions would have to be taken into account. The decision as to what represents a good standard of control would be for ACTS and its scientific subcommittee to make, informed by:

A. knowledge of the standards of control currently being achieved in different industry sectors using the substance
B. the potential for improving standards
C. the potential health impacts of the substance.

Criteria for setting WELs WELs are derived by the following criteria:

- The WEL value would be set at a level at which no adverse effects on human health would be expected to occur based on the known and/or predicted effects of the substance. However, if such a level cannot be identified with reasonable confidence, or this level is not reasonably achievable, then
- The WEL value would be based at a level corresponding to what is considered to represent good control, taking into account the severity of the likely health hazards and the costs and efficacy of control solutions. Wherever possible, the WEL would not be set at a level at which there is evidence of adverse effects on human health.

Applying workplace exposure limits
Scope of the limits
The list of WELs, unless otherwise stated, relates to personal exposure to substances hazardous to health in the air of the workplace, that is, the limits cannot be adapted readily to evaluate or control non-occupational exposure (levels in the neighbourhood of an industrial plant). WELs are approved for use only where the atmospheric pressure is between 90 and 110 kPa. To enable WELs to be applied in hyperbaric conditions the limits should be expressed as a partial pressure or mass/volume concentration at higher pressures.

Long-term and short-term limits
Some effects require prolonged or accumulated exposure to manifest themselves. The **long-term (eight-hour TWA) exposure limit** is intended to control such effects by restricting the total intake by inhalation over one or more workshifts. Other effects may be seen after a brief exposure. **Short-term exposure limits (usually 15 minutes)** may be applied to control these effects. For those substances for which no short-term limit is specified it is recommended that a figure of three times the long-term limit be used as a guideline for controlling short-term peaks in exposure.

Units of measure
In WELs, concentrations of airborne particles (fume, dust, etc.) are usually expressed in $mg\,m^{-3}$. In the case of dusts, the limits refer to the 'inhalable' fraction unless specifically stated otherwise, that is, 'respirable'. Exceptionally, the limits for machine-made mineral fibres (MMMFs) and for refractory ceramic fibres

(RCFs) can be expressed either as milligrams per cubic metre ($mg\,m^{-3}$) or as fibres per millilitre of air ($fibres\,ml^{-1}$). WELs for volatile substances are usually expressed in both parts per million by volume (ppm) and $mg\,m^{-3}$. For these substances, limits are set in ppm and a conversion to $mg\,m^{-3}$ is calculated.

$$\text{WEL in mg m}^{-3} = \frac{\text{WEL in ppm} \times \text{MW}}{24.05526}$$

where MW is the molecular weight (molar gas in $g\,mol^{-1}$) of the substance. (Note that $24.05526\,l\,mol^{-1}$ is the molar volume of an ideal gas at 20 °C and 1 atm pressure [760 mmHg, 101 325 Pa, 1.01325 bar].)

Unfortunately, it is rare for an individual to be exposed to only a single substance. Mixed exposures are much more common. The ways in which the constituent substances of a mixed exposure interact vary considerably. Some mixed exposures involve substances that act on different body tissues or organs, by different toxic mechanisms or by causing various effects that are independent of each other. Other mixtures will include substances that act on the same organs, or by similar mechanisms, so that the effects reinforce each other, and the substances are additive in their effect. In some cases, the overall effect is considerably greater than the sum of the individual effects, and the system is synergistic. This may arise from the mutual enhancement of the effects of the constituents because one substance potentiates another.

The main types of interaction are given below.

1. *Synergistic substances.* Cases of synergism (asbestos and smoking) and potentiation (methylethylketone [MEK] and *n*-hexane) are rare, but serious. Seek specialist advice.
2. *Additive substances.* Where there is reason to believe that the effects of the constituents are additive, and where the exposure limits are based on the same health effects, the mixed exposure should be assessed by means of the formula:

    $$C_1/L_1 + C_2/L_2 + C_3/L_3 \ldots < 1$$

    where C_1, C_2, etc. are the TWA concentrations of the constituents in air and L_1, L_2, etc. are the corresponding exposure limits. The use of this formula is only applicable where the additive substances have been assigned WELs and L_1, L_2, etc. relate to the same reference period in the list of approved WELs. Where the sum of the C/L fractions does not exceed unity, the exposure is considered not to exceed the notional exposure limits. If one of the constituents has been assigned an MEL, the additive effect should be taken into account in deciding the extent to which it is reasonably practicable to reduce exposure further.
3. *Independent substances.* Where no synergistic or additive effects are known or considered to be likely, the constituents can be regarded as acting independently. It is then sufficient to ensure compliance with each of the exposure limits individually.

Complicating factors

Several factors that complicate the assessment and control of exposure to individual substances will also affect cases of mixed exposures and will require similar special consideration. These factors include:

- the relevance of factors such as alcohol, medication or smoking
- absorption via the skin or by ingestion, as well as by inhalation
- substances in mixtures may mutually affect the extent of their absorption, as well as their health effects, at a given level of exposure.

8.2 Monitoring of the workplace environment

Given all that has been said above, basic techniques for measuring the airborne concentration of a specific chemical or particle are only mentioned briefly in this chapter, under the particular substance. It must be pointed out that these are not necessarily the definitive techniques, as often more than one is available, and new methods are continually being developed. Many analytical chemists also have their own preferences, and they should always be consulted before embarking upon a particular method of sampling. The HSE publishes guidance for the analysis of certain substances in the series Methods for the Determination of Hazardous Substances (MDHS). Where appropriate, the MDHS numbers are quoted.

8.3 Toxic gases

Although many organic compounds may be inhaled in vapour or gaseous form, the toxic gases per se are usually deemed to include compounds such as methane, sulphur dioxide and hydrocyanic acid. It is instructive to note how many of these gases are now recognised as being endogenously produced and for several to be of significant physiological importance – toxicology connotes physiology!
  In general, these gases may be classified as:

- simple asphyxiants, e.g. nitrogen, carbon dioxide and methane
- chemical asphyxiants, e.g. carbon monoxide, hydrogen sulphide and hydrogen cyanide
- upper respiratory tract irritants, e.g. ammonia and sulphur dioxide
- lower respiratory tract irritants, e.g. oxides of nitrogen and phosgene.

Simple asphyxiants

These gases are only likely to be a danger when their concentration in inhaled air is sufficient to cause a diminution in oxygen levels. Levels of oxygen below 14% lead to pulmonary hyperventilation and tissue anoxia.

Nitrogen (N_2)

Nitrogen is the main constituent of air and is also present in high concentrations in some mines ('choke damp'). Indeed, the miner's canary and safety lamp were, in the main, introduced to detect such asphyxiating underground environments. In addition, nitrogen has industrial uses in ammonia production as an inert atmosphere and as a freezing agent (boiling point, −195.8 °C). In hyperbaric work, such as diving, nitrogen becomes toxic, causing narcosis and 'the bends' (see Section 9.5). It is normally detected chemically by eliminating other gases: what remains as an inert gas is assumed to be nitrogen.

Methane (CH_4)

Methane is the product of the anaerobic decay of organic matter. Hence, it is found in sewers and wherever biodegradable organic matter is stored or dumped, such as farm slurry pits. It is also a natural constituent of fossil fuel reserves, and is frequently found in coal mines and, occasionally, in other mines. Natural gas, used as a fuel in the UK, contains a large percentage of methane. It is explosive and lighter than air, and therefore, in a concentrated form, will rise to make layers in unventilated ceilings and roofs, thus posing an explosive hazard. Explosive concentrations depend upon the percentage of oxygen present, but, in fresh air, 5.2% is the lower explosive limit and 14% is the upper explosive limit. Methods of detection started with the simple Davy lamp introduced in 1816, which, in modified form, is still used underground in coal mines today. The principle of detection involves a 'halo' of blue above the wick of a lowered flame, the shape of which indicates the concentration of methane. A double wire gauze prevents the heat igniting methane outside the lamp. The latest instruments use solid-state sensors.

Carbon dioxide (CO_2)

Carbon dioxide occurs naturally as a product of combustion and of gradual oxidation, and hence can occur wherever combustible or organic materials are to be found. Industrially, it is found as a by-product of brewing, coke ovens, blast furnaces and silage dumps. It has a wide use as an industrial gas, for example in the carbonisation of drinks, brewing and refrigeration. It is heavier than air and, in concentrated form, can produce 'pools' of inert atmosphere in low, unventilated places such as sumps and sewers. It occurs in mines in conjunction with nitrogen as a gas known as 'blackdamp', and in the aftermath of explosions as a gas known as 'afterdamp'.

Workplace exposure limits. HSE WEL: eight-hour TWA, $9150 \, \text{mg} \, \text{m}^{-3}$ and $5000 \, \text{ppm}$; 15-minute STEL, $27400 \, \text{mg} \, \text{m}^{-3}$ and $15000 \, \text{ppm}$.

Carbon dioxide, unlike methane and nitrogen, is capable of stimulating the medullary respiratory centre to produce hyperpnoea. This begins to occur at a concentration of 3%, while at concentrations of 10–29% it leads to convulsions and coma and at concentrations of 30% or more it acts rapidly, leading to loss of consciousness in seconds and death. At these higher concentrations reversal of effects often does not occur on removal and this indicates that there is more than a simple asphyxiant effect. Electrocardiogram changes have also been found in victims of massive over-exposure.

The 'weights' of the gases will determine the least hazardous approach by the rescue team to the stricken patient. Methane is lighter than air, carbon dioxide is heavier and nitrogen, constituting 80% of normal air, is approximately the same density as air. This characteristic of nitrogen, plus its inability to stimulate the respiratory centre, makes it a clinically inappropriate replacement for carbon dioxide as an inert gas for the transportation of other products. Nevertheless, this is exactly what is happening in many industries today.

Chemical asphyxiants

Carbon monoxide (CO)
Occurrence. Produced by the incomplete combustion of carbonaceous compounds; also from the metabolism of methylene chloride.

Properties. Colourless, odourless gas; burns with a blue flame. MW, 28.0. Density, lighter than air.

Uses. By-product of mining, smelting, foundry work, petrochemical processes and many processes involving combustion. In combination with hydrogen for synthesising chemicals as 'syngas'.

Metabolism. High affinity of absorbed gas for haem proteins, e.g. haemoglobin, leading to elevated carboxyhaemoglobin levels and diminished oxygen-carrying capacity of blood and cytochromes. Excreted through the lung. Non-cumulative poison. There is endogenous production of CO from haem by the haem oxygenase enzymes (HMOX1 and HMOX2). CO is a neurotransmitter and has immunomodulatory and coagulatory physiological and pathophysiological effects.

Health effects. Acute: insidious onset with giddiness, headache, chest tightness and nausea. Unconsciousness rapidly supervenes at concentrations in excess of 3500 ppm. No cyanosis (indeed, the patient [at post-mortem!] frequently has a deceptive healthy pink complexion due to carboxyhaemoglobin). Chronic: headache. Organic brain damage if asphyxiation is prolonged. Parkinsonism may occur in up to 10% post CO poisoning, starting within one month but most cases resolve spontaneously in one year.

Biological monitoring. Carboxyhaemoglobin levels in blood. Levels also raised in smokers and following exposure to methylene chloride. The biological monitoring guidance value (BMGV) is 30 ppm at end-tidal breath for CO at end of shift.

Measurement. Normally an immediate indication of concentration is required for safety reasons, and hence it is measured by direct reading instruments, using a variety of principles. It can be sampled over a long period by slowly filling a container for subsequent analysis through a direct reading instrument. Colorimetric detector tubes are also available.

Workplace exposure limits. HSE WEL: eight-hour TWA, 35 mg m^{-3} and 30 ppm; 15-minute STEL, 232 mg m^{-3} and 200 ppm; BMGV 35 mg m^{-3} and 30 ppm at end of eight-hour shift; 15-minute STEL, 117 mg m^{-3} and 100 ppm.

Legal requirements. Coal and Other Mines (Locomotives) Regulations 1956 (SI 1956 No. 1771). Limits applicable to underground mining and tunnelling industries until 21 August 2023.

Hydrogen cyanide (HCN)

Occurrence. Gas emanates from contact of cyanide salts with acid.

Properties. Colourless gas with a bitter almond smell.

Uses. Precious metal extraction, particularly the plating industry. Fumigant and steel hardener.

Metabolism. HCN binds to and inhibits the action of cytochrome oxidase, thus disrupting cellular respiration.

Health effects. Acute: rapid onset of headache, hypopnoea, tachycardia, hypotension, convulsions and death. The rapidity of the onset of symptoms necessitates immediate treatment. Chronic: none, except from dietary consumption of cyanogenic plants, e.g. cassava.

Biological monitoring. Blood thiocyanate (SCN) and cyanide (CN) blood levels, or urine sample end of shift, end of working week for SCN. Note that smoking can affect SCN levels.

Measurement. Sampled through a filter (to remove particulate cyanide interference) into a midget bubbler containing $0.1\,mol\,l^{-1}$ potassium hydroxide at an air flow rate of $2\,l\,min^{-1}$. The solution is analysed using a cyanide ion-selective electrode. Colorimetric detection tubes are also available.

Workplace exposure limits. HSE WEL: eight-hour TWA, $1\,mg\,m^{-3}$ and $0.9\,ppm$; 15-minute STEL, $5\,mg\,m^{-3}$ and $4.5\,ppm$ (skin notation).

Hydrogen sulphide (H₂S)

Occurrence. Wherever sulphur and its compounds are being used or disposed of, significant component of sewer and farm slurry gas, 'sour gas' in oil and gas operations.

Properties. Colourless gas with the smell of rotten eggs perceived around $0.02\,ppm$ but becomes imperceptible at levels higher than $100\,ppm$; a toxicity akin to hydrogen cyanide. Heavier than air.

Uses. None of major importance.

Metabolism. In over-exposure inhibition of cytochrome oxidase (see HCN) causes increase in sulphmethaemoglobin. Endogenous production by three enzymes: cystathionine β-synthase (CBS), cystathionine γ-lyase (CSE) and 3-mercaptopyruvate sulphurtransferase (3-MST). A gasotransmitter with vasoactive and neuromodulatory functions.

Health effects. Rapid respiratory absorption. Acute: lacrimation, photophobia and mucous membrane irritation in low concentrations. In high concentrations, headache, dizziness and rapid breathing with paralysis of the respiratory centre can cause sudden unconsciousness. At greater than $1000\,ppm$: immediate collapse and respiratory paralysis. Sequelae may include neurocognitive effects due to hypoxia or possibly other mechanisms. Chronic: keratitis. No cumulative effects.

Biological monitoring. Urine thiosulphate sampled post shift, or post incident, it is important to note that levels rise two hours post exposure with elimination inside 24 hours; it is important to record the time post exposure.

Measurement. Sampled onto a molecular sieve tube via a desiccant tube of sodium sulphate at an air flow rate of $150\,ml\,min^{-1}$ for subsequent analysis using gas chromatography. Colorimetric detection tubes are also available.

Workplace exposure limits. HSE WEL: eight-hour TWA, $7\,mg\,m^{-3}$ and $5\,ppm$; 15-minute STEL, $14\,mg\,m^{-3}$ and $10\,ppm$

Irritants

The irritant gases, as their name implies, are not respirable without discomfort. The somewhat artificial division into upper and lower respiratory tract irritants is largely on the basis of solubility. Thus, the highly soluble gases, such as ammonia, sulphur dioxide and chlorine, exert their principal irritant effect on the upper respiratory tract, which, unless the exposure is prolonged and severe, saves the lungs. Conversely, gases of low solubility, such as oxides of nitrogen and phosgene, have little effect on the upper respiratory tract; their effect is delayed and the main brunt of the damage is borne by the lungs.

Ammonia (NH_3), anhydrous
Properties. Colourless gas with pungent odour. Lighter than air.

Uses. Widely used industrial gas. Manufacture of fertilisers, refrigerants and as a catalyst and reagent.

Metabolism. Extremely soluble in water, producing a caustic alkaline solution of ammonium hydroxide. Detectable to most humans at 30–50 ppm.

Health effects. At concentrations above 50 ppm, the gas is an irritant to the eyes, mucous membranes and upper respiratory tract, but can be tolerated up to 100 ppm. Exposure is not voluntarily tolerated above 500 ppm. At 5000–10000 ppm, severe, and often fatal, respiratory tract damage occurs, with denuded bronchial epithelium and pulmonary oedema. There is some evidence of long-term respiratory damage following acute exposure.

Biological monitoring. None of relevance.

Measurement. Sampled onto silica gel treated with sulphuric acid at a flow rate between 0.1 and $0.2\,l\,min^{-1}$. Extracted with deionised water and analysed with visible absorption (US National Institute for Occupational Safety and Health [NIOSH] 6015).

Workplace exposure limits. HSE WEL: eight-hour TWA, $18\,mg\,m^{-3}$ and $25\,ppm$; 15-minute STEL, $25\,mg\,m^{-3}$ and $35\,ppm$.

Chlorine (Cl_2)
Properties. Greenish-yellow gas of pungent odour, over twice as heavy as air. Chlorine is released from hypochlorite solutions when mixed with acids, often inadvertently.

Uses. Chemical and pharmaceutical production; water disinfection in swimming pools; plastics manufacture.

Metabolism. Releases nascent oxygen from water and forms hydrochloric acid, which can cause severe protoplasmic damage in high concentrations.

Health effects. Acute: severe eye and upper respiratory tract irritation, leading to pulmonary oedema and death in those unable to escape its effects. A level of 0.2 ppm can cause eye irritation whereas 500 ppm inhaled for 5–10 minutes is reported to be fatal. Recovery from an acute exposure may be prolonged.

Chronic: chronic bronchitis. Adequate early warning of chlorine's presence is provided by its odour, but it can also cause olfactory fatigue or adaptation that can reduce an individual's awareness to prolonged exposures.

Biological monitoring. None of relevance.

Measurement. Sampled by passing air through a fritted bubbler containing 100 ml of dilute methyl orange at an air flow rate of around 1.5 l min^{-1} for subsequent colorimetric analysis. Colorimetric detector tubes are also available.

Workplace exposure limits. HSE WEL: 15-minute STEL, 1.5 mg m^{-3} and 0.5 ppm.

Fluorine (F$_2$)

Properties. A greenish-yellow gas with a pungent odour. One of the most chemically active elements.

Uses. Fluorides are used as metal fluxes; uranium hexafluoride is used to separate isotopes of uranium. Glass etching; pottery; refrigeration (organic fluorides). Fluorides added to drinking water prevent dental caries.

Metabolism. Gaseous fluorine is not much encountered but, in contact with mucous membranes, it will react with water and be rapidly reduced to form fluoride, in particular hydrogen fluoride (HF). Fluoride is excreted in three phases with just under half of a dose excreted as fluoride in the urine within four hours; the remainder enters the bone pool, with a small proportion excreted over two to three weeks and the rest with a half-life of about eight years.

Health effects. Acute: severe, penetrating, painful skin burns with HF. Severe inhalational effects, including laryngeal spasm, oedema and haemoptysis in higher concentrations (>50 ppm). Below 10 ppm exposure may be tolerated without immediate symptoms. Chronic: skin scarring. Pulmonary fibrosis. Fluorosis of the bones. Systemic effects of hydrofluoric acid exposure are related to the disturbance of calcium and magnesium metabolism. Cardiac arrhythmias may follow lowered levels of these elements in the blood. Serum electrolyte estimation may indicate the need for calcium supplements.

Biological monitoring. Urine sample end of shift for fluoride; pre-shift samples after a weekend/48 hour break may be useful for comparison.

Workplace exposure limits. HSE WEL: eight-hour TWA 1.6 mg m^{-3} and 1 ppm; and 15-minute STEL 1.6 mg m^{-3} and 1 ppm.

Nickel carbonyl (Ni(CO)$_4$)

Occurrence. Generated during nickel refining (Mond process).

Properties. Colourless, odourless gas to some but 'brick dust-like' odour for others.

Uses. The unique properties of nickel carbonyl enable nickel to be extracted from the ore and subsequently released from the carbonyl gas in nearly 100% pure form.

Metabolism. Similar to carbon monoxide.

Health effects. Acute: headache, nausea, vomiting, unconsciousness. These symptoms may subside and be followed up to 36 hours later with fever, chest pain, pulmonary irritation and oedema. Leucocytosis on blood count. Skin contact with nickel compounds can cause sensitisation and allergic dermatitis can develop. Chronic: cancer of nasal sinuses and lungs (International Agency for Research on Cancer [IARC] group 1), although it is not clear which form(s) of nickel are responsible for the cancers.

Biological monitoring. Urine nickel end of shift, end of the working week. Urinary nickel around eight hours after acute exposure to nickel carbonyl can help guide therapy.

Measurement. Sampled through an impinger containing a reagent at an air flow rate of $2 \, l \, min^{-1}$ for subsequent analysis using atomic absorption spectrophotometry. Colorimetric detector tubes are also available.

Occupational exposure limits. HSE WEL: 15-minute STEL $0.24 \, mg \, m^{-3}$ and $0.1 \, ppm$.

Oxides of nitrogen (N_2O, NO, NO_2)

Properties. NO_2 is the gas of greatest occupational health importance here and is reddish-brown with a pungent odour. Nitrous oxide (N_2O) is an anaesthetic gas. Nitric oxide (NO) is a colourless gas, of great physiological importance with gasotransmitter, neuromodulator, immunomodulator and vasoactive roles.

Uses. NO_2 is used in the manufacture of nitric acid, explosives and jet fuel. It is generated during welding (some types), silo storage, blasting operations and diesel engine operation.

Health effects. NO_2 exposure. Acute: insidious, owing to the slow progression of pulmonary irritation some 8–24 hours after exposure. Severe exposure can result in death from pulmonary oedema within 48 hours. NO_2 is the aetiological agent in silo-filler's disease with airway hydrolysis to nitrous and nitric acids. Chronic: brown discoloration of teeth. Transient patchy lung opacities on chest radiography. N_2O over-exposure in healthcare workers has been associated with neurological symptoms owing to inhibition of vitamin B12 metabolism.

Biological monitoring. In some jurisdictions urine N_2O has been used for healthcare worker monitoring.

Measurement. Sampled onto impregnated molecular sieve tubes in tandem at an air flow rate of between 25 and $50 \, ml \, min^{-1}$ for subsequent spectrophotometric analysis. Colorimetric detector tubes are available for nitrogen dioxide and nitrous fumes ($NO + NO_2$).

Occupational exposure limits. Nitrous oxide, HSE WEL: eight-hour TWA, $183 \, mg \, m^{-3}$ and $100 \, ppm$. Nitrogen dioxide, HSE WEL: eight-hour TWA, $0.96 \, mg \, m^{-3}$ and $0.5 \, ppm$; 15-minute STEL $1.91 \, mg \, m^{-3}$ and $1 \, ppm$. Nitrogen monoxide, HSE WEL: eight-hour TWA, $2.5 \, mg \, m^{-3}$ and $2 \, ppm$.

Legal requirements. Limits of $30 \, mg \, m^{-3}$ and $25 \, ppm$ will be applicable to underground mining and tunnelling industries beginning 21 August 2023.

Ozone (O_3)

Properties. Gas generated during arc welding (especially when the weld creates very little fume, that is, metal inert gas [MIG] and aluminium) and from the photochemical oxidation of automobile exhaust gases.

Uses. Oxidising agent; water fumigant; bleaching agent.

Health effects. Respiratory tract and mucosal irritant. Exposure to high concentrations (>50 ppm) can lead to pulmonary oedema.

Measurement. Colorimetric detection tubes are available.

HSE guidance. EH38.

Workplace exposure limits. HSE WEL: 15-minute STEL, 0.4 mg m^{-3} and 0.2 ppm.

Phosgene (carbonyl chloride) (COCl$_2$)

Properties. Sweet-smelling at around 0.5 ppm and 'mouldy hay' at around 1 ppm; highly toxic gas. MW, 98.93. Heavier than air.

Uses. Source of chlorine in industry; war gas. Evolution of phosgene is a hazard of burning chlorinated hydrocarbons, including many plastics.

Metabolism. Poor solubility in water means that most phosgene reaches the alveoli and there reacts with proteins undergoing hydrolysis to form hydrochloric acid and carbon dioxide.

Health effects. Acute: mild early symptoms include coughing and eye irritation followed by insidious onset of severe pulmonary oedema within the succeeding 24–48 hours. Chronic: chronic bronchitis may follow lung damage in acute exposure survivors.

Measurement. Air is drawn into a midget impinger containing nitrobenzylpyridine at an air flow rate of 1000 ml min^{-1} for subsequent colorimetric analysis. Colorimetric detector tubes are available.

Workplace exposure limits. HSE WEL: eight-hour TWA, 0.08 mg m^{-3} and 0.02 ppm; 15-minute STEL, 0.25 mg m^{-3} and 0.06 ppm.

Sulphur dioxide (SO$_2$)

Properties. Colourless gas with pungent odour of 'burnt matches' and a density twice that of air. Constituent of air pollution.

Uses. Chemical and paper industries; bleaching; fumigation; refrigeration; and preservative. A common by-product of smelting sulphide ores.

Metabolism. Produces sulphurous acid on solution in water, leading to acidosis. Activation of vagal transduced acid-sensing ion channels and capsaicin receptors may trigger bronchoconstriction.

Health effects. Acute: acute mucous membrane irritant. The respiratory tract irritation is so severe that escape from the gas is imperative. Failure to escape leads to severe pulmonary oedema and death. May trigger asthmatic attacks in susceptible individuals at levels below those set for workplace exposure. Corneal ulceration and scarring following prolonged eye irritation. Chronic: diminution in olfactory and gustatory senses. Chronic bronchitis.

Biological monitoring. None of relevance.

Measurement. Sampled onto an impregnated cellulose filter containing potassium hydroxide through a cellulose acetate pre-filter to collect particulate sulphates and sulphites at an air flow rate of 1.5 l min^{-1}. The impregnated filter is extracted with deionised water for subsequent anion exchange chromatography. Direct reading instruments and colorimetric detector tubes are also available; can also be sampled using a bubbler containing hydrogen peroxide for wet chemical analysis.

Workplace exposure limits. HSE WEL: eight-hour TWA, 1.3 mg m^{-3} and 0.5 ppm; 15-minute STEL, 2.7 mg m^{-3} and 1 ppm.

Arsine (AsH$_3$), phosphine (PH$_3$) and stibine (SbH$_3$)

Arsenic, phosphorus and antimony are unique among the elements in producing hydride gases. Apart from the use of arsine in semi-conductor technology, all are of little or no commercial importance, but are evolved when the elements are exposed to nascent hydrogen, as when metal dross is in contact with acidic water.

Arsine and stibine are both powerful haemolytic agents and can cause massive intravascular haemolysis, leading to acute oliguric renal failure. Phosphine produces gastrointestinal and neurological symptoms. Long-term sequelae may be the result of the effects of the hydrides or the release of the elements themselves as a result of oxidation. High exposures to arsine gas can cause fatal haemolysis and multiorgan damage.

Workplace exposure limits. Arsine: HSE WEL: eight-hour TWA, 0.16 mg m^{-3} and 0.05 ppm. Phosphine: HSE WEL: eight-hour TWA, 0.14 mg m^{-3} and 0.1 ppm; 15-minute STEL, 0.28 mg m^{-3} and 0.2 ppm.

Legal requirements. Arsine (as a component of arsenic): The Factories (Notification of Diseases) Regulations 1966 (SI 1966 No. 1400). Arsine and phosphine (as compounds of arsenic and phosphorus): Factories Act 1961, Section 8.2.

HSE guidance. EH11 – Arsine: Health and Safety Precautions. EH12 – Stibine: Health and Safety Precautions. EH20 – Phosphine: Health and Safety Precautions.

8.4 Dusts and particles

Many occupational hazards occur as airborne particles: dust, fibres, mists, fume, radioactive particles, bacteria and viruses. A dispersed suspension of solid or liquid particles in a gas or mixture of gases (normally air) is known as an aerosol. The health risks from inhaling such an aerosol depend upon the nature and size of the particles, their airborne concentration and the part of the respiratory system in which they are deposited. The particle size and the position in the lung are related.

In order to define the size of particles found in the workplace, which are mainly irregular in shape, a convention is adopted that assigns a diameter to a particle based upon its aerodynamic properties, in particular its settling velocity in still air. This aerodynamic diameter is defined as the diameter of a unit density sphere, that is, water, which settles at the same velocity as the particle in question. A simple rule of thumb: the higher the energy imparted upon the source term, the smaller the particle generated.

This dimension is relevant to the way in which the particle is deposited in the lung, the method of sampling and air cleaning.

Typical airborne particles

- Dusts: 1–75 μm in diameter; sources: from attrition, for example cutting, grinding, sanding, finishing, transport, sieving, crushing, screening, blasting.
- Fibres: 1:3 aspect ratio; sources: natural mineral (asbestos), natural vegetable (jute, cotton), synthetic mineral (glass fibre, rockwool, ceramic), synthetic organic (nylon, Terylene).

- Fume: usually below 1 µm; sources: from the sublimation and oxidation of molten metal, for example lead, cadmium, chromium, iron, nickel.
- Mists: atmospheric: above 20 µm; sources: water droplets condensed on a particle nucleus from surfaces of open tanks.
- Smoke: mixture of particles and gases usually below 1 µm; sources: combustion.
- Biological: bacteria, viruses, fungi.
- Radiation: radioactive particles, α and β; sources: mining, manufacturing, power generation, research, investigations; also occurs naturally.

Particle size and respiratory penetration

Ill health from the inhalation of aerosols can be divided into three groups, depending upon the region of the respiratory system into which the particles are deposited:

1. extrathoracic (upper respiratory tract)
2. thoracic (bronchi and bronchioles)
3. alveolar (alveoli).

Extrathoracic. Certain bacteria, fungi and allergens may deposit in the upper respiratory tract, which may lead to inflammation of mucous membranes, for example rhinitis; particles such as wood dust, nickel and radioactive particles may lead to ulceration and nasal cancer.

Thoracic. Many particles that reach the tracheobronchial region (i.e. bronchi and bronchioles) may lead to bronchoconstriction, bronchitis and bronchial carcinoma.

Alveolar. Certain particles that reach the gas exchange region of the lung (i.e. alveoli) may lead to pneumoconiosis, emphysema, alveolitis and pulmonary carcinoma. Particles reaching this part of the lung are known as respirable. Certain fibres may be carried to the pleura, where they can cause mesothelioma.

International collaboration has led to agreement on the definitions of health-related aerosol fractions in the workplace. These had been defined as: *inhalable, thoracic* and *respirable*. They are published in British Standard BS EN 481 (also by ISO as ISO 7708) and are summarised in Figure 8.1, which relates the aerodynamic diameter of the particle to the percentage of particles penetrating the three regions.

The respirable fraction curve (E_R) is defined as the mass fraction of inhaled particles that penetrates to the unciliated airways of the lung, and is given by a cumulative log-normal curve with a median aerodynamic diameter of 4.25 µm and a geometric standard deviation of 1.5. The thoracic fraction curve (E_T) is defined as the mass fraction of inhaled particles penetrating the respiratory system beyond the larynx, and is given by a cumulative log-normal curve with a median aerodynamic diameter of 11.64 µm and a geometric standard deviation of 1.5. The inhalable fraction curve (E_I) is defined as the mass fraction of total

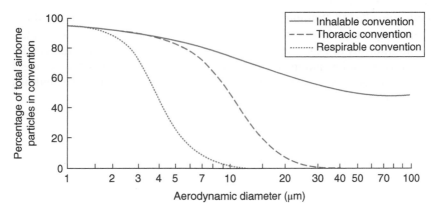

FIGURE 8.1   International Organization for Standardization (ISO)/European Committee for Standardization (CEN)/American Conference of Governmental Industrial Hygienists (ACGIH) sampling conventions for health-related aerosols. Source: BS EN 481:1993, Workplace atmospheres. Size fraction definitions for measurement of airborne particles (British Standard), British Standards Institution (BSI).

airborne particles that is inhaled through the nose and/or mouth. It was derived from wind tunnel measurements of the sampling efficiency of full-sized tailor's mannequins and replaces the very loosely defined 'total' aerosol fraction used previously. For industrial workplaces it is given by:

$$E_1 = 50\left(1 + \exp\left(-0.06D\right)\right)$$

Respirable fibres are defined as having an aspect ratio (length to width) of 3:1, a length of more than 5 µm and a diameter of less than 3 µm.

Asbestos

Occurrence. Naturally occurring fibrous silicates – either serpentine (chrysotile) or amphibole (crocidolite, amosite and anthophyllite).

Properties. Highly resistant to temperature, pressure and acids, but these properties vary with the variety of asbestos. Serpentine varieties are also capable of being woven into cloth.

Uses. Many and varied, including asbestos cement, building and insulation materials, brake lining and fire-proofing devices.

Health effects. Acute: none of note. Chronic: chronic fibrotic lung disease – asbestosis. Pleural plaque formation and calcification. Diffuse pleural thickening. Carcinoma of the lung (synergistic effect with cigarette smoking). Malignant mesothelioma of the pleura and peritoneum The IARC considers asbestos exposure an established carcinogen for the larynx and ovary. There is limited evidence for the association of asbestos with cancers of the gastrointestinal tract. 'Asbestos corns' on the skin.

Health surveillance. Pulmonary function tests, including spirometry and gas diffusion. Frequent serial chest radiology is of limited value. Factors such as the nature and intensity of exposure and time since first exposure should inform the periodicity. A major limitation of these procedures is that, while they may detect pulmonary effects of asbestos exposure, there are at present no effective methods for treatment or reversal of most of these effects.

Treatment. Removal from exposure. Clinical management of chronic fibrotic lung disease and malignancies. Treatment is often palliative rather than curative.

Exposure measurement. It is necessary to determine the number of airborne respirable fibres by sampling onto a cellulose acetate filter for subsequent microscopic analysis and counting. Sampling should be carried out in accordance with HSE Guidance Note EH10 and MDHS 39/4. Workplace exposure standards typically rely on 'regulated' fibres, meaning asbestos particles with a length-to-diameter ratio greater than 3 to 1, a length greater than 5 μm and a diameter less than 3 μm. It should be noted, though, that smaller fibres have been associated with health risks and standards may change to account for them.

Workplace exposure limits. HSE control limits:

a. For the control of asbestos fibres in any localised atmosphere, the limit below is not to be considered as a 'safe' level and work should be designed to achieve exposure levels as far below the control limit as possible:
   i.   0.1 fibres per millilitre of air averaged over any continuous period of four hours;
b. For work involving some lower risk asbestos-containing materials (e.g. asbestos cement products and textured decorative coating, among others):
   i.   0.6 fibres per millilitre of air averaged over any continuous period of 10 minutes.

Legal requirements. The Control of Asbestos at Work Regulations 2012.

HSE guidance. EH10 (Rev) Asbestos – Control Limits, Measurement of Airborne Dust Concentrations and the Assessment of Control Measures.

Coal dust

(See also Section 3.3 on lung diseases.)

Occurrence. Mainly underground and worldwide. Formed as a result of the prehistoric accumulation of rotting vegetation.

Properties. Vary with the type and rank of coal.

Uses. Combustion; petrochemicals.

Health effects. Acute: none. Chronic: pulmonary fibrosis ranging from simple pneumoconiosis to progressive, massive fibrosis, which is a frequent precursor of death from respiratory failure.

Health surveillance. Lung function tests, especially spirometry. Serial chest radiography is of limited value and should be discontinued. Comments regarding limitations of health surveillance for asbestos exposure also apply to coal dust.

Treatment. Removal from exposure. Management of chronic respiratory disease.

Exposure measurement. Sampled for airborne respirable fraction by drawing a known volume of air through a pre-weighed filter for reweighing and analysis. Respirable size selection for personal exposure is undertaken by means of a cyclone separator at an air flow rate of 2.21min^{-1} (SIMPEDS) or, for static sampling, by means of a horizontal parallel plate elutriator, as in the MRE 113A sampler, at an air flow rate of 2.51min^{-1}. As quartz dust is often found with coal, it may be necessary to determine the respirable quartz content. Therefore, the following filters may be required: for gravimetric analysis alone, glass fibre; for X-ray diffraction analysis for silica, silver membrane; and for infrared analysis for silica, polyvinyl chloride (PVC).

Workplace exposure limits. Permitted levels of respirable dust in coalmines are laid down in the regulations given below. Exposure limits for workplaces other than coalmines: coal dust containing less than 5% quartz: TWA, 2mg m^{-3} respirable dust; coal dust containing more than 5% quartz: see silica below.

Legal requirements. The Coal Mines (Control of Inhalable Dust) Regulations 2007. The Mines Regulations 2014 (SI 2014/3248).

Cotton dust

(See also Section 3.3 on lung diseases.)

Occurrence. Cotton occurs on the plant as a 'boll', which is picked either by hand or by machine, and usually contains some stem and leaves. The bolls pass through a 'ginning' process, which separates the seeds and other materials from the raw cotton. The cotton is then baled for transportation. The ginning process usually occurs close to the cotton fields. At the mills, the bales are opened and the cotton is mechanically cleaned by blowing. It is then combed or 'carded' before being spun, dyed and woven. The dustiest areas are the blowing, blending and carding rooms, where the dust consists of 'fly', that is, large fibres of cotton (up to 3 cm in length) that are too large to be inhaled, 'trash', which is a mixture of plant debris and soil, and fine, inhalable cotton dust. The endotoxin content of cotton dust is an important factor.

Health effects. The health hazard is from byssinosis, with its characteristic cough, chest tightness and difficulty in breathing, which is particularly prevalent on the first day back to work after a break, for example Monday mornings. Schilling has graded the symptoms of byssinosis into five grades (0, 1/2, 1, 2, 3).

Health surveillance. Periodic review of respiratory symptoms, spirometry and serial peak flow rates when indicated.

Exposure measurement and standards. Many studies have shown a direct relationship between total airborne dust measured in milligrams per cubic metre and the prevalence of byssinosis. The standard is therefore gravimetric. The HSE WEL TWA for cotton dust is 0.5mg m^{-3} of collected dust less fly. Sampling is therefore based on gravimetric techniques using a specially designed apparatus unique to the cotton industry. It draws air at about 10 l min^{-1} through a glass-fibre filter paper, which is screened by a gauze of 2 mm mesh, using 0.2 mm wire, to eliminate the fly. During the sampling period, the screen has to be cleared of fly from time to time to prevent it from becoming a pre-filter, reducing the collected fibre amounts.

Legal requirements. The Cotton Cloth Factories Regulations 1929 (S, R and O 1929 No. 300), Cotton Cloth Factories Regulation Hygrometers Order 1926 (S, R and O 1926 No. 1582).

HSE guidance. EH25 Cotton Dust Sampling, MS9 Byssinosis.

Silica dust

Occurrence. Worldwide, as Earth's crust contains 28% silicon.

Properties. Silica (SiO$_2$) is a hard, rock-like compound capable of fragmentation into fine particles. It is a constituent of many ore-bearing rocks, coal seams, granites, china clay, sandstones and sand.

Uses. Abrasives; building materials; ceramics; foundry work; and road stone.

Health effects. Inhalation into the lungs triggers a florid fibrotic reaction from the pulmonary tissues. Acute: none. Chronic: nodular pulmonary fibrosis, mainly in the upper lung zone, which can be severe. 'Eggshell' calcification of lymph nodes may be evident. Chronic obstructive pulmonary disease (COPD). A predisposition to tuberculosis (TB) is a major health concern. Silica is considered to be a lung carcinogen where it is generated as a result of a work process.

Health surveillance. Pulmonary function tests, particularly spirometry. Serial chest radiography is of value, especially in high-burden TB countries, but the periodicity should take account of the intensity and duration of exposure and TB incidence. Limitations of these procedures, as outlined for asbestos and coal dust.

Treatment. Removal from exposure. Management of chronic pulmonary fibrosis.

Exposure measurement. Airborne dusts that may contain silica need to be analysed for crystalline silica. It is usual to collect the respirable fraction by drawing a known volume of air through a pre-weighed filter for reweighing and analysis. Respirable size selection for personal exposure is undertaken by means of a cyclone separator (Higgins and Dewell, SIMPEDS) at an air flow rate of 2.2 l min^{-1} or, for static sampling, by means of a horizontal parallel plate elutriator, as in the MRE 113A sampler, at an air flow rate of 2.5 l min^{-1}. The nature of the crystalline silica is determined by sampling onto a silver membrane filter for subsequent analysis using X-ray diffraction.

Workplace exposure limits. Silica, respirable crystalline WEL: eight-hour TWA, 0.1 mg m^{-3}; fused respirable dust WEL: eight-hour TWA, 0.08 mg m^{-3}.

HSE guidance. MDHS 51/2.

Synthetic mineral fibres (man-made mineral fibres, MMMFs)

Occurrence and uses. Manufactured by drawing, blowing, centrifuging and flame attenuation at very high temperatures, using various raw materials, and producing a range of fibres with differing diameters and properties.

Continuous filament: glass-drawn material, molten at 1000–1500 °C, 3–15 mm in diameter; product forms – yarn, roving, woven fabrics; uses – industrial textiles, glass-reinforced plastics.

Insulation wools: rockwool, slagwool, glass wool; basalt or dolerite rock, blast furnace slag, glass-blown or centrifuged material at 1000–1500 °C, 4–9 μm in diameter; product forms – bulk fibre, blanket, slab, board, mattress; uses – acoustic and thermal insulation.

Refractory fibres: ceramic materials or alumina drawn or blown at 1000–1500 °C, 2–3 μm in diameter; product forms – bulk fibre, needled blanket, board, paper, woven cloth, rope and specially moulded shapes; uses – high-temperature insulation for turbines, boilers, heat exchangers, fire protection, hot face linings in furnaces and kilns, seals, gaskets, expansion joints and high-temperature gas and liquid filters. Refractory fibres have a low thermal mass and thus furnaces can be lighter and respond more quickly.

Special purpose fibres: lime-free borosilicate glass flame attenuated; 0.1–3 μm in diameter; product forms – bulk fibre, felt mat, blanket; uses – aero-engine and rocket insulation, jet engine pipes and fuel systems.

Health effects. Fibres are not crystalline; they break transversely rather than longitudinally. Therefore, crushing and attrition do not yield smaller fibres. The larger fibres cause skin irritation, but there is no evidence of lung disease. Implantation and some inhalational studies on animals show that fibres below 0.25 μm in diameter produce tumours. The production of fibres below 1 μm in diameter is a recent development, and thus the effects on humans will not become apparent for many years. Recent international studies of MMMF workers have failed to resolve the question of whether MMMFs are human carcinogens. At present, there remains a serious suspicion of carcinogenicity – particularly for the ceramic fibres and, perhaps, the rockwool/slagwool fibres. Glass fibres appear to be less implicated.

Exposure measurements and standards. HSE has published a gravimetric standard, that is, an WEL of 5 mg m^{-3} and 2 fibres ml^{-1}. Sampling is by drawing a known volume of air through a pre-weighed glass-fibre filter mounted in a modified UK Atomic Energy Authority (UKAEA) or Institute of Occupational Medicine (IOM) sampling head; the weight gain in milligrams is divided by the volume of air sampled in cubic metres. For respirable fibres, the method is similar to that of asbestos sampling and is explained in MDHS 59. A respirable fibre is defined as one that is greater than 5 μm in length, with a length to breadth ratio of at least 3 : 1 and a diameter of less than 3 μm. See also MDHS 59.

HSE guidance. MDHS 59.

Wood dust

Wood dust causes irritation of the eyes, nose and throat. The particles generated by the machining and processing of timber are usually large particles that affect mucosal surfaces and the upper respiratory tract. Glues and wood preservatives can be used for timber products, and dust from such sources may release formaldehyde and organic solvents. Hardwoods are timbers from deciduous trees, such as beech, ash, oak, mahogany and teak. Softwoods are mainly from coniferous trees such as Scots pine, yew and cedar. Hardwood dusts are considered to be a sensitiser. Western red cedar wood dust has been associated with the development of occupational asthma. Iroko and pine have been known to cause irritant and allergic contact dermatitis. Chronic exposure to hardwood dusts in the furniture trade has been linked to the development of adenocarcinoma of the nasal sinuses. In the UK, a cluster of such cases in the High Wycombe area was described by Acheson. The exact chemical agent in hardwood dust responsible for this effect has not been identified.

Health surveillance. Advice to wood workers on the early recognition of relevant symptoms and clinical evaluation and follow-up of those with symptoms. Lung function tests indicated for those who are exposed to dusts and woods known to cause asthma.

Management. Reduction of exposure for those who develop occupational asthma or dermatitis. Medications may provide symptomatic relief. Job change to be considered for those with severe health effects.

Exposure measurement. Sampled by drawing a known volume of air through a pre-weighed glass fibre mounted in a modified UKAEA or IOM sampling head; the weight gain in milligrams is obtained by dividing by the total flow volume in cubic metres.

Workplace exposure limits. Hardwood dust (inhalable fraction) HSE WEL: $3\,mg\,m^{-3}$. Softwood dust HSE WEL: $5\,mg\,m^{-3}$. If hardwood dust is mixed with other wood dusts, the WEL shall apply to all the wood dusts present in the mixture.

HSE guidance. MDHS 14/3.

Dusts (other than those mentioned separately)

We are cautioned by the HSE that, although not all dusts have been assigned WELs, the lack of such limits should not be taken to imply an absence of hazard, and that exposure should be controlled to the minimum that is reasonably practicable. However, where there is no indication of the need for a more stringent standard, personal exposure should not exceed $10\,mg\,m^{-3}$ total dust and $4\,mg\,m^{-3}$ respirable (alveoli fraction) dust. Any airborne dust concentrations above these values should be regarded as 'substantial concentrations' for the purposes of Regulation 2 of COSHH and, as such, are substances hazardous to health.

HSE guidance. EH44. MDHS 14/3.

Fume

This is regarded as solid particles generated by chemical reactions or condensation from the gaseous state, usually from the volatilisation of molten metal. Often the particles are in the region of $1\,\mu m$ in diameter, unless oxidisation has taken place, as with zinc fume, and then the diameters will be larger.

Some welding processes generate fume that contains components which have specific WELs; these limits should be applied to control exposure if these substances are present in the fume. In any other case, HSE WEL: welding fume, $5\,mg\,m^{-3}$.

Table 8.1 shows the latest list of MDHSs.

TABLE 8.1

Health and Safety Executive (HSE) Methods for the Determination of Hazardous Substances (MDHS) guidance.

	Title	Last revision date	ISBN
3	*Generation of test atmospheres of organic vapours by the syringe injection technique* Portable apparatus for laboratory and field use.	May 1990 *reprint*	0-11-885632-4
4	*Generation of test atmospheres of organic vapours by the permeation tube method* Apparatus for laboratory use.	May 1986 *reprint*	0-11-885647-2
6/3	*Lead and inorganic compounds of lead in air* Laboratory method using flame or electrothermal atomic absorption spectrometry.	March 1998	0-7176-1517-0
10/2	*Cadmium and inorganic compounds of cadmium in air* Laboratory method using flame atomic absorption spectrometry or electrothermal atomic absorption spectrometry.	June 1994	0-7176-0676-7
12/2	*Chromium and inorganic compounds of chromium in air* Laboratory method using flame atomic absorption spectrometry.	May 1996	0-7176-1181-7
14/4	*General methods for sampling and gravimetric analysis of respirable and inhalable dust*	June 2014	
16/2	*Mercury and its inorganic divalent compounds in air* Laboratory method using Hydrar® diffusive badges or pumped sorbent tubes, acid dissolution and analysis by cold vapour atomic absorption spectrometry or cold vapour atomic fluorescence spectrometry.	April 2002	0-7176-2348-3
25/4	*Organic isocyanates in air* Laboratory method using sampling either onto 1-(2-methoxyphenyl) piperazine-coated glass-fibre filters followed by solvent desorption or into impingers and analysis using high-performance liquid chromatography.	January 1999	0-7176-1668-1

(Continued)

TABLE 8.1 (Continued)

	Title	Last revision date	ISBN
27	*Protocol for assessing the performance of a diffusive sampler*	February 1994	0-7176-0635-X
29/2	*Beryllium and beryllium compounds in air* Laboratory method using flame atomic absorption spectrometry or electrothermal atomic absorption spectrometry.	April 1996	0-7176-1130-2
30/2	*Cobalt and cobalt compounds in air* Laboratory method using flame atomic absorption spectrometry.	April 1996	0-7176-1128-0
32	*Dioctyl phthalates in air* Laboratory method using Tenax sorbent tubes, solvent desorption and gas chromatography.	December 1987 *reprint*	0-11-885619-7
33/2	*Sorbent tube standards* Preparation by the syringe injection technique.	January 1997	0-7176-1337-2
35/2	*Hydrogen fluoride and inorganic fluorides in air* Laboratory method using an ion-selective electrode or ion chromatography.	May 1998	0-7176-1558-8
39/4	*Asbestos fibres in air* Sampling and evaluation by phase contrast microscopy (PCM) under the Control of Asbestos Regulations.	November 1995	0-7176-1113-2
41/2	*Arsenic and inorganic compounds of arsenic (except arsine) in air* Laboratory method using continuous flow or flow injection analysis hydride generation atomic absorption spectrometry.	November 1995	0-7176-1008-X
42/2	*Nickel and inorganic compounds of nickel in air (except nickel carbonyl)* Laboratory method using flame atomic absorption spectrometry or electrothermal atomic absorption spectrometry.	March 1996	0-7176-1094-2
46/2	*Platinum metal and soluble platinum compounds in air* Laboratory method using electrothermal atomic absorption spectrometry or inductively coupled plasma–mass spectrometry.	December 1996	0-7176-1306-2

	Title	Last revision date	ISBN
47/3	*Determination of rubber process dust and rubber fume (measured as cyclohexane soluble material) in air* Laboratory method using filters, gravimetric determination and Soxhlet extraction.	March 2015	978 0 7176 6446 7
48	*Newspaper print rooms: measurement of total particulates and cyclohexane soluble material in air* Laboratory method using filters and gravimetric estimation.	December 1987 *reprint*	0-11-885 639-1
52/4	*Hexavalent chromium in chromium plating mists* Colorimetric field method using 1,5-diphenylcarbazide.	November 2014	0-7176-1520-0
53/2	*1,3-Butadiene in air* Laboratory method using pumped samplers, thermal desorption and gas chromatography.	August 2003	0-7176-2735-7
54	*Protocol for assessing the performance of a pumped sampler for gases and vapours*	August 1986 *reprint*	0-11-885649-9
56/3	*Hydrogen cyanide in air* Laboratory method using an ion-selective electrode.	December 2014	
57/2	*Acrylamide in air* Laboratory method using an impinger and analysis by high-performance liquid chromatography.	November 2014	
59/2	*Man-made mineral fibre* Airborne number concentration and classification by phase-contrast light microscopy.	June 2014	
61	*Total hexavalent chromium compounds in air* Colorimetric laboratory method using 1,5-diphenylcarbazide.	March 1988 *out of print; revision in draft*	0-7176-0302-4
62/2	*Aromatic carboxylic acid anhydrides in air* Laboratory method using glass-fibre filter with sorbent back-up tube and liquid chromatography.	November 2014	
63/2	*1,3-Butadiene in air* Laboratory method using diffusive samplers, thermal desorption and gas chromatography.	February 2005	0-7176-2898-1

(*Continued*)

TABLE 8.1 (Continued)

	Title	Last revision date	ISBN
70	*General method for sampling airborne gases and vapours*	October 1990 *reprint*	0-7176-0608-2
71	*Analytical quality in workplace air monitoring*	March 1991 *reprint*	0-7176-1263-5
72	*Volatile organic compounds in air* Laboratory method using pumped solid sorbent tubes, thermal desorption and gas chromatography.	March 1993	0-11-885692-8
75/2	*Aromatic amines in air and on surfaces* Laboratory method using pumped acid-coated filters, moistened swabs and high-performance liquid chromatography.	June 2014	
77	*Asbestos in bulk materials* Sampling and identification by polarised light microscopy (PLM).	June 1994	0-7176-0677-5
78	*Formaldehyde in air* Laboratory method using a diffusive sampler, solvent desorption and high-performance liquid chromatography.	May 1994	0-7176-0678-3
79/2	*Peroxodisulphate salts in air* Laboratory method using sample collection on filters and analysis by ion chromatography.	November 2014	
80	*Volatile organic compounds in air* Laboratory method using diffusive solid sorbent tubes, thermal desorption and gas chromatography.	August 1995	0-7176-0913-8
81	*Dustiness of powders and materials*	September 1996	0-7176-1268-6
82/2	*The dust lamp* A simple tool for observing the presence of airborne particles.	January 2015	
83/3	*Resin acids in rosin (colophony) solder flux fume* Laboratory method using gas chromatography.	March 2015	

	Title	Last revision date	ISBN
84/2	*Measurement of oil mist from mineral oil-based metalworking fluids* Laboratory method using inhalable sampler and gravimetric analysis.	November 2014	
85/2	*Triglycidyl isocyanurate (and coating powders containing triglycidyl isocyanurate) in air* Laboratory method using pumped filters, liquid desorption and liquid chromatography.	March 2015	
86/2	*Hydrazine in air* Laboratory method using sampling either onto acid-coated glass-fibre filters followed by solvent desorption or directly into modified impingers. Final analysis by liquid chromatography after derivatisation.	November 2014	
87	*Fibres in air* Guidance on the discrimination between fibre types in samples of airborne dust on fibres using microscopy.	November 1998	0-7176-1487-5
88	*Volatile organic compounds in air* Laboratory method using diffusive samplers, solvent desorption and gas chromatography.	December 1997	0-7176-2401-3
89	*Dimethyl sulphate and diethyl sulphate in air* Laboratory method using thermal desorption, gas chromatography–mass spectrometry.	March 1998	0-7176-1540-5
91/2	*Metals and metalloids in workplace air by X-ray fluorescence spectrometry*	February 2015	
92/2	*Azodicarbonamide in air* Laboratory method with sample collection onto filters, solvent desorption and liquid chromatography.	November 2014	
93	*Glutaraldehyde in air* Laboratory method using high-performance liquid chromatography.	November 1998	0-7176-1618-5
94/2	*Pesticides in air and/or on surfaces* Methods for the sampling and analysis of pesticides in air using pumped filters and sorbent tubes in series and on dermal surrogates using cotton pads and clothing. Analysis by gas chromatography.	March 2015	

(Continued)

TABLE 8.1 (Continued)

	Title	Last revision date	ISBN
95/3	*Measurement of personal exposure of metalworking machine operators to airborne water-mix metalworking fluids* Elemental marker method using flame atomic absorption spectrometry or inductively coupled plasma–atomic emission spectrometry.	February 2015	
96	*Volatile organic compounds in air* Laboratory method using pumped solid sorbent tubes, solvent desorption and gas chromatography.	March 2000	0-7176-1756-4
98/3	*Hydroquinone in air* Laboratory method using high-performance liquid chromatography.	November 2014	
100	*Surveying, sampling and assessment of asbestos-containing materials*	July 2001	0-7176-2076-X
101/2	*Crystalline silica in respirable airborne dusts* Direct-on-filter analyses by infrared spectroscopy and X-ray.	February 2015	
102	*Aldehydes in air – laboratory method using high performance liquid chromatography*	June 2010	
103	*Volatile organic compounds in air* Laboratory method using sorbent tubes, solvent desorption or thermal desorption and gas chromatography.	June 2016	

CHAPTER 9

Physical Hazards – Light, Heat, Noise, Vibration, Pressure and Radiation

9.1 Light

Many countries have regulations that relate to light in the working environment. In the UK this is covered under Regulation 8 of the Workplace (Health, Safety and Welfare) Regulations 1992, which requires that every workplace shall have suitable and sufficient lighting and the lighting shall, so far as is reasonably practicable, be by natural light.

Lighting levels at work can affect health and safety in a number of ways, notably the following.

- When people move about, they must be able to see obstacles that could lead to accidents from tripping, falling or by just walking into them.
- The tasks must be adequately lit so that workers can see enough detail to carry out these jobs correctly.

Pocket Consultant: Occupational Health, Sixth Edition. Kerry Gardiner, David Rees, Anil Adisesh, David Zalk, and Malcolm Harrington.
© 2022 John Wiley & Sons Ltd. Published 2022 by John Wiley & Sons Ltd.

- Operators of machinery must be able to see the controls, information dials and screens.
- Colours should be rendered correctly if that forms part of the work.
- Stroboscopic effects on rotating machinery must be minimised to prevent the moving part from appearing stationary.
- Items being worked on must have a three-dimensional shape and not appear flat.
- Glare must be minimised.

The above points imply that:

- the lighting levels falling on a work surface must be of the correct intensity
- the light must be positioned to provide good modelling
- the colour output of any artificial light source must not distort the colour of the item being worked on if that is important
- the background levels of light sources or the reflections from surfaces must not be too great to cause glare
- where rotating machinery is concerned, the source of illumination must not oscillate in time with the frequency of the electrical supply.

Units used in lighting

Luminous intensity. Unit, candela (cd); a measure of brilliance or brightness, which is the power of a source to emit light.
Luminous flux. Unit, lumen (lm); a measure of the total amount of light emitted within a unit solid angle (1 steradian [sr]) by a point source having a uniform luminous intensity of 1 cd. A lamp of 1 cd emits 4π lm.
Luminance. Unit, $cd\,m^{-2}$; the flow of light in a given direction.
Illuminance. Unit, lux (lx or $lm\,m^{-2}$); this is the unit that expresses the amount of light falling on a surface.

Recommended lighting standards

In the UK the Society of Light and Lighting (SLL) has published a significant number of SLL Lighting Guides:

- SLL Lighting Guide 0: *Introduction to Light and Lighting* (2017)
- SLL Lighting Guide 1: *The Industrial Environment* (updated 2018)
- SLL Lighting Guide 2: *Lighting for Healthcare Premises* (2019)
- SLL Lighting Guide 4: *Sports* (2006) (under review)
- SLL Lighting Guide 5: *Lighting for Education* (2011) (under review)
- SLL Lighting Guide 6: *The Exterior Environment* (2016)
- SLL Lighting Guide 7: *Offices* (2015)
- SLL Lighting Guide 8: *Lighting for Museums and Art Galleries* (2015)
- SLL Lighting Guide 9: *Lighting for Communal Residential Buildings* (2013) (under review)

TABLE 9.1	
Typical levels of suitable lighting.	
Area	**Recommended lighting level (lx)**
Circulation areas, e.g. corridors, stairs, lifts	100–150
Entrances, lobbies, waiting areas	150
Enquiry desks	500
Factories (dependent on the degree of detail to be viewed)	300–500
Offices, general at desk	500
Offices, drawing boards	750
Typical outdoor levels	10 000

- SLL Lighting Guide 10: *Daylighting – A Guide for Designers: Lighting for the Built Environment* (2014)
- SLL Lighting Guide 11: *Surface Reflectance and Colour* (2001)
- SLL Lighting Guide 12: *Emergency Lighting* (2015) (under review)
- SLL Lighting Guide 13: *Lighting for Places of Worship* (updated 2018)
- SLL Lighting Guide 14: *Control of Electric Lighting* (2016)
- SLL Lighting Guide 15: *Transport Buildings* (2017)
- SLL Lighting Guide 16: *Lighting for Stairs* (2017)
- SLL Lighting Guide 17: *Lighting for Retail Premises* (2018)
- SLL Lighting Guide 18: *Lighting for Licensed Premises* (updated 2018)
- SLL Lighting Guide 19: *Lighting for Extreme Conditions* (2019)
- SLL Lighting Guide 20: *Lighting and Facilities Management* (2020)
- *Guide to Limiting Obtrusive Light* (2012)

Some typical values for the most suitable lighting levels (illuminance) for many workplaces are given in Table 9.1.

Glare

As a result of the illumination of a task, it will reflect light to the eye at a certain level of luminance. Surrounding the task will be an immediate field and, in the background, will be yet another field, both of which emit light at a certain luminance. If any of these fields emit too much light into the eye, glare will occur. Where there is a direct interference with vision, as with an undipped car headlamp at night, the condition is known as *disability glare*. If there is no direct impairment of vision but there is discomfort or annoyance, it is known as *discomfort glare*. Where the task is satisfactorily illuminated but the surroundings are too bright, a distraction is caused that may lead to visual fatigue. Such a situation is often found in open-plan offices, where lines of lamps hanging below a ceiling appear to merge into the distance, creating one distracting source. This is prevented by recessing the light fittings into a false ceiling or by turning the worker's desk through 90°. Another example is where a computer screen is placed with a window as a background; the intensity of daylight seen around the screen is far greater than the intensity received from the screen and discomfort glare occurs.

To minimise glare, the ratio of task to immediate surround to background surround emission should be $10:3:1$. For example, if the task emits $500 \, \text{cd} \, \text{m}^{-2}$, the immediate surround should emit no more than $150 \, \text{cd} \, \text{m}^{-2}$ and the far background no more than $50 \, \text{cd} \, \text{m}^{-2}$.

Colour effects

No artificial lamp reproduces exactly the combination of light wavelengths that is found with daylight, and therefore colours seen under artificial light may appear to be different from those illuminated naturally.

Where the matching of colours is important, as with electronic assembly work, the fabric trade and interior decorating, it is essential that any artificial light uses lamps that are as close to the daylight frequencies as possible.

Stroboscopic effects

Lamps that operate from the mains electrical supply in the UK, which is at a frequency of 50 Hz, turn on and off 100 times per second whereas in the USA it is 60 Hz, meaning the turning on/off would occur 120 times per second. With certain fluorescent lamps, the light output, in effect, ceases at that frequency. If a piece of machinery rotates as an exact function of the mains supply frequency and is illuminated by such a lamp, it may appear to be stationary, which could lead to an accident. Filament lamps glow even when the supply is off and thus their light output is continuous.

Lighting surveys

A full lighting survey will provide details of any defects in the lighting system and of any potentially acute or chronic occupational health problems. However, some basic information, collected on the report sheet shown in Figure 9.1, will probably highlight the more obvious problems; where detailed measurements are required, it is suggested that an occupational/industrial hygienist with comprehensive knowledge of this field is utilised.

For a much more detailed description of light, its measurement and control see Chapter 19 by N. Alan Smith in *Occupational Hygiene* (Smith 2005).

Lighting survey sheet

Date .... Time ....

Location Address ....

Survey Person ....

Reason for Survey ....

> Room Dimensions:　L = ...　　W = ...　　　H = ...
>
> Window Dimensions: H = ...　　W = ...

Daylight Availability:　Side Glazing .... Roof Glazing ....

Artificial Lighting:　Luminaires/Lamps ....

　　　　　　　　　Luminaire Type ....

　　　　　　　　　Lamp Type ....

　　　　　　　　　Lamp Rating ....

　　　　　　　　　Date of Lamp Change ....

Condition of Equipment and Room Fabrics:

　　　　　　　　　Ceiling ....

　　　　　　　　　Walls ....

　　　　　　　　　Floor ....

　　　　　　　　　Windows ....

　　　　　　　　　Luminaires ....

Pirincipal Visual Tasks ....

Pirincipal Planes of interest ....

CIBSE Recommended illuminance Values ....

FIGURE 9.1　Typical lighting preliminary report sheet.

9.2 Heat

Health effects

Body temperature is maintained within close limits by an efficient homeostatic mechanism, although diurnal variation is observed over a range of 0.5–1 °C. Physical exercise will increase body temperature in proportion to oxygen consumption, the range being 0.5 °C for moderate exercise up to 4 °C for marathon running. Under normal conditions, however, the body temperature stays within the range 36–39 °C as a balance is struck between the following:

- metabolic heat (M)
- evaporation (E)
- convection (C)
- conduction (K)
- radiation (R)
- storage (S).

Traditionally, this is expressed as:

$$M = E \pm C \pm K \pm R \pm S$$

Diving in a full suit or working in hot, humid conditions can greatly alter this homeostasis. For example, sweating ceases to be an effective means of heat loss at ambient temperatures above 37 °C with a relative humidity of 80% or greater. Against this is the fact that acclimatisation to heat is possible over a period of 10 days and is facilitated by a greatly increased sweating rate. Furthermore, physical fitness improves an individual's ability to cope with the stresses of heat.

The severity of health effects from heat increases with the temperature, humidity and duration of exposure. In order of increasing seriousness, these effects are:

- lassitude, irritability, discomfort
- lowered work performance and lack of concentration
- heat rashes
- heat cramps
- heat exhaustion
- heat stroke.

Any effect up to heat cramps is readily amenable to cooling and the administration of salt and water supplements. Heat exhaustion and heat stroke signify the onset of the failure of the thermoregulatory mechanism; this demands rapid and effective cooling, with fluid and electrolyte replacement by parenteral routes if necessary. Complete recovery of homeostasis may take a further week.

Environmental monitoring

The four means of heat exchange are: conduction, convection, radiation and evaporation; however, these are not measured directly. The thermal environment around the body, which affects the rate of heat flow, is instead expressed by the following four parameters:

- the dry bulb temperature of the air
- the moisture content or water vapour pressure of the air
- the air velocity
- the radiant heat exchange between the skin and surrounding surfaces.

The relationship between the dry bulb temperature and the moisture content is shown in the psychrometric chart given in Figure 9.2. The two conditions that can be measured and plotted on this chart are the ventilated wet bulb and dry bulb temperatures, as measured by the sling or aspirated psychrometer. Other factors, such as the moisture content, percentage saturation (approximately the same as the relative humidity), specific enthalpy and specific volume, can be read from the appropriate scales from the point of intersection of the wet and dry bulb temperatures, as shown in Figure 9.3. The air velocity is measured by an air flow meter (such as a cup anemometer or rotating vane anemometer), unless the value is low, in which case a kata thermometer is used. The air velocity is obtained from the cooling time of the kata thermometer, using the nomograms given in Figures 9.4 and 9.5.

The radiant heat exchange is obtained from the globe thermometer, which integrates the radiant heat flux from all the surfaces that surround it. As the instrument is affected by the air temperature and velocity, a correction is made, using the nomograms given in Figure 9.6a–d, to provide the mean temperature of the surroundings (mean radiant temperature).

Other factors that affect body heat gains and losses are:

- the metabolic rate of the subject due to the degree of activity
- the type of clothing worn
- the duration of exposure to the heat or cold.

Typical metabolic rates for different activities are shown in Table 9.2. Work rates tend to be self-regulating because workers will voluntarily reduce their rate if they feel overheated; the exception is in firefighting and rescue work, where psychological pressures may overcome normal scruples.

Clothing assemblies have varying resistances to heat flow, expressed by the unit 'Clo' ($1\,\text{Clo} = 0.155\,°\text{C}\,\text{m}^2\,\text{W}^{-1}$). Typical Clo values for various clothing assemblies are given in Table 9.3.

External factors, such as moisture content and wind, will influence the resistance of clothing to heat flow. Moist clothing will have a lower resistance. Higher air velocities tend to collapse clothing, reducing its thickness and hence its resistance, while with open weave clothing wind can remove the inner layers of warm air. Except when used as a protection against chemicals or other hazards,

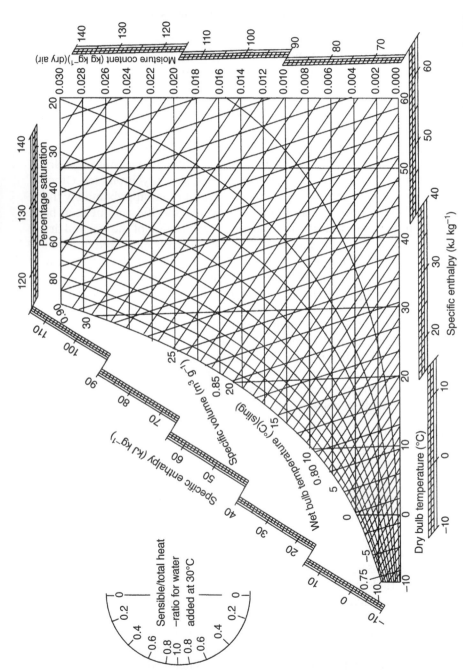

FIGURE 9.2 Psychrometric chart. Pads of 50 A3-sized charts suitable for permanent records are available from the Chartered Institution of Building Services Engineers (CIBSE) (https://www.cibse.org). Source: PC01 CIBSE Psychrometric Chart (−10 to +60 degree C) 50 charts, The Chartered Institution of Building Services Engineers (CIBSE).

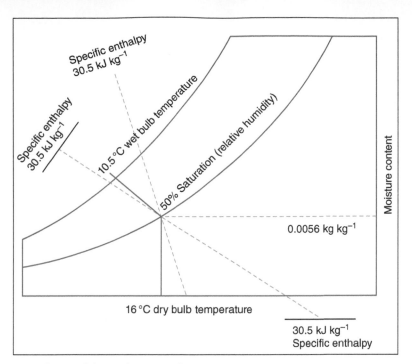

FIGURE 9.3 The use of the psychrometric chart.

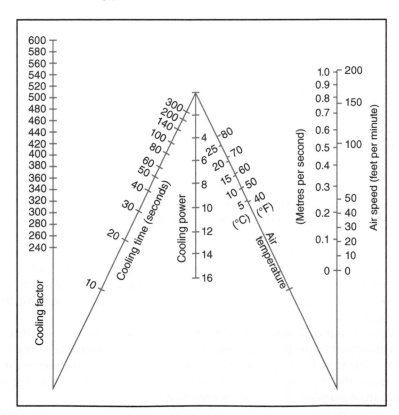

FIGURE 9.4 Kata thermometer chart for the temperature range 38–35 °C. Source: BS 3276: 1960, Thermometers for Measuring Air Cooling Power, British Standards Institution (BSI).

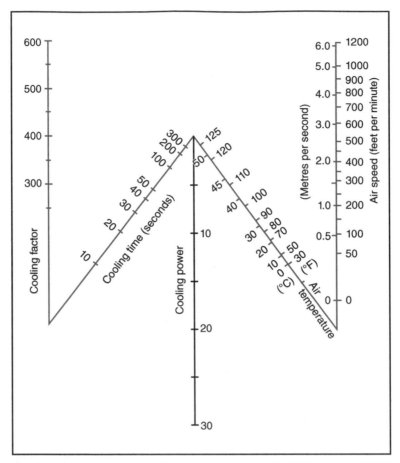

FIGURE 9.5   Kata thermometer chart for the temperature range 54.5–51.5 °C. Source: BS 3276: 1960, Thermometers for Measuring Air Cooling Power, British Standards Institution (BSI).

personal insulation tends to be self-regulating, people adding or removing layers of clothing according to their feelings of comfort.

The *duration of exposure* can be varied by work/rest regimes, preferably with the rest period being taken in a less extreme environment. In certain circumstances, such as in hot mines and places of extreme climate, it may not be possible to remove the worker from the environment. This also occurs with rescue work, where the motive to continue the work at all costs is uppermost in the worker's mind.

It is usually either ill-advised or not possible to assess hazards/risks in a thermal environment by the use of just one of the parameters mentioned previously; therefore, attempts have been made to bring together these parameters into a single index representing a thermal environment, from which the degree of hazard can be assessed. Some indices are given below.

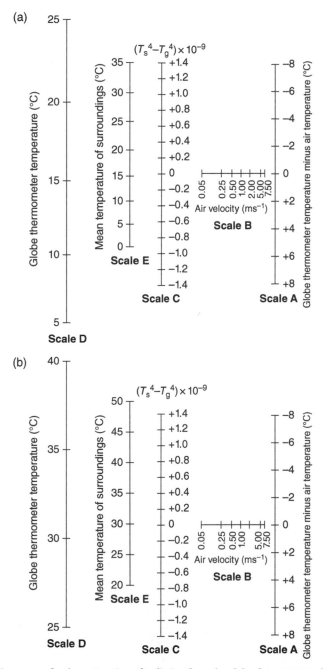

FIGURE 9.6 Nomogram for the estimation of radiation from the globe thermometer. (a) Range 5–25 °C; (b) range 25–30 °C; (c) range 40–55 °C; (d) range 50–65 °C.

(c)

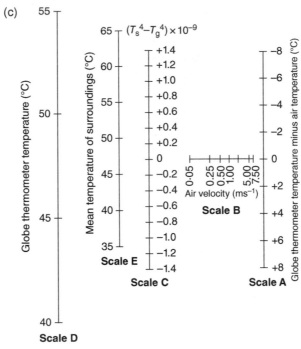

(d)

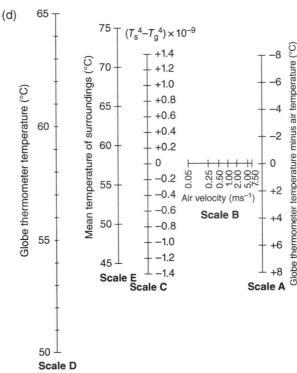

FIGURE 9.6 (Continued)

TABLE 9.2	

Typical metabolic rates.

Activity	Metabolic rate (W)
Sitting	95
Standing	115
Walking at $4\,km\,h^{-1}$	260
Standing: light hand work	160–210
Standing: heavy hand work	210–260
Standing: light arm work	315
Standing: heavy arm work (e.g. sawing)	420–675
Work with whole body: light	315
Work with whole body: moderate	420
Work with whole body: heavy	560

TABLE 9.3	

Typical clothes thermal insulation (Clo) values.

Clothing assembly	Clo
Naked	0
Shorts	0.1
Light summer clothing	0.5
Typical indoor clothing	1.0
Heavy suit and underclothes	1.5
Polar clothing	3–4
Practical maximum	5

Wet bulb globe temperature (WBGT)
For indoor use:

$$\text{WBGT}\left(^\circ\text{C}\right) = 0.7t_n + 0.3t_g$$

For outdoor use:

$$\text{WBGT}\left(^\circ\text{C}\right) = 0.7t'_n + 0.3t_g + 0.1t$$

where t'_n is the natural or unventilated wet bulb temperature, t_g is the globe temperature and t is the dry bulb temperature.

Note that the ventilated wet bulb can be used instead of the natural wet bulb according to the following rules:

> ### TABLE 9.4
>
> **Wet bulb globe temperatures (WBGTs) and recommended work/ rest regimes (°C).**
>
> | | Workload (total) | | |
> |---|---|---|---|
> | | **Light** | **Moderate** | **Heavy** |
> | Continuous | 30.0 | 26.7 | 25.0 |
> | 75% work, 25% rest each hour | 30.6 | 28.0 | 25.9 |
> | 50% work, 50% rest each hour | 31.4 | 29.4 | 27.9 |
> | 25% work, 75% rest each hour | 32.2 | 31.1 | 30.0 |
>
> Workload: light, 230 W; moderate, 230–400 W; heavy, 400–580 W. For example, at a WBGT of 30 °C, a person could undertake continuous light work, but if heavy work was involved he/she could only maintain it for 25% of the time in any hour.

- If the relative humidity of the air is below 25%, add 1 °C to the ventilated wet bulb temperature.
- If the relative humidity of the air is between 25% and 50%, add 0.5 °C to the ventilated wet bulb temperature.
- If the relative humidity of the air is above 50%, use the ventilated wet bulb temperature.

Recommended work/rest regimes for various wet bulb globe temperatures (WBGTs) are given in Table 9.4.

Clothing correction for WBGT
Corrections should be made to Table 9.4 to allow for the type of clothing worn as follows:

- light summer clothing, 0
- cotton overalls, −2
- winter clothing, −4
- water barrier (permeable), −6.

Hence, Table 9.4 is suitable only for persons wearing light summer clothing; a new table would have to be drawn up for each clothing type by applying the correction given above to all values in the table.

Effective and corrected effective temperatures (ET and CET)
The three charts in Figure 9.7a–c give the 'basic', 'normal' and 'adjusted' scales of the (corrected) effective temperature. The 'basic' scale refers to a worker stripped to the waist; the 'normal' scale refers to a worker lightly clothed; and the 'adjusted' scale takes into account the work rate.

(a)

ft min⁻¹	m s⁻¹	m s⁻¹ Plotted	m s⁻¹ Error
20	0.1016	0.100	0.0016
100	0.508	0.500	0.008
200	1.015	1.000	0.016
300	1.524	1.500	0.024
400	2.032	2.000	0.032
500	2.540	2.500	0.040
600	3.048	3.000	0.048
700	3.556	3.500	0.056

Conversion factor
$$\text{ft min}^{-1} \times 0.00508 = \text{m s}^{-1}$$
Factor used
$$\text{ft min}^{-1} \times 0.005 \text{ (error 1.6\%)}$$

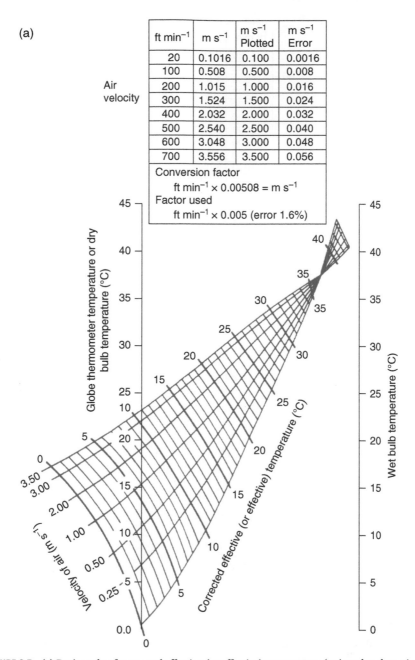

FIGURE 9.7 (a) Basic scale of corrected effective (or effective) temperature (stripped to the waist). (b) Normal scale (lightly clothed). (c) Normal scale with additional nomogram including work rates.

(b)

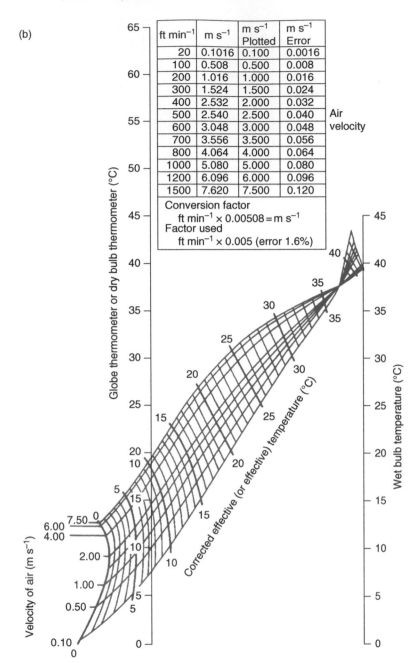

ft min^{-1}	m s^{-1}	m s^{-1} Plotted	m s^{-1} Error
20	0.1016	0.100	0.0016
100	0.508	0.500	0.008
200	1.016	1.000	0.016
300	1.524	1.500	0.024
400	2.532	2.000	0.032
500	2.540	2.500	0.040
600	3.048	3.000	0.048
700	3.556	3.500	0.056
800	4.064	4.000	0.064
1000	5.080	5.000	0.080
1200	6.096	6.000	0.096
1500	7.620	7.500	0.120

Conversion factor
ft min^{-1} × 0.00508 = m s^{-1}
Factor used
ft min^{-1} × 0.005 (error 1.6%)

Air velocity

FIGURE 9.7   (Continued)

(c)

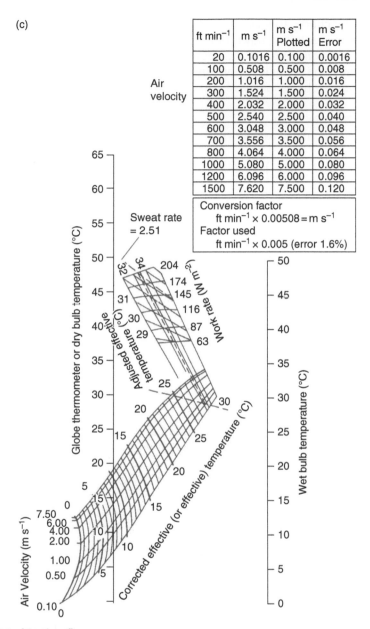

ft min⁻¹	m s⁻¹	m s⁻¹ Plotted	m s⁻¹ Error
20	0.1016	0.100	0.0016
100	0.508	0.500	0.008
200	1.016	1.000	0.016
300	1.524	1.500	0.024
400	2.032	2.000	0.032
500	2.540	2.500	0.040
600	3.048	3.000	0.048
700	3.556	3.500	0.056
800	4.064	4.000	0.064
1000	5.080	5.000	0.080
1200	6.096	6.000	0.096
1500	7.620	7.500	0.120

Air velocity

Conversion factor
$ft\ min^{-1} \times 0.00508 = m\ s^{-1}$
Factor used
$ft\ min^{-1} \times 0.005\ (error\ 1.6\%)$

Sweat rate = 2.51

Globe thermometer or dry bulb temperature (°C)

Air Velocity (m s⁻¹)

Adjusted effective temperature (°C)

Work rate (W m⁻²)

Corrected effective (or effective) temperature (°C)

Wet bulb temperature (°C)

FIGURE 9.7 (Continued)

To use the charts, it is necessary to join the globe or dry bulb temperature reading to the wet bulb temperature with a straight line. The ET or CET can be read from the nomogram at the point of intersection of the line with the air velocity line. If the dry bulb temperature is used, it will provide the answer as ET, whereas if the globe temperature is used the answer will be CET.

Heat stress index (HSI)

This index is calculated as follows:

$$\text{HSI} = \left(E_{req} / E_{max} \right) \times 100\%$$

where $E_{req} \left(\text{W} \right) = M + R + C$. For lightly clothed persons: $E_{max} \left(\text{W} \right) = 12.5 v^{0.6} \left(56 - \rho_s \right)$

$M \left(\text{W} \right) = $ metabolic rate of the worker

$R \left(\text{W} \right) = 7.93 \left(t_r - 35 \right)$

$C \left(\text{W} \right) = 8.1 v^{0.6} \left(t - 35 \right)$

For persons stripped to the waist:

$$E_{max} \left(\text{W} \right) = 21 v^{0.6} \left(56 - \rho_s \right)$$
$$R \left(\text{W} \right) = 13.2 \left(t_r - 35 \right)$$
$$C \left(\text{W} \right) = 13.6 v^{0.6} \left(t - 35 \right)$$

where ρ_s is the water vapour pressure in millibars, an approximate value of which can be found by reading across horizontally from the dry bulb/wet bulb intersection (on the psychrometric chart) until it meets the air moisture content in kg kg^{-1} and multiplying that value by 1560; t_r is the mean radiant temperature (°C); t is the dry bulb temperature (°C); and v is the air velocity (m s^{-1}). A work/rest regime can be calculated from:

$$\text{Exposure time} \left(\text{min} \right) = \frac{4400}{E_{req} - E_{max}}$$

$$\text{Rest time} \left(\text{min} \right) = \frac{4400}{E_{max} - E_{req}}$$

Note that, for the rest time, E_{max} and E_{req} refer to the thermal environment in the rest area, if one is used, and normally the work rate will be less.

The upper limit for safety is if the HSI reaches 100%. Any value above this will result in an increase in the deep body temperature, which, if allowed to continue for any length of time, may lead to stress. A negative value indicates cold stress.

One very useful aspect of the HSI is that, if an environment has been found to be unacceptable, potential values to control the environment can be tried in the

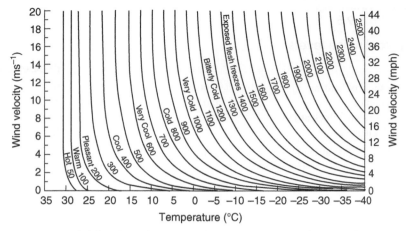

FIGURE 9.8 The wind chill index. Values marked against the curves are the rates of cooling in kcal h^{-1} m^{-2} (multiply by 1.16 to convert to W m^{-2}) at different combinations of wind velocity (m s^{-1}) and temperature (°C).

equation; for example, if the real work environment has a wind velocity of 0.5 m s^{-1}, a value of 1 m s^{-1} can be tried in the equation. If this is still not satisfactory, and 1 m s^{-1} is the maximum value that can be used but the water vapour pressure can be changed, the combined effect of these can be tried until a satisfactory outcome is achieved.

The *required sweat rate*, the most comprehensive HSI published to date, is given in detail in ISO 7933. It takes into account potential heat stress from the acclimatised and non-acclimatised worker. However, the equations are complex and are best suited to computer solutions; ISO 7933 provides a computer program for their solution.

Wind chill index

In a cold environment, the effect of wind is important. Figure 9.8 shows the equivalent still-air temperatures of various wind velocities. The curves are labelled with a heat loss value in kilocalories per hour per square metre. At a heat loss of 1750 kcal h^{-1} m^{-2} exposed flesh freezes in approximately 20 minutes, but at 2800 kcal h^{-1} m^{-2} it freezes in 1 minute.

For a much more detailed description of the thermal environment, its measurement and control see Chapter 20 by Anthony Yule in *Occupational Hygiene* (Youle 2005).

9.3 Noise

Sound involves pressure changes in the air that are picked up by the eardrum and transmitted to the brain. Pressure is measured in pascals (Pa). The threshold of human hearing is at approximately 0.00002 Pa, but at 25 m from a jet aircraft taking off the pressure is 10^7 times greater at 200 Pa. The expression of such a

TABLE 9.5

Typical noise levels.

	Pressure (Pa)	Decibel (dB)
Threshold of hearing	0.00002	0
Quiet office	0.002	40
Ringing alarm clock at 1 m	0.2	80
Ship's engine room	20	120
Turbojet engine at 25 m	200	140

wide range of sound is simplified with the decibel scale, which compares the actual sound with the reference value of 0.00002 Pa using a logarithmic scale (to base 10) as follows:

$$\text{Decibel (dB)}, 20 \log_{10} \frac{P_a}{P_r}$$

where P_a is the pressure of the actual sound and P_r is the reference sound pressure at the threshold of hearing.

Typical sound intensities are given in Table 9.5.

Addition of sounds

If two sounds are being emitted at the same time, their total combined intensity is not the numerical sum of the decibel levels of each separate intensity. Because of the logarithmic nature of the decibel scale, they must be added according to the graph given in Figure 9.9.

Sound spectrum

The lowest frequency sound that can be detected by the human ear is about 20 Hz, and the highest, for a young person, is up to 18 kHz. With age, the ear becomes less sensitive to the higher frequencies. A doubling of the frequency raises the pitch of the note by one octave. The ear is most receptive to sounds between 500 Hz and 4 kHz; indeed, 500 Hz to 2 kHz is the frequency range of speech. Unless a sound is a pure tone, which is unusual (most noises are made up of sounds of many frequencies and intensities) when assessing the intensity, it may be necessary to discover the intensity values over the whole range of frequency, i.e. to measure the sound spectrum. This is especially useful for controlling noise. For convenience, it is usual to divide the sounds into octave bands and to use a measuring instrument that assesses the intensity of all notes

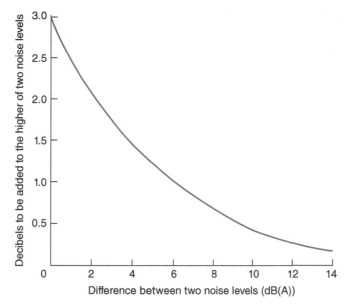

FIGURE 9.9   Graph for adding two unequal noise levels.

between the octaves and expresses it as a mid-octave intensity. The mid-octave frequencies chosen for this analysis are: 62.5, 125, 250, 500 Hz, 1, 2, 4, 8 kHz and, sometimes, 16 kHz. Thus, a spectrum of noise will quote the intensities at each of these mid-octave band frequencies.

Noise rating

Because of the sensitivity range of the ear, it can tolerate louder sounds at lower frequencies than at higher ones. A range of octave band curves, known as 'noise rating (NR) curves', that indicate the recommended octave band analyses for various situations has been produced. The curve lying immediately above the measured octave band analysis of the noise in question represents the NR of that noise. Figure 9.10 gives a range of NR curves as well as the recommended ratings for various situations.

Decibel weightings

As noise is a combination of sounds at various frequencies and intensities, the noise intensity can be expressed either as a spectrum, mentioned previously, or as a combination of all frequencies summed together in one value. As the human ear is more sensitive to certain frequencies than others, it is possible to make allowances for this in the electronic circuitry of a sound level meter, i.e. certain frequencies are suppressed as others are boosted, in order to approximate to the response of the ear.

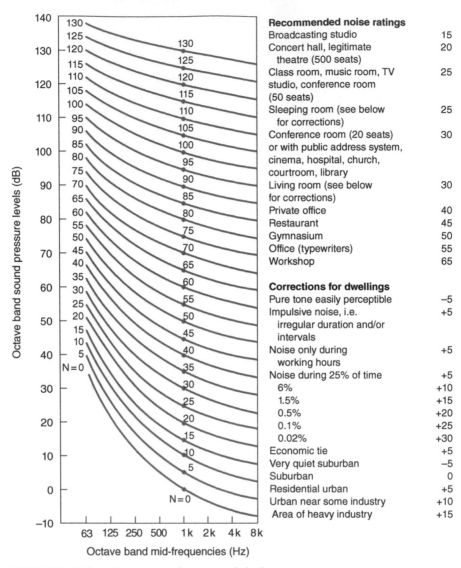

Recommended noise ratings

Broadcasting studio	15
Concert hall, legitimate	20
theatre (500 seats)	
Class room, music room, TV	25
studio, conference room	
(50 seats)	
Sleeping room (see below	25
for corrections)	
Conference room (20 seats)	30
or with public address system,	
cinema, hospital, church,	
courtroom, library	
Living room (see below	30
for corrections)	
Private office	40
Restaurant	45
Gymnasium	50
Office (typewriters)	55
Workshop	65

Corrections for dwellings

Pure tone easily perceptible	−5
Impulsive noise, i.e.	+5
irregular duration and/or	
intervals	
Noise only during	+5
working hours	
Noise during 25% of time	+5
6%	+10
1.5%	+15
0.5%	+20
0.1%	+25
0.02%	+30
Economic tie	+5
Very quiet suburban	−5
Suburban	0
Residential urban	+5
Urban near some industry	+10
Area of heavy industry	+15

FIGURE 9.10   Noise rating curves and recommended values.

This technique is known as weighting, and there are A, B, C and D weightings available for various purposes. Figure 9.11 shows the A, B and C weighting networks. That which is most usually quoted is the A weighting, and instruments measuring sound intensity with that weighting give readings in dB(A). The weightings given to the mid-octave band frequencies for the dB(A) scale are shown in Table 9.6.

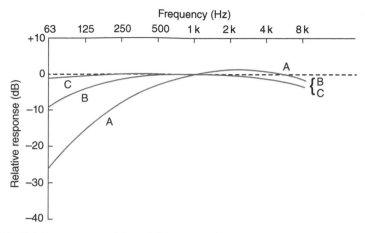

FIGURE 9.11 Relative responses of the weighting networks.

TABLE **9.6**

Mid-octave band frequency corrections for the dB(A) weighting.

Frequency (Hz)	62.5	125	250	500	1000	2000	4000	8000
Correction (dB)	−26	−16	−9	−3	0	+1	+1	−1

Noise dose and L_{eq}

Exposure to noise normally varies in intensity over a working period and, in order to estimate an equivalent noise level that would give the same total amount of sound energy as the fluctuating noise, the unit L_{eq} has been devised. In order to measure the L_{eq}, personal noise dosemeters are used; these are convenient, as they fit into the worker's pocket, and the read-out (depending on type) is directly in percentage dose, L_{eq}, maximum peak, Pa² h, etc.

Guidance for the UK Control of Noise at Work Regulations 2005 recommends that measurement should be made in the 'undisturbed field'; however, results are unlikely to be significantly affected by reflections if the microphone is kept at least 4 cm away from the operator (it should also be placed on the side of the subject likely to receive most noise) (Figure 9.12). Therefore, most dosemeter microphones are provided with a clip to hold them onto the brim of a safety helmet or overall lapel. Thus, the expectation/aspiration is that the microphone receives the same sound pressure as the worker's ear, which the dosemeter 'A' weights, and then, after squaring, totals over the measurement period and displays the value as the noise dose.

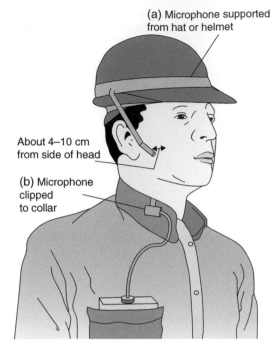

FIGURE 9.12   Location of a microphone for dosemeters: (a) head-mounted microphone; (b) collar- or shoulder-mounted microphone. Source: Health and Safety Executive (HSE), 1990. Licensed under OGL (crown copyright).

The recommended maximum noise doses for the unprotected ear are given in Table 9.7. Each of the doses shown represents the same amount of sound energy and is regarded as 100% noise dose. Noise dosemeters sold on the British market are set to indicate a percentage dose based on this value. For example, if a dose-meter were placed on an unprotected worker for a period of time and the reading showed 150%, the recommended dose would have been exceeded, but if it showed 30% it would not.

This degree of energy does not fully protect some people from suffering noise-induced hearing loss if exposed day after day; a more suitable dose is 85 dB(A) for eight hours. A slightly modified version of these two noise doses is now written into the UK Control of Noise at Work Regulations 2005 as the 'first action level' (80 dB(A) $L_{EP,d}$) and the 'second action level' (85 dB(A) $L_{EP,d}$). The term $L_{EP,d}$ refers to a daily dose rather than one of eight hours. The Control of Noise at Work Regulations 2005 are summarised below. These regulations are published together with two Health and Safety Executive (HSE) Noise Guides; a further five Noise Guides are published separately. All are available from The Stationery Office (TSO; formerly HMSO).

The noise dose for workers exposed to reasonably steady sources of sound can be estimated from the chart in Figure 9.13, which is taken from HSE Noise Guide 3. By drawing a line joining the duration of exposure on the right-hand side of the

TABLE 9.7	

Noise exposures equivalent to 85 dB(A) for 8 h.

Limiting dB(A) (L_{eq})	Maximum duration of exposure
85	8 h
88	4 h
91	2 h
94	1 h
97	30 min
100	15 min
103	7 min
106	4 min
109	2 min
112	1 min
115	30 s

chart to the intensity of steady noise on the left-hand side, the $L_{EP,d}$ can be read from the centre line of the chart. Also shown on the centre line are numbers marked f, which represents the fraction of 100% dose mentioned above. If a worker moves into other noisy areas, f numbers can be added from each to give a total fractional dose for the day.

Example.

An unprotected worker works in a steady 105 dB(A) for 10 minutes, 95 dB(A) for four hours and 88 dB(A) for three hours. What is the noise dose?

Answer.

$$105 \text{ dB}(A) \text{ for 10 min: } f = 0.7.$$
$$95 \text{ dB}(A) \text{ for 4 h: } f = 1.5.$$
$$88 \text{ dB}(A) \text{ for 3 h: } f = 0.25.$$
Total: $f = 2.45$ or 245% dose.

This level of noise is equivalent to a daily exposure of 94 dB(A), which is in excess of the 'second action level' as defined in the Control of Noise at Work Regulations 2005.

The US Occupational Safety and Health Administration (OSHA) regulatory standard has a permissible exposure limit (PEL) of 90 dB(A) for an eight-hour day. The OSHA standard utilises a 5 dB(A) exchange rate. As hearing damage to the ear can be considered proportional to the acoustic energy received, a given level of noise exposure for four hours can result in comparable damage to hearing as a noise exposure 5 dB lower for eight hours. This means that for every 5 dB(A) increase to exposure levels the acceptable time-weighted average (TWA) is halved. Therefore,

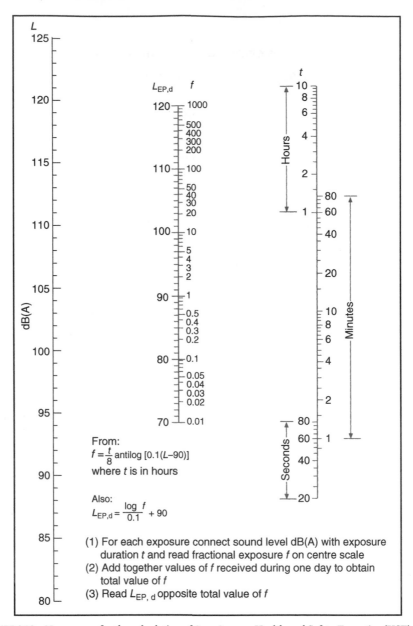

FIGURE 9.13 Nomogram for the calculation of $L_{EP,d}$. Source: Health and Safety Executive (HSE) Noise Guide 3, 1990. Licensed under OGL (crown copyright).

US OSHA would consider 95 dB(A) to be acceptable at less than four hours, 100 dB(A) for two hours, etc. The US National Institute for Occupational Safety and Health (NIOSH) does not have regulatory standing but recommends an occupational noise exposure limit of 85 dB(A) as an eight-hour TWA using a 3-dB exchange rate. The American Conference of Governmental Industrial Hygienists (ACGIH) threshold limit value (TLV) for audible sound is 85 dB(A), which also has a 3-dB exchange rate, halving the acceptable exposure for every 3-dB increase. This is not considered a regulatory requirement in the USA; however, many countries throughout the world have incorporated the ACGIH TLVs into their health and safety national regulations. The US OSHA standard does have a regulatory requirement to implement a hearing conservation programme when noise exposure is at or above 85 dB(A) for an eight-hour TWA. Hearing conservation programmes are intended to prevent the onset of occupational hearing loss to protect and preserve hearing capabilities and afford workers the knowledge and controls necessary to provide safeguards from further hearing loss.

Control of noise exposure levels

As with the control of all situations in the working environment, one must attempt to prevent rather than control exposure and, if prevention/elimination is not possible, to descend the hierarchy of acceptable/effective control measures (see Chapters 15 and 16). The control of noise exposure provides the classic example of viewing the work environment in three distinct sections: source, transmission path and receiver (Figure 9.14).

Noise reduction at source

Because movement causes vibration, which is passed on to air particles and perceived as sound, the minimisation of movement in any process will achieve a measure of noise control at source. A number of methods of preventing noise generation are given below:

- substitution of a quieter process, i.e. welding not riveting
- avoid or cushion impacts
- introduction of or increase in the amount of damping
- reduction of turbulence of air exhausts and jets by silencers, either of the 'absorption' type, where the attenuation (insertion loss) is achieved by a lining of absorbent material, or of the 'expansion chamber' type, where the insertion loss is achieved by acoustic mismatch between the volume of the chamber and inlet/outlet pipe (a number are now a hybrid of these two types)

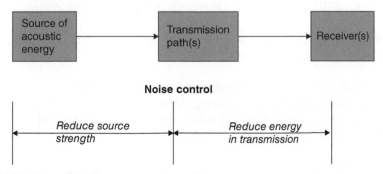

FIGURE 9.14   Energy flow diagram.

- use of low-noise air nozzles and pneumatic ejectors
- matching the pressure of the supplied air to the needs of the air-powered equipment
- avoidance of 'chapping' airstreams by rotating components
- improved design of fans, fan casings, compressors, etc.
- dynamic balancing of rotating parts
- use of better quality control in design and manufacturing procedures to obviate the need for post hoc rectification
- better machine maintenance
- limiting the duration for which a noisy machine or part of a machine is used.

Control of the transmission path

Having made every effort to control the noise exposure at the source, the next most appropriate course of action is to minimise the progress of the energy from the source to the receiver. A number of examples are given below:

- use of correctly chosen reflecting and absorbent barriers for the direct component
- use of correctly chosen absorbent material on surrounding surfaces to minimise the reflected component
- use of anti-vibration mountings under machines
- enclosure of the source
- provision of a noise refuge
- increasing the distance between the source and receiver
- segregation of noisy processes
- use of remote control
- use of flexible exhaust hoses to ensure that the exhaust is discharged away from the operator(s)
- active noise control, where the addition of a second source with the same amplitude, but with reversed phase, causes destructive superposition.

Control of noise exposure for the receiver

Other than a reduction in the time for which a worker is exposed, ear protection is the main means of control. This is discussed in much more detail in Chapters 15 and 16.

The UK control of noise at work regulations 2005

The following is a summary of Regulation 4; the wording is that of the authors, not the Health and Safety Executive (HSE).

Regulation 4 – exposure limit values and action values

1. The lower exposure action value (EAV)s are:
   a. a daily or weekly personal noise exposure of 80 dB(A); and
   b. a peak sound pressure of 135 dB(C).

2. The upper EAVs are:
   a. a daily or weekly personal noise exposure of 85 dB(A);
   b. a peak sound pressure of 137 dB(C).

3. The exposure limit values (ELVs) are:
   a. a daily or weekly personal noise exposure of 87 dB(A);
   b. a peak sound pressure of 140 dB(C).

4. Where the exposure of an employee to noise varies markedly from day to day, an employee may use weekly personal noise exposure in place of daily personal noise exposure for the purpose of compliance with these regulations.
5. In applying the ELVs in paragraph (3), but not in applying the lower and upper EAVs in paragraphs (1) and (2), account shall be taken of the protection given to the employee by any personal hearing protectors provided by the employer in accordance with Regulation 7(2).

Auditory health effects

The ear is not well equipped to protect itself from the deleterious effects of noise. Admittedly, a sudden loud sound is rapidly followed by a reflex contraction of muscles in the middle ear, which can limit the amount of sound energy transmitted to the inner ear. Nevertheless, in the occupational setting, such circumstances are relatively rare. Most workers exposed to noise suffer prolonged exposure, which may be intermittent or continuous. Such energy transmission, if suffi-ciently prolonged and intense, will damage the organ of Corti and eventually can lead to permanent deafness.

Noise-induced hearing loss differs from presbycusis in being primarily cen-tred on the ear's ability to hear sound at around 4 Hz – the upper level of speech appreciation. With time, this loss extends over the range 3–6 kHz, and this has the effect of removing the sibilant consonants and, thereby, diminishing the hearer's appreciation of the spoken word. Unlike presbycusis, noise-induced hearing loss is not improved by the use of a hearing aid. The degree of hearing loss is related to the level of noise and the duration of exposure, hence the attempt to establish a maximum permissible exposure level for dB(A), L_{eq}, with time, as outlined above. Figure 9.15 shows the progressive stages of noise-induced hearing loss.

For a much more detailed description of noise, its measurement and its con-trol see Chapter 17 by Kerry Gardiner in *Occupational Hygiene* (Gardiner 2005).

9.4 Vibration

Vibration is oscillatory motion about a point. In occupational health terms, workers may be exposed to two types.

1. *Hand-transmitted vibration* is the vibration that passes to the hands from a source of vibration. This occurs where (i) hand-held vibrating tools are used to smooth out rough surfaces of an object such as a metal casting or (ii) work pieces are held by the hands or fingers and pushed against a rotating grinding wheel. Examples of such tools are drills, chain saws, concrete

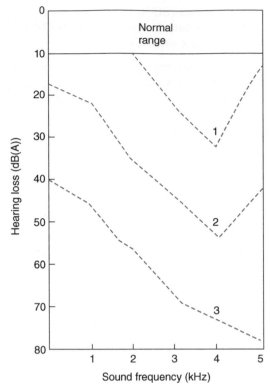

FIGURE 9.15 Audiogram showing the progressive stages of noise-induced hearing loss.

breakers and grinders (Table 9.8). Industries where significant exposure of this nature occurs include agriculture, mining, construction, forestry and fishing.

2. *Whole-body vibration* occurs when the body is supported on a surface that is vibrating (e.g. sitting on a seat that vibrates, standing on a vibrating floor or lying on a vibrating surface). Examples of occupations where this is an issue are tractor cab drivers and helicopter pilots. Whole-body vibration occurs in all forms of transport and when working near some industrial machinery.

Characteristics of vibration

Vibration magnitude

During the oscillatory displacements of an object, it has alternately a velocity in one direction and then a velocity in the opposite direction. This change in velocity means that the object is constantly accelerating and decelerating, first in one direction and then in the opposite direction. Figure 9.16 shows the displacement

TABLE **9.8**	

Tools and processes potentially associated with vibration injuries.

Type of tool	Examples of tool type
Percussive metalworking tools	Riveting tools Caulking tools Chipping tools Chipping hammers Fettling tools Hammer drills Clinching and flanging tools Impact wrenches Swaging Needle guns
Grinders and other rotary tools	Pedestal grinders Hand-held grinders Hand-held sanders Hand-held polishers Flex-driven grinders/polishers Rotary burring tools
Percussive hammers and drills used in mining, demolition and road construction	Hammers Rock drills Road drills, etc.
Forest and garden machinery	Chainsaws Anti-vibration chainsaws Brush saws Mowers and shears Barking machines
Other processes and tools	Nut runners Shoe-pounding-up machines Concrete vibro-thickeners Concrete levelling vibro-tables Motorcycle handlebars

Source: Griffin (1990).

waveform, the velocity waveform and the acceleration waveform for a movement occurring at a single frequency (i.e. a sinusoidal oscillation). Vibration can be quantified by its displacement, its velocity or its acceleration. The magnitude of vibration is presently expressed in terms of the acceleration and measured using accelerometers. The units of acceleration are metres per second per second (i.e. $m\,s^{-2}$). For comparison, the acceleration due to gravity on Earth is approximately $9.81\,m\,s^{-2}$.

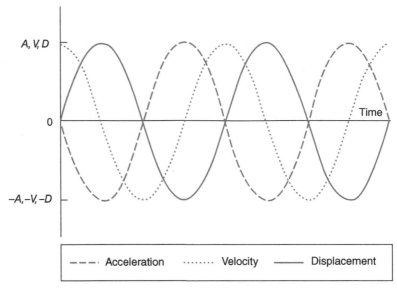

FIGURE 9.16   Displacement, velocity and acceleration waveforms for a sinusoidal vibration. If the vibration is of frequency f and peak displacement D, the peak velocity $V = 2\pi f D$ and the peak acceleration $A = (2\pi f)^2 D$.

The magnitude of vibration is expressed in terms of an average measure of the acceleration of the oscillatory motion, usually the root-mean-square value (i.e. $m\,s^{-2}$ r.m.s.). (For a sinusoidal motion, the r.m.s. value is the peak value divided by 2.)

Vibration frequency

The frequency of vibration is expressed in cycles per second using the SI unit hertz (Hz). The frequency of vibration determines the extent to which vibration is transmitted to the surface of the body (e.g. through seating), the extent to which it is transmitted through the body and the response to vibration within the body. Oscillations at frequencies below about 0.5 Hz can cause motion sickness. The frequencies of greatest significance to whole-body vibration are usually at the lower end of the range from 0.5 to 100 Hz; for hand-transmitted vibration, frequencies as high as 1000 Hz or more may have detrimental effects.

Vibration direction

The responses of the body differ according to the direction of the motion. Vibration is usually measured at the interfaces between the body and the vibrating surfaces in three orthogonal directions. Figure 9.17 shows a coordinate system used when measuring vibration in contact with a hand holding a tool.

The three principal directions for seated and standing persons are: fore and aft (x-axis), lateral (y-axis) and vertical (z-axis). Figure 9.18 illustrates the translational

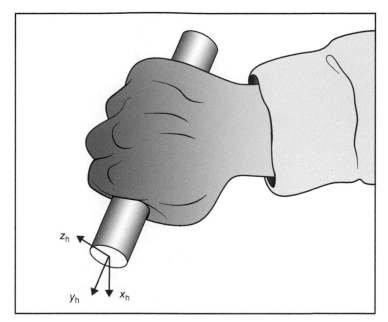

FIGURE 9.17 Axes of vibration used to measure hand-transmitted vibration.

and rotational axes for an origin at the ischial tuberosities of a seated person. A similar set of axes is used to describe the directions of vibration at the back and feet of seated persons.

Vibration duration

The effects of vibration are dependent on the total duration of vibration exposure. Additionally, the duration of measurement may affect the measured magnitude of the vibration. The r.m.s. acceleration may not provide a good indication of vibration severity if the vibration is intermittent, contains shocks or otherwise varies in magnitude from time to time.

Hand-transmitted vibration

Aspects of exposure to the risk factors for hand-transmitted vibration include:

- the nature and extent of exposure to vibration (magnitude, frequency, direction and duration)
- continuous or intermittent exposure
- method of work and ergonomic factors
- workplace temperature
- individual susceptibility.

The effects on the hands are due to damage to the nerve and blood supply to the digits. The main effects are vascular, sensorineural and musculoskeletal, and

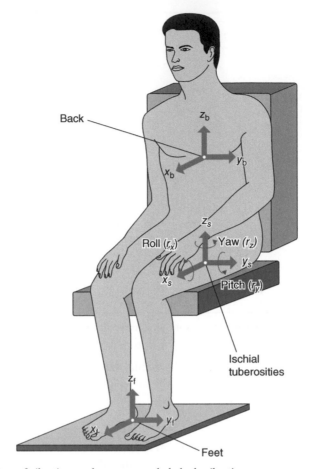

FIGURE 9.18   Axes of vibration used to measure whole-body vibration.

the term 'hand and arm vibration syndrome' (HAVS) is used for the clinical entity caused by hand-transmitted vibration.

Vascular effects – vibration white finger

Vibration white finger (VWF) is a secondary onset of Raynaud's disease characterised by intermittent blanching of the fingers and/or thumbs, with the tips usually being the first to blanch. Attacks of blanching are precipitated by cold (i.e. cold weather or handling cold objects). Hence, attacks may occur at or away from work. The affected digits initially turn white, then blue (from cyanosis) and then red as the blood supply returns to normal, often following warming of the hands. Return of digital blood flow is often accompanied by discomfort in the digits. Episodes of blanching last from 10 to 30 minutes or longer depending on severity. Early cases have symptoms mainly during cold weather (winter), and severe cases can be affected by temperature changes throughout the year.

Cold provocation tests under specific conditions of testing can be used to demonstrate prolonged finger re-warming times or reduced finger systolic blood pressure. However the aim of such tests is not to elicit finger blanching.

Sensorineural effects

Neurological effects of hand-transmitted vibration present as numbness, tingling, loss of tactile discrimination (often manifesting as inability to handle and distinguish small objects such as coins, needles, screws and buttons) and elevated sensory thresholds for touch and temperature. These effects can be determined by clinical examination and the use of special devices such as Semmes–Weinstein monofilaments (for sensory perception), the Purdue pegboard and standardised tests of vibrotactile and thermotactile perception. Some centres use current perception thresholds. There is also a higher risk of carpal tunnel syndrome, which is not itself a component of HAVS, in those exposed to hand-transmitted vibration; electromyography should be used for confirmation.

Musculoskeletal effects

These effects include weakness in the hands; joint pain and stiffness; Dupuytren's contracture; bony exostoses; and cysts in the wrist bones. Special tests include the use of a dynamometer for reduced grip strength, whereas the Purdue pegboard provides additional information on hand function.

Diagnosis of hand and arm vibration syndrome (HAVS)

The criteria for diagnosing a case of HAVS are:

1. Evidence of sufficient exposure to a source of hand-transmitted vibration. Exposure to hand-transmitted vibration can be measured using an accelerometer. Typical exposure levels in the use of various tools are available online from https://www.karla-info.de/en. A vibration exposure calculator is also available from the HSE website (www.hse.gov.uk/vibration). In the UK, the Control of Vibration at Work Regulations 2005 gives an EAV of $2.5\,\mathrm{m\,s^{-2}}$ A(8) and an ELV of $5.0\,\mathrm{m\,s^{-2}}$ A(8). These limit values refer to r.m.s. triaxial measurements, whereas in some jurisdictions maximal uniaxial values may be used. Levels above the ELV indicate an unacceptable level of risk and that urgent control measures are needed. Levels between the EAL and the ELV indicate a significant level of risk and require control measures and health surveillance.
2. Episodic pallor of digits and/or sensorineural effects.
3. Relevant time interval between exposure and effect (usually between 5 and 10 years but can range from 6 months to 20 years). Effects that appear more than two years after cessation of exposure to vibration are unlikely to be HAVS.
4. Consideration of differential diagnosis:
   - Primary Raynaud's disease also presents as episodic digital pallor. However, the onset tends to be earlier and bilateral, and the feet may also

be affected. There is often a family history in cases of primary Raynaud's disease.

- Autoimmune diseases such as rheumatoid arthritis, polyarteritis nodosa, scleroderma, dermatomyositis, the CREST syndrome (calcinosis, Raynaud's phenomenon, oesophageal dysmotility, sclerodactyly and telangiectasia) and hypofibrinogenaemia can present with Raynaud's phenomenon.
- Other systemic disorders include diabetes mellitus, hypothyroidism, vitamin B12 deficiency, Buerger's disease, polyneuropathy associated with hepatitis and leukaemia.
- Medications such as beta-blockers, vinblastine, bleomycin and ergot alkaloids can cause similar vascular effects. Streptomycin, chloramphenicol, indometacin, isoniazid, metronidazole and nitrofurantoin are recognised causes of similar sensorineural effects.
- Occupational neurotoxins to be considered include n-hexane, acrylamide, methyl n-butyl ketone, carbon disulphide, inorganic lead and vinyl chloride monomer. Inorganic lead exposure tends to cause motor rather than sensory or mixed neuropathy.

5. Other supporting evidence, or indications of alternative causes:
   - Examination of the hands may show digital pallor, although it is more likely that the patient may have available images taken on a cell phone; callosities; Dupuytren's contracture; reduced radial and/or ulnar pulses; loss of light touch and temperature perception; loss of two-point discrimination; and poor grip strength.
   - A range of clinical tests can also be considered to rule out other causes of the vascular effects, e.g. Allen's test (to indicate patency of the palmar arches), Adson's test (to detect the thoracic outlet syndrome also with vascular and sensorineural presentations), Tinel's test over the median and ulnar nerves and Phalen's test, which is suggestive of carpal tunnel syndrome.
   - Findings from other standardised tests. While a positive result from one or more special tests may be supportive, a negative result does not rule out a diagnosis of HAVS.

The most important criteria remain the history of sufficient exposure and relevant effect.

Staging of HAVS

Several scoring systems are used to stage the severity of HAVS.

- The Griffin method provides a numerical score out of a maximum of 33 for each hand, depending on the number of phalanges affected by finger blanching (Figure 9.19). The blanching scores for the hands shown in Figure 9.19 are 4/33 for the right hand and 16/33 for the left hand. The scores correspond to areas of blanching on the digits, commencing with the thumb. On the fingers, a score of 1 is given for blanching on the distal phalanx; a score of 2 for blanching on the middle phalanx; and a score of 3 for blanching on the

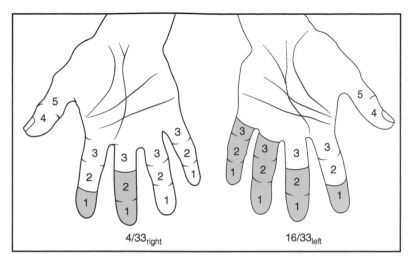

FIGURE 9.19   Method of scoring the areas of the digits affected by blanching. Source: From Griffin (1990).

proximal phalanx. On the thumbs, the scores are 4 for the distal phalanx and 5 for the proximal phalanx. The scores can be used to track the progression or regression of finger blanching. They do not take into account frequency of attacks, or functional disability.

- The Stockholm Workshop Scale provides a separate staging for the vascular and the sensorineural component of HAVS (Table 9.9). If a person has stage 2 vascular with three fingers of the left hand affected and stage 1 vascular with three fingers on the right hand, the condition is reported as 2VL(3)/1VR(3) with a separate staging for any sensorineural component according to the Stockholm Workshop Scale. Lawson and McGeogh proposed further subdivision of the vascular and sensorineural stage 2 into 'early' and 'late' stages and this has been adopted by the UK HSE. Individuals at late stage 2 are more likely to progress to functional incapacity, and this staging can be used to indicate when removal from further exposure may prevent significant disability.

Management of HAVS

- The principle underlying prevention of HAVS is a reduction in exposure to hand-transmitted vibration. This may be done through engineering control measures, better maintenance of machinery, selection of appropriate tools and providing information, instruction and training for exposed workers. The main emphasis on management should be prevention of new cases and prevention of deterioration of current cases. A clear policy for HAVS and vibration exposure in the workplace is essential.
- Health surveillance is required when the risk assessment indicates a risk to workers' health. This must be instituted for workers exposed regularly to vibration levels above the EAV (2.5 m s^{-2} A(8)). This should also be

TABLE 9.9

Stockholm Workshop Scale.

(a) Vascular effects

Stage	Grade	Description
0		No attacks
1	Mild	Occasional attacks affecting only the tips of one or more fingers
2	Moderate	Occasional attacks affecting the distal and middle (rarely also proximal) phalanges of one or more fingers
3	Severe	Frequent attacks affecting all phalanges of most fingers
4	Very severe	As in stage 3, with trophic skin changes in the fingertips

(b) Sensorineural effects

Stage	Symptoms
0_{SN}	Exposed to vibration, but no symptoms
1_{SN}	Intermittent numbness with or without tingling
2_{SN}	Intermittent or persistent numbness, reduced sensory perception
3_{SN}	Intermittent or persistent numbness, reduced tactile discrimination and/or manipulative dexterity

considered for workers with lower vibration exposures and those diagnosed with HAVS, even if their exposures are below the EAV. Hand-transmitted vibration exposures of less than $1\,m\,s^{-2}$ A(8) are generally considered to be without adverse effects. The HSE suggests a tiered system for health surveillance that includes monitoring by individuals with different levels of competence and expertise, with activities ranging from use of a simple questionnaire (pre-placement and screening questionnaires), through clinical history and examination to diagnosis and optional special standardised tests.

- Clinical treatment of the affected individual. Pharmacological (e.g. nifedipine or amlodipine, both of which are calcium antagonists, used orally or topically, and rarely prostaglandin analogues) are of limited value and can make assessment of progression more difficult. Cessation or reduction of cigarette smoking is advisable.

Tools and processes causing hand-transmitted vibration

Table 9.8 lists the processes and tools that are often associated with vibration injuries.

Whole-body vibration

Various industrial machines and all forms of transport cause whole-body vibration.

Vibration magnitude

The absolute threshold for the perception of vertical whole-body vibration in the frequency range 1–100 Hz is approximately $0.01\,\mathrm{m\,s^{-2}}$ r.m.s.; a magnitude of $0.1\,\mathrm{m\,s^{-2}}$ r.m.s. will be easily noticeable; magnitudes around $1\,\mathrm{m\,s^{-2}}$ r.m.s. are usually considered to be uncomfortable; and magnitudes of $10\,\mathrm{m\,s^{-2}}$ r.m.s. are usually dangerous. The precise values depend on the vibration frequency and exposure duration and are different for other axes of vibration. A doubling of the vibration magnitude (expressed in $\mathrm{m\,s^{-2}}$) produces an approximate doubling of discomfort. A halving of the vibration magnitude can therefore produce a considerable improvement in comfort.

Vibration frequency and direction

The dynamic responses of the body and the relevant physiological and psychological processes dictate that subjective reactions to vibration depend on the vibration frequency and vibration direction.

Vibration duration

Vibration discomfort tends to increase with increasing duration of exposure to vibration. The precise rate of increase may depend on many factors, but a simple 'fourth power' time dependence is sometimes used to approximate how discomfort varies with exposure duration from the shortest possible shock to a full day of vibration exposure (i.e. [acceleration]^4 × duration = constant).

Health effects

The most consistent health effect reported is low back pain. Other symptoms with varying supportive evidence include headaches and motion sickness, sleep and visual disturbances, and urinary and abdominal symptoms.

Control of exposure to whole-body vibration

Wherever possible, elimination or the reduction of vibration at source is preferred. Methods of reducing the transmission of vibration to operators – whether it be a reduction in the amplitude or alteration of the frequency of that vibration – requires an understanding of the characteristics of the vibration environment and the route for the transmission of vibration to the body. Preventive measures include the appropriate design and selection of seats for vehicles; the selection of commensurate vibration damping material and suspension options for vehicular seats; maintenance of seats and vehicles; consideration of good ergonomics and posture for drivers; and medical advice to exposed individuals (Griffin 2005).

9.5 Pressure

Within the Earth's atmosphere, humans are exposed to atmospheric or barometric pressure – variously measured in pounds per square inch, millimetres of mercury or in SI units: newtons per square metre (pascals). Conveniently, the atm unit of measure equates to the pressure at sea level: 1 atm, 1 bar, 14.7 lb in^{-2} or 101 kPa (1 Pa = 1 N m^{-2}). One metre of sea water (1 msw) is equal to 0.1 bars. Pressure varies with the altitude from the surface, and the depth of the water column. At the sea water surface, pressure is 1 atm and increases by 1 atm for every 10 m depth, so at 10 msw/33 feet seawater (fsw)/29.4 psi = 2 atm. Exposure to rapid changes in pressure can be rapidly fatal, but, in occupational health, the main occupational groups exposed to controlled pressure changes are:

- divers – scientific and archaeological; media, e.g. photographers and journalists; offshore oil and gas workers; inshore civil engineering, marine project or aquaculture workers; diving instructors; members of the police and armed forces
- caisson (tunnel) workers
- high-flying aviators.

The first two groups (divers, caisson workers) experience *increased* pressures; the last (aviators) *decreased* pressures. Most of the ill effects of pressure in working environments result from decompression stress. These are as follows:

- Direct effects due to barotrauma (Boyle's law) related to gas expansion: ruptured tympanic membrane, ruptured alveoli, sinus pain and dental cavity pain, arterial gas embolism (AGE).
- Indirect effects due to nitrogen dissolved in the blood at increased pressure, potentially causing narcosis (Dalton's law), and being released as bubbles on rapid decompression (Henry's law); the myriad of potential manifestations that occur as nitrogen bubbles form, and potentially block blood vessels and damage tissues through complex mechanisms, is called *decompression sickness*. Decompression sickness has historically been classified as type I or type II (neurological) but, in practice, it is often more practical to consider a description of the clinical manifestations, which can include pulmonary, cutaneous, spinal, cerebral, inner ear and lymphatic presentations.
- Other associated effects, e.g. immersion pulmonary oedema, hypothermia, the effects of medications under pressure, dysbaric osteonecrosis, high-pressure neurological syndrome associated with HeliOx diving (Table 9.10).

The nature of decompression sickness depends on the rate and degree of decompression and on the site of nucleation or impaction of bubbles; the effects can range from minor discomfort to death. Symptom onset occurs within hours post surfacing for most cases and within 24 hours for almost all cases. Dive tables are used to guide the rate of resurfacing for divers, who should follow varying rates of ascent or add pauses (decompression stops) dependent on the depth and time dived in order to allow dissolved gas to be expelled slowly instead of expanding to form bubbles. For compressed air tunnelling work decompression tables are used that vary by country, with most now requiring the use of oxygen

TABLE **9.10**		

The symptoms of decompression sickness types I and II.

Presentation	
Type I	Mild to severe limb pain
	Skin itching
	Skin mottling – 'marbling' (cutis marmorata)
	Swelling and pain in lymph nodes
Type II	Weakness or fatigue
	Sensory or motor nerve effects to the limbs
	Dizziness – 'staggers'
	Headaches
	Breathlessness
	Chest pains – 'chokes'
	Convulsions
	Coma
Sequelae	Permanent neurological or cerebral effects
	Aseptic bone necrosis

during the latter part of decompression. Treatment of decompression sickness involves recompression in a hyperbaric chamber. This has the effect of squeezing bubbles down in size, relieving local pressure effects and restoring blood flow, which allows time for bubble resorption and increases both the blood oxygen content and tissue delivery. Hyperbaric treatment uses tried and tested treatment tables that govern the exact times and 'depths' for repressurisation. These are often based on those of the US Navy, Royal Navy or the Canadian Defense and Civil Institute of Environmental Medicine (DCIEM).

The assessment of workers for diving requires careful selection and medical surveillance, which in the UK must be carried out by medical practitioners approved by the HSE. Requirements vary by international jurisdiction but physicians should have training to at least Level 1 – Medical assessment of divers (Medical Examiner of Divers). Particular attention is paid to the previous medical history, medications, dental and otological health, assessment of cardiorespiratory fitness and spirometry with additional examination or investigation as required. A return-to-work medical assessment requires specific examination of the possible effects of the particular illness or injury on diving safety and the ability to undertake diving work. Return to work following decompression illness (DCI) requires careful risk assessment. The relationship between a patent foramen ovale or other right-to-left shunts and neurological, vestibular, cutaneous and cardiorespiratory DCI is increasingly well understood and additional assessment for PFO as an underlying contributor, might be worthy of consideration particularly in severe cases.

9.6 Radiation

Radiation is energy that is transmitted, emitted or absorbed in the form of particles or waves. The effect of such radiation on living tissue is variable, but the ability of this energy to ionise the target tissue distinguishes the two main sections of the electromagnetic spectrum: ionising radiation and non-ionising radiation. The range of the whole spectrum is enormous (Figure 9.20).

Ionising radiation

Ionising radiation is of two main types: electromagnetic and particulate. The electromagnetic group includes X-rays and gamma (γ) rays, and the particulate group includes electrons (beta [β] particles), protons, neutrons and alpha (α) particles. The degree of activity is measured in units of disintegration per second (becquerels, Bq), while the effects of radiation, such as the absorbed radiation dose, are measured in grays (Gy). To compare the effects of different radiations with a reference standard, the absorbed dose is multiplied by a weighting factor. The product is called the equivalent dose and is measured in sieverts (Sv).

The health effects of ionising radiation can be divided into non-stochastic and stochastic, i.e. effects for which there is a threshold (and thus a progression of severity of effect with dose) and effects for which there is no threshold. These are as follows.

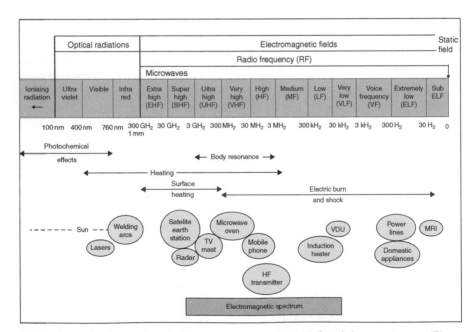

FIGURE 9.20 The electromagnetic spectrum. By convention, wavelength (nanometres to millimetres) is used for optical radiation and frequency (gigahertz to hertz) for electromagnetic fields. MRI, magnetic resonance imaging; VDU, video display unit.

Non-stochastic:
- acute radiation syndrome – gut, blood, central nervous system (CNS)
- delayed – cataracts, dermatitis.

Stochastic:
- cancer, genetic damage.

The major consequence of radiation exposure is a shortening of life, acutely so for doses in excess of 5–10 Gy, whereas lower doses will produce late effects, such as cancer one to four years after exposure. There are three clinically important radiation syndromes following acute exposure:

- 30–100 Gy – CNS damage leading to death from cerebral oedema within hours
- 10–30 Gy – gastrointestinal syndrome with nausea, vomiting and diarrhoea; dehydration and overwhelming infection lead to death within days
- 1–10 Gy – haemopoietic damage, with loss of peripheral cellular components and destruction of stem cells; death occurs within a few weeks from bleeding and overwhelming infection.

Occupational exposures are at lower levels, but are more prolonged. Thus, it is the neoplastic risk that is uppermost in most people's minds. The tumour site will depend on whether the source of radiation 'seeks' out a particular organ (e.g. iodine-131 and the thyroid, strontium-90 and bone) and on the site irradiated. Rapidly dividing cells are particularly radiosensitive; hence, the bone marrow, gonads and gastrointestinal mucosa are at particular risk. Additionally, care must be taken to protect target organs incapable or only slowly capable of repair (e.g. the ocular lens and nerve tissue).

Safe dose limits are recommended by the International Commission on Radiological Protection (ICRP), and have been adopted by the HSE, as published in the Ionising Radiations Regulations 2017.

SCHEDULE 3 – Dose limits
PART 1 Classes of persons to whom dose limits apply
Employees and trainees of 18 years of age or above

1. For the purposes of regulation 12(1), the limit on effective dose for any employee or trainee, being of 18 years of age or above, is 20 mSv in any calendar year.
2. Without prejudice to paragraph 1–
   a. the limit on equivalent dose for the lens of the eye is–
      i. 20 mSv in a calendar year; or
      ii. in accordance with conditions approved by the Executive from time to time, 100 mSv in any period of five consecutive calendar years subject to a maximum equivalent dose of 50 mSv in any single calendar year;
   b. the limit on equivalent dose for the skin is 500 mSv in a calendar year as applied to the dose averaged over any area of 1 cm^2 regardless of the area exposed;
   c. the limit on equivalent dose for the extremities is 500 mSv in a calendar year.

Trainees aged under 18 years

3. For the purposes of regulation 12(1), the limit on effective dose for any trainee under 18 years of age is 6 mSv in any calendar year.
4. Without prejudice to paragraph 3–
    a. the limit on equivalent dose for the lens of the eye is 15 mSv in a calendar year;
    b. the limit on equivalent dose for the skin is 150 mSv in a calendar year as applied to the dose averaged over any area of 1 cm^2 regardless of the area exposed;
    c. the limit on equivalent dose for the extremities is 150 mSv in a calendar year.

Other persons

5. Subject to paragraph 6, for the purposes of regulation 12(1) the limit on effective dose for any person other than an employee or trainee referred to in paragraph 1 or 3, including any person below the age of 16, is 1 mSv in any calendar year.
6. Paragraph 5 does not apply in relation to any person (not being a carer and comforter) who may be exposed to ionising radiation resulting from the medical exposure of another and in such a case the limit on effective dose for any such person is 5 mSv in any period of five consecutive calendar years.
7. Without prejudice to paragraphs 5 and 6–
    a. the limit on equivalent dose for the lens of the eye is 15 mSv in any calendar year;
    b. the limit on equivalent dose for the skin is 50 mSv in any calendar year averaged over any 1 cm^2 area regardless of the area exposed;
    c. the limit on equivalent dose for the extremities is 50 mSv in a calendar year.

PART 2

8. For the purposes of regulation 12(2), the limit on effective dose for employees or trainees of 18 years or above is 100 mSv in any period of five consecutive calendar years subject to a maximum effective dose of 50 mSv in any single calendar year.
9. Without prejudice to paragraph 8–
    a. the limit on equivalent dose for the lens of the eye is–
        i.   20 mSv in a calendar year; or
        ii. in accordance with conditions approved by the Executive from time to time, 100 mSv in any period of five consecutive calendar years subject to a maximum equivalent dose of 50 mSv in any single calendar year;
    b. the limit on equivalent dose for the skin is 500 mSv in a calendar year as applied to the dose averaged over any area of 1 cm^2 regardless of the area exposed;
    c. the limit on equivalent dose for the extremities is 500 mSv in a calendar year.

10. The employer must ensure that any employee in respect of whom regulation 12(2) applies is not exposed to ionising radiation to an extent that any dose limit specified in paragraphs 8 or 9 is exceeded.

11. An employer must not put into effect a system of dose limitation pursuant to regulation 12(2) unless–
    a. the radiation protection adviser and any employees who are affected have been consulted;
    b. any employees affected and the approved dosimetry service have been informed in writing of the decision and of the reasons for that decision; and
    c. notice has been given to the appropriate authority at least 28 days (or such shorter period as the appropriate authority may allow) before the decision is put into effect giving the reasons for the decision.

12. Where there is reasonable cause to believe that any employee has been exposed to an effective dose greater than 20 mSv in any calendar year, the employer must, as soon as is practicable–
    a. undertake an investigation into the circumstances of the exposure for the purpose of determining whether the dose limit referred to in paragraph 8 is likely to be complied with; and
    b. notify the appropriate authority of that suspected exposure.

13. An employer must review the decision to put into effect a system of dose limitation pursuant to regulation 12(2) at appropriate intervals and in any event not less than once every five years.

14. Where as a result of a review undertaken pursuant to paragraph 13 an employer proposes to revert to a system of annual dose limitation pursuant to regulation 12(1), the provisions of paragraph 11 apply as if the reference in that paragraph to regulation 12(2) was a reference to regulation 12(1).

15. Where an employer puts into effect a system of dose limitation in pursuance of regulation 12(2), the employer must record the reasons for that decision and must ensure that the record is preserved until any person subject to the system of dose limitation under regulation 12(2) has or would have attained the age of 75 years but in any event for at least 30 years from the making of the record.

16. In any case where–
    a. the dose limits specified in paragraph 8 are being applied by an employer in respect of an employee; and
    b. the appropriate authority is not satisfied that it is impracticable for that employee to be subject to the dose limit specified in paragraph 1 of Part 1 of this Schedule, the appropriate authority may require the employer to apply the dose limit specified in paragraph 1 of Part 1 with effect from such time as the appropriate authority may consider appropriate having regard to the interests of the employee concerned.

17. In any case where, as a result of a review undertaken pursuant to paragraph 13, an employer proposes to revert to an annual dose limitation in accordance with regulation 12(1), the appropriate authority may require the employer to defer the implementation of that decision to such time as the appropriate authority may consider appropriate having regard to the interests of the employee concerned.

To put this in perspective, let us consider the average person's dose in the UK (which is probably less than 2 mSv). This is made up of the following radiation components:

- cosmic 13%
- gamma (γ) 16% (mainly building materials)
- radon 33%
- medical 20.7%
- fall-out 0.4%
- occupational 0.4%
- discharges 0.1%
- miscellaneous 0.4%.

Occupational exposure is not therefore a major factor in normal radiation dosage, but it is a potential danger for a large number of workers (estimated to be in excess of seven million workers in the USA).

- *Justification*. No practice shall be undertaken involving radiation unless it is likely to bring net benefit.
- *Optimisation*. Radiation doses and risks should be kept 'as low as reasonably achievable' (ALARA).
- *Dose limits*. No individual shall be exposed to radiation in excess of that recommended by the ICRP.

Various instruments are available for radiological protection. They include:

- ionisation chambers
- Geiger–Müller tubes
- scintillation counters
- proportional counters
- film badges
- thermoluminescent dosemeters.

All the above are capable of being portable. Whereas the first four are electronic, measure current radiation levels and are capable of giving audible and visible warning signals, the last two are measures of cumulative exposure and are the usual devices worn by radiation workers. No one instrument is capable of detecting or measuring all forms of radiation – α, β, γ and X-rays. Most are usually designed to monitor the most penetrating radiations, such as γ or X-rays.

Control can be summarised in three words:

- time
- distance
- shielding.

The first is obvious; the second is important because, for radiation, the inverse square law applies, i.e. trebling the distance from the source reduces the radiation dose to one-tenth. Shielding will vary with the type of radiation source. Paper or water may be effective enough for α and β rays, but thicker, denser materials, such as lead or concrete, may be required for X-rays.

All that has gone before relates mainly to external sources of radiation. 'Internal' radiation must also be considered; thus it is important to make sure that the radiation source cannot penetrate the skin, be inhaled or be swallowed. Once inside, so to speak, removal of the source of radiation is a complicated and frequently incomplete procedure. Thus prevention of absorption is of paramount importance.

The legal requirements are listed below.

- Radioactive Material (Road Transport) Regulations 2002
- Ionising Radiations Regulations 1999
- Working with ionising radiation. Ionising Radiations Regulations 2017. Approved Code of Practice and guidance.

For a much more detailed description of ionising radiation, its measurement and control, see Chapter 22 by Ronald Clayton in *Occupational Hygiene* (Clayton 2005).

Non-ionising radiation

For practical purposes, the two most important sources of non-ionising radiation are lasers and microwaves. Both are capable of producing localised heating of tissues, which may be intense and dangerous, and both may be either continuous wave or pulsed.

The instrumentation required for the measurement of *laser radiation* is complex owing to the wide range of wavelengths and energies exhibited by commercial laser systems. Control measures largely revolve around instrument shielding and/or personal protective clothing, such as goggles.

Microwave exposure limits vary in different countries. Table 9.11 provides a summary of those that have set standards. The devices used to monitor such radiations are usually small dipoles consisting of a diode or thermocouple device for converting microwave energy into electrical energy, which can then be measured by a voltmeter. Control measures to limit exposure consist of effective containment of the microwaves within the apparatus concerned. Mesh screens or even concrete may occasionally be used, but personal protective clothing is rarely involved.

During the past few years, great interest has been created over the possible health effects of radiowaves and electric power lines. The frequency ranges from 30 Hz to 30 GHz, an enormous spectrum. For electric power lines, the range is 50–300 Hz and, because of the increasing exposure of the general public and occupational groups alike, recent epidemiological studies provide some cause for concern. The putative health risks are leukaemia and brain cancer. However, the most recent studies of electricity generation and transmission workers have failed to resolve the issue. Some suggest modest rises in risk for brain cancer,

TABLE 9.11

Exposure (Wm⁻²).

Country	Continuous	Intermittent	Maximum
UK	100	$10\,(0.1\,h^{-1})$	500
USA	100	$10\,(0.1\,h^{-1})$	250
Poland	2	32	100
Sweden, Czech Republic and Canada		$Time = \dfrac{32}{\left(power\ surface\ density\right)^2}$	
Russia	0.1	–	10

Power surface density levels are set in units of watts per square metre.

others for acute myeloid leukaemia, but pooling the data does not lead to any clear-cut excess risk (similar conclusions are obtained for studies of children and adults living near overhead power lines).

One of the problems is the poor quality of retrospective exposure assessments. Another problem relates to the immense complexity of finding a valid exposure measure – or even an instrument that will accurately assess exposures. Indeed, it is not clear whether the relevant exposure is the electric field or the magnetic field, or a combination of the two. There is no doubt that occupational exposures can be higher in certain industrial processes – such as electric arc furnaces, welding or induction heating processes.

Exposures to radiowaves were, in the past, largely restricted to radiomast maintenance personnel, but the explosion in the growth of cellular telephone communication has highlighted the risk of exposure. The risk to mobile phone users is unquantified at present, but the dose is clearly concentrated close to the brain – and, indeed, the salivary glands.

A much more detailed description of non-ionising radiation, its measurement and control is given in Chapter 21 by Philip Chadwick in *Occupational Hygiene* (Chadwick 2005).

References

Chadwick, P. (2005). Non-ionizing radiation: electromagnetic fields and optical radiation. In: *Occupational Hygiene*, 3e (eds. K. Gardiner and J.M. Harrington), 307–327. Oxford: Blackwell Publishing.

Clayton, R. (2005). Ionizing radiation: physics, measurement, biological effects and control. In: *Occupational Hygiene*, 3e (eds. K. Gardiner and J.M. Harrington), 328–343. Oxford: Blackwell Publishing.

Gardiner, K. (2005). Noise. In: *Occupational Hygiene*, 3e (eds. K. Gardiner and J.M. Harrington), 222–249. Oxford: Blackwell Publishing.

Griffin, M.J. (1990). *Handbook of Human Vibration*. London: Academic Press.

Smith, N.A. (2005). Light and lighting. In: *Occupational Hygiene*, 3e (eds. K. Gardiner and J.M. Harrington), 268–285. Oxford: Blackwell Publishing.

Youle, A. (2005). The thermal environment. In: *Occupational Hygiene*, 3e (eds. K. Gardiner and J.M. Harrington), 286–306. Oxford: Blackwell Publishing.

Further Reading

Divers Alert Network. www.dan.org. Accessed 26 November 2021.

Diving Medical Advisory Committee. www.dmac-diving.org. Accessed 26 November 2021.

Griffin, M., Bovenzi, M., Seidel H., Lundstrom, R., Hulshof, C, Donati, P. (2007). *Risks of Occupational Vibration Exposures: VIBRISKS*. EC FP5 project no. QLK4–2002-02650. Quality of Life and Management of Living Resources Programme, January 2003 to December 2006. http://www.vibrisks.soton.ac.uk.

CHAPTER 10

Musculoskeletal Disorders

10.1 Introduction

Musculoskeletal disorders include conditions that are caused, or aggravated, by work and the way in which it is performed. Work-related musculoskeletal disorders can be considered to be those where the work environment and the way in which work is performed contribute significantly but to differing degrees to the causation of the condition. Although the locomotor system gives rise to these symptoms both their onset and persistence can be multifactorial, meaning that it is important to consider biopsychosocial factors and to address these as necessary. Musculoskeletal disorders are among the most common reasons for sickness absence and occupational insurance claims. Back pain and problems affecting the upper limbs are most common, although the lower limbs can also be affected. Since these conditions can be chronic the prevalence is high; there are also a significant number of new cases annually. The discipline of ergonomics is important in the design of workplaces as well as in the recognition and remediation of poor workplace practices and environments.

10.2 Low back pain

Pain experienced on the dorsum from the lower margin of the 12th ribs to the lower gluteal folds is considered to be lower back pain. It may or may not be accompanied by pain referred to the legs. Although most people with new-onset

Pocket Consultant: Occupational Health, Sixth Edition. Kerry Gardiner, David Rees, Anil Adisesh, David Zalk, and Malcolm Harrington.
© 2022 John Wiley & Sons Ltd. Published 2022 by John Wiley & Sons Ltd.

low back pain get better in a few weeks, up to one-third experience symptoms for more than one year. For those people who experience symptoms for longer than three months there is a 50% chance that they will still have pain one year later. Early intervention when back pain has lasted for 6–12 weeks is therefore important.

Low back pain may result from a specific incident at work (or outside of work) or it may be insidious and appear gradually without an identified incident. Contributory factors are:

- trauma to the lower back
- poor posture
- poor techniques for lifting or carrying heavy objects
- exposure to whole-body vibration.

Clinical assessment

- The single best predictor of future low back pain and associated sickness absence is a previous history of the same.
- Individual psychosocial factors contribute to a small risk for onset of low back pain in those not previously affected. A patient's positive expectations of recovery are related to a higher likelihood of returning to work. Other aspects of personal function, limitations in activity and pain experience are also related to recovery. Tools such as the Örebro Musculoskeletal Pain Questionnaire can help in the assessment of these 'yellow flags' (Table 10.1).
- Clinical examination can be an important component of treatment for patient reassurance as well as for detecting any unsuspected medical conditions. A useful sequence of examination is given by the Institute for Work & Health (https://www.iwh.on.ca/publications/3-minute-primary-care-low-back-pain-examination).

TABLE 10.1

Yellow flags – recognition.

Questions to ask:	Look for:
'Do you think your pain will improve or become worse?'	Belief that back pain is harmful or potentially severely disabling.
'Do you think you would benefit from activity, movement or exercise?'	Fear and avoidance of activity or movement.
'How are you emotionally coping with your back pain?'	Tendency to low mood and withdrawal from social interaction.
'What treatments or activities do you think will help you recover?'	Expectation of passive treatment(s) rather than a belief that active participation will help.

Source: Centre for Effective Practice, https://cep.health/tool/download/19.

TABLE 10.2

Red flags – recognition and action.

Cause (mnemonic 'NIFTI')	Presentation	Investigation and referral
Neurological	Cauda equina syndrome	MRI indicated EMERGENCY referral within hours
	Diffuse motor/sensory loss, progressive neurological deficits, age of onset >50 for first ever episode of serious back pain	MRI indicated SOON referral within weeks
Infection	Fever, IV drug use, immune suppressed	X-ray and MRI URGENT referral within 24–48 hours
Fracture	Trauma, osteoporosis risk/fragility fracture	X-ray and may require CT scan URGENT referral within 24–48 hours
Tumour	History of cancer, unexplained weight loss, significant unexpected night pain, severe fatigue	X-ray and MRI URGENT referral within 24–48 hours
Inflammation	Chronic low back pain >3 months, age of onset <45, morning stiffness >30 minutes, improves with exercise, disproportionate night pain	Rheumatology consultation and guidelines

CT, computed tomography; IV, intravenous; MRI, magnetic resonance imaging. Sources: Adapted from McMaster University and CEP, Clinically Organized Relevant Exam (CORE) Back Tool.

- Assessment should include evaluation for the presence of 'red flags' (Table 10.2).

Investigations

- The use of imaging and blood tests should be guided by the presence of red flags. In chronic low back pain, radiographs of the lumbar spine are very poor indicators of serious pathology.
- Functional testing by machine does not correlate well with sustained return to work.

Clinical and occupational management of cases

- Evaluation should include assessment for psychosocial risk factor 'yellow flags' to identify those at risk to allow early intervention both clinically and in the workplace as this has shown substantially improved outcomes.
- Paracetamol (acetaminophen) and/or non-steroidal anti-inflammatory drugs (NSAIDs) should be sufficient for most causes of mechanical low back pain, although patients with radiculopathy may require opioids for a brief period if the pain does not respond to initial treatment. However opioids have not led to benefit greater than that of NSAIDs, and opioids cause the most harms.
- Advice should encourage activity and exercises, which can be tailored according to the type of lower back pain.
- Continuing at, or returning to, work within the limitations of discomfort with appropriate work modifications should be considered and discussed.
- Being off work for a protracted period for low back pain reduces the likelihood of permanent and full return to work duties.
- Multidisciplinary biopsychosocial rehabilitation for people with low back pain lasting 6–12 weeks results in less pain and disability, increased likelihood of return to work and fewer sick leave days at 12-month follow-up.

Prevention

- Following treatment for low back pain, exercises can reduce both the rate and the number of recurrences of back pain.
- For healthy people changing work break frequencies or types of breaks does not seem to be effective in changing reported musculoskeletal pain, discomfort and fatigue.
- Lumbar supports (back braces or corsets) are not a useful preventive measure for people with low back pain.

10.3 Work-related upper limb disorders

Work-related problems of the shoulders, arms, wrists, hands and fingers are one type of work-related musculoskeletal disorder (WRMSD) and are frequently referred to as 'repetitive strain injury' (RSI) by both patients and healthcare providers. The latter term is problematic because there is often no evidence of 'injury', while 'strain' implies excessive tensile force subjected onto the muscle and movements do not have to be 'repetitive' since prolonged static loading can also cause discomfort. It is also sometimes used when a more precise diagnosis can, and should, be made.

Synonyms

- Repetitive motion injuries
- Cumulative trauma disorder (CTD)
- Occupational overuse syndrome (OOS)
- Work-related repetitive movement injury (WRRMI)

Presentation

Patients may present with a variety of soft tissue complaints, including swelling, paraesthesiae, tenderness, stiffness, fatigue, sleep problems and mood changes. There may be some overlap of symptoms with those of fibromyalgia. However the prevalence of these conditions declines at older ages and they predominantly affect the 30–49 years age group.

Some work-related upper limb disorders (WRULDs) are ill-defined presentations of forearm pain or cramp; also included in this grouping are clinically well-recognised conditions that are broadly tendon-related disorders and peripheral nerve entrapment disorders:

- tenosynovitis (trigger finger)
- de Quervain's disease (thumbs)
- carpal tunnel syndrome (wrists)
- cubital tunnel syndrome (elbows)
- epicondylitis (elbows).

Risk factors

The main workplace physical risk factors are outlined in Box 10.1; however, there may be other contributory elements.

- *Non-occupational factors*. Where repetitive movements and other relevant exposures also occur from non-occupational activity, such as hobbies or household chores, these exposures can contribute to the clinical effects. However, with hobbies in particular, there is a degree of control over discontinuation of these non-occupational activities if necessary. Similar discretionary control may not be available in carrying out work tasks.
- *Previous injury* affecting the same sites may predispose to pain and discomfort. This depends on the nature and severity of the previous injury.
- *Individual susceptibility*. Some cases have been described in part-time rather than full-time workers, and sometimes in those with relatively minor manual tasks but not in others with considerable physical effort in the performance of work duties. This suggests that work activity is not the only determining factor in the development of WRULDs.
- *Psychosocial* – especially with monotonous work, where a bonus is paid depending on work output, e.g. 'piece work', or if work performance is affected

by peer pressure from supervisors or team members. High workloads, tight deadlines and lack of control over the work and working methods may make people more likely to develop and report WRULDs. Consider the applicability of the 'yellow flags' (Box 10.1).

Box 10.1 | Risk Factors for Work-Related Upper Limb Disorders (WRULDs)

Repetition

Repetitive elements in a task for more than approximately two hours per shift
Repeating the same movements every few seconds
Repeating a sequence of movements more than twice per minute
More than half of the time spent on that task involves performing the same sequence of movements

Postures

Awkward working postures for more than approximately two hours per shift
Large range of joint movements, e.g. side to side or up and down
Awkward or extreme joint positions
Joints held in fixed positions
Stretching to reach items or controls
Twisting or rotating items or controls
Working with hands above shoulder height

Force

Sustained or repeated forces for more than approximately two hours per shift
Pushing, pulling or moving things, including with the fingers or thumb
Grasping or gripping, including twisting and squeezing
Pinch grips, i.e. holding or grasping objects between thumb and finger
Steadying or supporting items or workpieces
Shock and/or impact being transmitted to the body from tools or equipment, including hands being used as a hammer
Equipment or work items creating concentrated pressure on any part of the upper limb, including pressure from a trigger or button

Vibration

Hand-transmitted vibration from any powered, hand-held or hand-guided tools, or hand-feed workpieces to vibrating equipment regularly (at some point during most shifts)

Source: Adapted from UK Health and Safety Executive 'Simple filter for identifying risks of upper limb disorders'.

- *Financial compensation.* Schemes for providing monetary benefits for work-related illnesses have been thought to contribute to the reporting of cases. This includes state-administered schemes as well as civil court claims. The extent may also be related to the perceived difficulty or ease of obtaining benefits.

Extent of the problem

The prevalence of WRULDs varies between countries: ranging from 4% to 28% in one European Union survey, with 10% of Canadians in a household survey reporting an upper limb condition, of which 55% were said to be work related. Of the estimated 480 000 workers affected by work-related musculoskeletal disorders in 2019–2020 the UK Health and Safety Executive reports that 44% affected the upper limbs or neck and that this accounted for 50% of the working days lost at 20.8 days per case. Across a number of studies from the general and working populations the point prevalence was reported as 1.6–53% and the 12-month prevalence was 2.3–41%. In the USA, an estimate of 8.23% or approximately 11.2 million workers were reported as having a WRULD in a 30-day period. In this group, 1.24% (1.7 million) said it affected their work. There is a lack of data for low- and middle-income countries, which probably relates to issues of case definition, a lack of national statistics, lack of regulatory support and the low availability of qualified occupational and safety professionals.

Some occupations and industries with a high prevalence of WRULDs are:

- poultry processing
- construction and mining
- electronics assembly
- textile workers
- mechanical components assembly line
- data processing
- telephonists
- checkout operators at supermarkets and stores.

WRULDs are more prevalent in women and in blue-collar workers.

Treatment

Clinical treatment provides varying degrees of relief from persistent symptoms. Treatment regimes vary depending on the severity, site and clinical findings. Procedures that have been tried include:

- surgery, e.g. carpal tunnel syndrome
- splinting during the acute stages, e.g. de Quervain's disease
- physiotherapy
- analgesics and NSAIDs
- local injection with hydrocortisone, e.g. lateral elbow epicondylitis

- ultrasound
- infrared and laser treatment
- acupuncture.

Where there are workplace risk factors including yellow flags, these treatment procedures are less likely to be effective unless accompanied by improvements in job design, psychosocial factors or ergonomics of the workplace.

Further Reading

Centre for Effective Practice (March 2016). Clinically Organized Relevant Exam (CORE) Back Tool. Toronto: Centre for Effective Practice. https://cep.health/tool/download/19

Choi, B.K.L., Verbeek, J.H., Tam, W.W.S., and Jiang, J.Y. (2010). Exercises for prevention of recurrences of low-back pain. *Cochrane Database of Systematic Reviews* (1): CD006555. https://doi.org/10.1002/14651858.CD006555.pub2. Accessed 30 December 2020.

Hayden, J.A., Wilson, M.N., Riley, R.D. et al. (2019). Individual recovery expectations and prognosis of outcomes in non-specific low back pain: prognostic factor review. *Cochrane Database of Systematic Reviews* (11): CD011284. DOI: https://doi.org/10.1002/14651858.CD011284.pub2. Accessed 30 December 2020. https://www.cochranelibrary.com/cdsr/doi/10.1002/14651858.CD011284.pub2/full.

Huisstede, B.M., Bierma-Zeinstra, S.M., Koes, B.W., and Verhaar, J.A. (2006). Incidence and prevalence of upper-extremity musculoskeletal disorders. A systematic appraisal of the literature. *BMC Musculoskeletal Disorders* 7: 7. https://doi.org/10.1186/1471-2474-7-7.

Luger, T., Maher, C.G., Rieger, M.A., and Steinhilber, B. (2019). Work-break schedules for preventing musculoskeletal symptoms and disorders in healthy workers. *Cochrane Database of Systematic Reviews* (7): CD012886. https://doi.org/10.1002/14651858.CD012886.pub2. Accessed 30 December 2020.

Marin, T.J., Van Eerd, D., Irvin, E. et al. (2017). Multidisciplinary biopsychosocial rehabilitation for subacute low back pain. *Cochrane Database of Systematic Reviews* (6): CD002193. DOI: https://doi.org/10.1002/14651858.CD002193.pub2. Accessed 30 December 2020. https://www.cochranelibrary.com/cdsr/doi/10.1002/14651858.CD002193.pub2/full.

CHAPTER 11

Psychosocial Aspects of the Workplace

11.1 Introduction

The benefits of work are recognised, as is the premise that work, in and of itself, should not harm workers. However, the increasing complexity, inclusive of ongoing change, of the structure of work, organisations and the work environment, has affected the psychological well-being of workers. Common mental health disorders, causing mild to moderate mental ill health, affect up to 20% of the working population and were estimated as costing 3.5% of gross domestic product (GDP) in European Union countries, with similar findings for the USA and Australia. Occupational health, in its practice and research, has a key role in supporting and sustaining workers' mental health. The occupational health role operates under a wider remit of

Pocket Consultant: Occupational Health, Sixth Edition. Kerry Gardiner, David Rees, Anil Adisesh, David Zalk, and Malcolm Harrington.
© 2022 John Wiley & Sons Ltd. Published 2022 by John Wiley & Sons Ltd.

11.6 Bullying, mobbing and harassment at work

What is workplace bullying?; Identifying workplace bullying; Who gets bullied and who does the bullying?; How can bullying affect your health?; Mental health effects of bullying

11.7 Gender at work

Gender-sensitive OSH practice; A continuing focus on gender mainstreaming

11.8 Role of occupational health practitioners in managing occupational stress

occupational safety and health (OSH), which has standards on workers' treatment and of what constitutes a healthy workplace. As such, a safe and healthy work environment considers 'psychosocial hazards' or 'work stressors' (to describe any factor that may be mentally distressing) that exist and is active in reducing their impact or removing them from the workplace. Employers have a duty of care to maintain the mental and physical health of their workforce. Despite this requirement, the available data and research around work hazards and stressors show that the work environment continues to cause workers to experience mental ill health and poorer psychological wellbeing. The work-relevant mental ill-health conditions that continue to prevail are occupational stress (work-related stress), anxiety and depression. It is useful to note that work-related fatigue is on the increase. This chapter focuses on occupational stress as it continues to have a major impact on workers and workplaces, and is well known as a workplace issue, both within and outside of organisations.

11.2 Occupational stress

The *biopsychosocial model* provides more context towards an understanding of occupational stress. It proposes less reliance on the biomedical model, i.e. acknowledging a direct disease-to-body connection, but rather accepts that psychosocial factors can adversely affect ill health as well. It proposes that the occurrence of 'somatic' and 'mental' disorders are not distinct, that they do interconnect and that they are influenced by social, psychological, behavioural and biological factors. This approach accepts the importance of considering the many and varied factors that can impinge on workers' mental health.

Occupational stress is not a condition that has a clear medical definition. It is accepted as a multifaceted condition that does not arise from one specific hazard or displays one specific symptom. It has a code in the 10th revision of the International Statistical Classification of Diseases and Related Health Problems (ICD-10) (Z56.6 – Other physical and mental strain related to work), thereby allowing its categorisation as a health-related problem, although it is not a diagnosis. The nature and proliferation of the condition has led to a plethora of models, theories and strategies on how best it could be defined, assessed and supported. These tend to focus on specific hazards or stressors, as identified within any particular context. However, one definition that is useful to highlight is that given in guidance on work-related stress prepared by the European Commission (2000), which states that it is:

> the emotional, cognitive, behavioural and physiological reaction to aversive and noxious aspects of work, work environments and work organisations. It is a state characterised by high levels of arousal and distress and often by feelings of not coping.
>
> *p. 3*

Responses to stress vary among individuals, even if the stressful situations appear the same for them; there is no universal profile of what would constitute a stressful situation for everyone. Occupational stress can often affect people when the demands placed upon them outweigh their ability to meet those demands. Demands arise from personal and occupational sources; when they occur in tandem without appropriate support systems in place, they may deplete coping mechanisms. For example, workers' personal circumstances, e.g. needing to look after a sick child or going through a divorce when dealing with a demanding workload with limited control on how to manage this, are important contributors to their ability to deal with occupational stressors effectively. Stress can also arise when workers are under-utilised – boredom and lack of challenge can be just as harmful as high demands. Such an imbalance can happen in all spheres of life, not just on the job, although workplaces are the most common arenas where individuals will have high demands or endure boredom.

The types of demands that can cause stress responses in workers can be either psychological or physical, or both. An added complication to this is that many individuals who are struggling with high job demands may hesitate to request support, preferring to try to complete the demands, and may ignore increasing signs of occupational stress until their behaviours or actions are raised with them. In addition to potential problems brought about by demands, a second important factor relates to how much control people have in meeting such demands. Many jobs may be highly demanding, but if employees have the resources, inclusive of autonomy, to manipulate how they can best meet such demands, this support system aids in creating jobs that can be rewarding and productive. Senior managers and executives may operate in these circumstances. Those jobs where individuals have limited autonomy in deciding their assigned workload and how to best manage high demands with which they are tasked are ones that could be seen as being stressful and could cause harm to the worker. Jobs with limited autonomy and no control over how workers choose to perform their tasks, conducted in an environment where workers may have little control over their surroundings (such as noise, lighting or temperature), are ones that could contribute to occupational stress. Junior doctors in hospitals and workers on factory lines are examples of individuals in these situations.

Sources of stress

Several factors can be identified in the workplace as stressors for individual workers. Some of these problems are potentially solvable and can be remedied by modifications to the workplace. Such causes can be categorised as shown in Table 11.1.

TABLE 11.1	
Potential workplace stressors.	
Content of job	*Workplace culture*
Overload of work	Poor and infrequent communication (management/workers)
Time pressures	Low involvement in decision-making
Deadlines	Infrequent and inconsistent feedback
Difficulty of work	Resources not provided
Under-loading (work too easy)	Poor support (management/workers)
Organisation of work	*Relationships*
Shift work	Poor and infrequent communication
Long working hours	Harassment
Unsociable working hours	Bullying
Unpredictable working hours	Verbal abuse
Restructuring	Physical abuse/intimidation
Non-consulted change	*Structure*
Constant change	Over-promotion (of self and others)
Work role	Under-promotion (of self and others)
Lack of clarity of job	Redundancy threats and precarious work arrangements
Conflict of interests	Pay structure/inequalities and imbalances in reward for effort
Conflict of beliefs	Unfairness of policies or their application
Environment	*Home–work interface*
Noise	Childcare issues
Temperature	Transport problems
Lighting	Commuting
Space	Relocation
Ergonomics	Housing issues
Hazard exposure	

The effects of stress

It can be difficult to always ascribe specific health problems confidently and clearly to the presence of psychosocial hazards in individuals' workplaces, although large-scale epidemiological evidence has demonstrated the contributory role of stress in the development of ill health. The health effects of occupational stress can be viewed as occurring on three distinct levels: psychological effects (such as worry, anxiety or depression), behavioural effects (drinking, eating or smoking more, arguing with colleagues and increased risk-taking) and physical effects (cardiovascular problems, a potential for musculoskeletal problems). It must be remembered that health effects attributed to stress can be either direct effects, such as decreases in cardiovascular wellbeing due to prolonged physiological changes in the stressed person, or indirect effects, such as lung cancer, exacerbated by the (behavioural) effects of smoking more while stressed.

The number and type of psychological or emotional symptoms exhibited by stressed individuals can vary greatly from person to person, as can the behaviours they may indulge in as a way of coping with increasing stress levels. Symptoms induced by stress are shown in Table 11.2.

TABLE 11.2

Common symptoms induced by stress.

Physical symptoms	Mental symptoms	Changes in behaviour
Aching muscles	Concentration problems	Avoiding specific places or people
Back pain	Constantly worrying	Carelessness or recklessness
Chest pain	Feeling overwhelmed	Confidence problems
Difficulty waking up	Forgetful	Eating too much or too little
Dizziness	Indecisive	Increased aggression
Fatigue	Nervousness	Increased irritation
Headaches	Obsessive thoughts	Increased use of alcohol, cigarettes or drugs
Immune system suppression	Struggling to make decisions	Insomnia
Loss of sexual interest		Poor time-keeping
Loss of appetite		Relationship difficulties
Nausea		Withdrawn
Palpitations		
Stomach problems		
Sweating		
Tiredness		
Tremor		

Some of the symptoms listed in Table 11.2 are known as non-specific symptoms and are often not directly related to the obvious psychosocial hazard in question. Many additional factors can affect the presence and severity of such symptoms in stressed workers. These can include perceptions and beliefs about the management and/or the organisation, as well as perceptions of intrusion by any investigation into the causes of the stress or by any interest shown by health experts, nurses or doctors. These influences upon symptomology can often heighten and exacerbate workers' stress levels, further increasing their susceptibility to potential hazards in the workplace.

Managing occupational stress

The management of occupational stress is likely to be unsuccessful unless a clear understanding of what may be causing the stress is gained. Many organisations and workplaces conduct surveys and interviews with their employees to ascertain the sources of stress and the workforce stress levels. Surveys are easily developed, tested, administered and analysed using electronic communication and appropriate software packages. This allows a fairly quick understanding of those stressors in the work environment that are affecting workers. It is essential that any workers who do not have access to electronic communication are provided with paper copies of the relevant survey to allow them to contribute. There are many freely available stress assessment tools that most organisations can use (see Section 11.5 for more quantitative objective measures).

Poor response rates to these questionnaires are not infrequent, so incentives to promote their completion by staff need to be considered. Senior management commitment to the entire process has to be obtained and communicated across the organisation at the start, with their guarantee to address any issues that arise from the research as soon as possible.

The best management of potential psychosocial problems in the workplace will contain the three types of interventions that are described below.

Primary interventions

Primary interventions occur at the organisational level and involve assessing the work environment to understand the preventative measures that should be put in place to eliminate or mitigate the occurrence of occupational stress. When sources of stress are identified that are potentially avoidable, they should always be addressed through the relevant organisational changes that tackle the specific cause or source of stress. In addition, organisational measures can reduce problems that may be intrinsic to the operations of concern to the organisation (e.g. in jobs with a realistic threat of customer-to-employee violence, the introduction of call-back procedures and buddy systems may help reduce employee stress). Primary interventions can include reduction of stressors external to the workplace, such as the provision of childcare facilities.

Secondary interventions

Secondary interventions are those that target teams or groups within organisations. They aim to detect those concerns that are more specific to teams rather than the wider organisation. Secondary interventions could include providing any required training to the team members, understanding the support systems within the teams to determine if anything else is required and/or implementing a peer support system. For example, resilience training might prove useful when jobs are expected to be inherently stressful, such as the emergency services or those that involve working with members of the public; in these cases, it is often appropriate to train workers in specific stress management or avoidance techniques. Some training is designed as a resource to manage stressful situations better when they develop, or to help employees better control such situations, such as aggression management or assertiveness skills. Other training can be aimed at enhancing individual coping techniques, such as personal stress management training or relaxation skills to minimise some of the effects of stress. Such training is useful, but is not a substitute for any primary intervention measures that could reasonably be taken.

Tertiary interventions

Tertiary interventions focus on the worker and treatment of the effects that arise from experiencing occupational stress. Organisations should consider having appropriate services in place, such as occupational health services and employee assistance programmes (EAPs), which workers can access as and when needed; also managers should consider seeking advice when they identify possible concerns. Workers may wish to see their physician/general practitioner at the onset to discuss their concerns and explore possible ways to deal with them.

For those who have suffered stress and may go on to exhibit severe effects, counselling services and specific medical treatment, e.g. for anxiety and depression, should be explored, and this may also be useful for unusual or dangerous incidents that could result in post-traumatic stress disorder (PTSD) for some individuals. Organisations may wish to consider incorporating specific interventions into their occupational health services/EAPs to address non-occupational difficulties that may be affecting an individual's work performance, such as substance misuse or relationship difficulties.

11.3 Potential long-lasting ill-health conditions

Post-traumatic stress disorder

While the occurrence of PTSD is rare in most jobs, it is a disorder that will have a devastating impact on those it affects. Despite the histories of shell shock and battle fatigue, PTSD was originally conceived by psychiatrists as a 'political' diagnosis specific to military personnel returning from the Vietnam War, but, in recent years, the diagnosis of PTSD has become widely recognised in non-military spheres. In some occupations, such as the emergency or uniformed services, individuals are increasingly likely to be exposed to traumatic or disturbing events and incidents. Such exposure could also occur in other occupations where traumatic incidents are not routinely expected. PTSD is listed by the International Labour Organization (ILO) as an occupational disease and is compensable in some jurisdictions. The occurrence of such unpredictable incidents can produce equally devastating effects for individuals. Some workers may, as a result of exposure to such events, suffer from this anxiety disorder, which is caused when individuals experience very stressful, frightening or distressing events, characterised by the following diagnostic criteria:

- experience of intense fear
- persistent re-experience of fearful event
- avoidance of associations with fearful event
- persistent increased arousal
- flashbacks to traumatic event
- hyperarousal – sleep and concentration problems; irritability.

PTSD, as a recognised and diagnosable psychiatric condition, can become chronic and disabling in individuals. Several types of interventions are worth considering for such affected individuals, such as those that utilise cognitive, behavioural and pharmaceutical help. These interventions should be conducted by appropriately trained professionals. Any treatment that individuals consider will depend on the severity of symptoms and how soon after the traumatic event they occurred.

Watchful waiting. Individuals monitor their symptoms to see whether they improve or get worse without treatment.

Eye movement desensitisation and reprocessing (EMDR). This requires individuals to recall a traumatic event while receiving bilateral stimulation. Bilateral stimulation involves receiving a stimulus that is heard, seen or felt in a rhythmic left–right pattern. It could involve individuals moving their eyes from side to side, tapping movements on opposite sides of their body or listening to tones through one ear then the other while wearing headphones. This treatment might not suit everyone.

Talking therapies. This would involve encouraging the sufferer (if willing or able) to talk through what has happened to them – either soon after the incident or after some time has elapsed; the timing is best dictated by the sufferer. Evidence for this can be mixed – it might work for those sufferers who want to talk about their experience but not for those who do not. A single talking session may be more harmful than helpful; a programme of therapy is therefore recommended.

Tackling avoidance issues. Tackling avoidance issues can be done by discussing and planning a gradual increase in activities with which the sufferer has problems, for example slowly returning to road travel after a car crash, by using graduated steps of exposure to road travel; again, the level of gradation is best dictated by the sufferer.

Coping with anxiety. Anxiety management techniques can be used to help the sufferer control their fears and stress level. Such techniques include learning methods of relaxation, distraction techniques and self-hypnosis.

Dealing with anger. Dealing with anger is a cognitive technique aiming to encourage the sufferer to discuss feelings concerning what has happened, and to make sure the sufferer does not blame him/herself unduly.

Overcoming sleep problems. In order to overcome sleep problems, the importance of regular sleep habits in coping with any distress should be emphasised, and the avoidance of excessive caffeine and alcohol use should be encouraged.

Treating associated depression. There may be a limited but crucial role for the use of antidepressants, hypnotics and anti-anxiety medication immediately after the traumatic incident.

Burnout

Burnout is a 'known' phenomenon in the workplace, with increased interest in its occurrence in recent times. There has been debate on how it should be categorised, and its inclusion in ICD-11 as an occupational phenomenon, but not as a medical condition, supports its relevance to the work environment. The World Health Organization (WHO) defines burnout as '. . .a syndrome conceptualised as resulting from chronic workplace stress that has not been successfully managed'. It notes that those who suffer from the syndrome display or have three sets of behaviours or attitudes: they feel that their energy is depleted or they feel exhausted; they feel mentally distant from their job, or they feel negative or cynical about their job; and they display reduced professional effectiveness. It is anticipated that burnout's established link to the occupational context, along with its clear definition, would help to remove some of the stigma associated with the phenomenon.

Burnout occurs when psychosocial hazards and stressors within the work environment are continuous and become more intense, and individuals do not have the resources in place to manage the stressors or are denied the resources to cope with the stressors. The work stressors that are most relevant to the syndrome are unfair treatment at work, an unmanageable workload and a lack of clarity about work role. Burnout can be reversed by taking appropriate action. This can entail taking an individual approach by leaving the organisation that is causing the burnout; changing job or position; seeking help from occupational health professionals; seeing a physician/general practitioner; or practising self-care: better sleep, nutrition, work–life balance, health and fitness. Other ways to improve those working conditions that are contributing to and causing the burnout are to change work patterns (e.g. by working fewer hours, taking more breaks, not working overtime, ensuring a balance between work and life); to develop a range of coping skills (these could include, for example, cognitive restructuring, conflict resolution, time management); to increase the social support that is available to the individual at work and at home; and to learn and use various relaxation strategies.

It is useful to note that the interventions to address burnout can occur at the individual, team/group or organisation level. However, most interventions tend to take place at the individual level, rather than eliminating or mitigating the psychosocial hazards at an organisational level. This is despite the research evidence of the benefits of focusing on situational factors at the onset, rather than on those personal or social factors that are secondary to the issue.

Moral injury

Similar to PTSD and burnout, moral injury tends to occur when a worker experiences traumatic or extremely stressful events. While moral injury is not considered as a mental illness, it can cause psychological distress. Workers may suffer moral injury when they commit, do not prevent or witness an event that goes against their deeply held moral beliefs, values, expectations or ethical codes of conduct. The experience of betrayal of what the worker considers as right by someone in 'legitimate authority' could also contribute to moral injury. Workers may feel shame, disgust, guilt or anger along with attributing negative self-beliefs because of their actions, and they may engage in maladaptive coping, such as substance abuse. It is these perceptions, beliefs and behaviours that are seen as contributing factors to succumbing to mental ill-health conditions, which could manifest as distress, depression and suicidality. It is important to note that a defined and valid treatment for moral injury is lacking at present, with an acknowledgement that the treatments and methods that are in place for mental ill health may not be suitable for this condition. Those techniques that are likely to support workers in this aspect of psychological distress are those that focus on moving forward positively, including taking a spiritual perspective, such as self-forgiveness, acceptance and self-compassion, and making amends for the wrong, if possible.

Moral injury has been mainly considered in military personnel and veterans, but can happen within other jobs, such as with healthcare workers during disasters and pandemics.

Severe fatigue/chronic fatigue syndrome

Severe fatigue, a serious inability to function both physically and mentally, can occur in as many as 3% of the working population at any one time. Chronic fatigue syndrome (CFS) was formerly known as myalgic encephalomyelitis or ME and is now often termed systemic exertion intolerance disease. It is a more contentious condition, with conflicting ideas about its cause, definition and even its existence. Similar to this condition is that of 'burnout', which is seen as being an extremely severe fatigue response to prolonged exposure to stress in the workplace. Possible causes of severe fatigue-type responses include viral infections, muscular problems, immune system problems and even psychological distress. Most evidence suggests that there are usually multiple causes of severe fatigue and chronic fatigue, with physical causes rarely being solely involved. As such, severe fatigue and chronic fatigue are seen as occurring more commonly in individuals who may be 'psychologically vulnerable' and who may also often be working under conditions they find stressful. CFS is a condition that can be very difficult to manage, and usually requires sensitive specialist psychiatric involvement.

Musculoskeletal disorders

The translation of many psychological stressors into physical disorders, such as cardiovascular disease and immunological disorders, is well documented. In addition, it can be seen that the amount of work may correlate with the severity of musculoskeletal complaints. However, much research indicates this this is too simplistic an explanation and that there are more complex mechanisms involved which link psychosocial hazards in the workplace with musculoskeletal problems. Some research has found musculoskeletal problems to be completely unrelated to the amount of physical exertion involved in a job, with such physical factors seemingly unimportant in comparison with the role psychosocial hazards play as predictors of musculoskeletal problems. Psychosocial hazards that have been linked with increased musculoskeletal problems are monotonous work, perceived high work load, lack of control, lack of social support and time pressures. For further discussion of musculoskeletal problems see Chapter 10.

11.4 Individual resources

External/internal locus of control

Individuals with a highly developed internal locus of control are those people who have a strong belief in the influence of their own decisions upon their personal circumstances. An internal locus of control can be seen as a hallmark of those who see themselves as self-motivated and believe they do things for themselves. In contrast, those individuals who believe that their situations are determined largely by other people or by chance, and who have a tendency towards powerlessness in their lives, are seen as having an external locus of control. It is those individuals with an external locus of control who are often psychologically vulnerable when faced with highly stressful situations, while those with an internal locus of control tend to be generally hardier and more resilient.

Coping mechanisms

The way in which individuals cope (wittingly or unwittingly) with a stressful or traumatic occupational situation will often be determined by their personality type as well as by other intrinsic psychological factors. Some types of coping can be seen to be *adaptive* in that they are positive steps to confront any problem and to seek a genuine long-term solution. Other types of coping may be seen as *maladaptive*, in that the individual may try to cope by drinking, smoking or eating more, or taking excessive sickness absence. Such maladaptive strategies can be seen as offering merely temporary or short-term solutions to any problem and may themselves result in further health problems. Stress management training and other forms of secondary intervention (as discussed in Section 11.2) tend to emphasise the use of adaptive strategies.

Self-efficacy

Self-efficacy is a construct that focuses on the belief that people have the capability to influence events that affect their lives, whether they are in their personal or work lives. It involves having the ability to regulate the self, by influencing how the individual feels, thinks, motivates themselves and behaves. An individual's level of self-efficacy could determine how effectively they cope with adverse experiences and challenges through the amount of effort they are willing to expend, and how long they will be able to sustain this effort, when faced with difficult situations. It has been shown to be a useful personal resource in increasing motivation and wellbeing, and in reducing the impact of mental ill health. Overall, individuals with high self-efficacy are more likely to attain daily benefits. These include being able to cope more effectively when faced with adversity and stress, developing healthy lifestyle habits, improving their performance, achieving educational goals and having a sense of personal accomplishment.

11.5 Psychological assessment of stress

There are many self-stress assessments that workers can complete by themselves. After simplicity of completion, the two most important aspects of any stress assessment are those of *validity* (in that the assessment actually measures work-related stress and not something else, for example a mental health problem) and *reliability* (if the assessment were to be completed a number of times by the same person, the outcome measure/stress score would be essentially similar). Results obtained from stress assessments can be very useful, not only in understanding what various sources of stress may be for workers but also in understanding what a sensible and effective solution would be. It is recommended that the results of stress assessments are not used in isolation, but in combination with other information that can be indicative of stress, such as sickness absence patterns, productivity or turnover. Some common examples of popular stress assessments are given below.

The Life Events Inventory

The Life Events Inventory (LEI) is a 55-item checklist that consists of potential stressful events that individuals may have experienced in the previous six months of taking the test. It is a self-complete test with respondents having to select a 'true positive' response if they had experienced any of the 55 listed events. The events in the LEI cover potentially distressing events from both the domestic and occupational domains, thereby providing a more holistic 'whole person' approach in determining psychological distress. Some example items (stated as an event) from the LEI are relevant to: 'Change in hours or conditions in present job', 'Getting into debt beyond means of repayment' and 'Trouble with superiors at work'.

The Copenhagen Psychosocial Questionnaire

The Copenhagen Psychosocial Questionnaire (COPSOQ) is widely used globally and has been validated in several countries. It is revised periodically; version III is the latest (COPSOQ-ISTAS is a Spanish adaptation). COPSOQ is an international instrument designed for the assessment and improvement of psychosocial conditions in workplaces and for research purposes. The COPSOQ guidance states that 'COPSOQ is designed as a tool for workplace psychosocial risk assessment and for organizational development. It is a generic tool, which can be used for all kind of jobs, in any industry and for workplaces of different sizes (private or public). From an operational perspective, it provides useful information for the prioritization of risk factors and to prompt preventive actions in workplaces.' It has short, middle and long versions for different settings, e.g. workplace surveys or formal research. Advantageous features are guidelines for its use and benchmark scores to compare workplace questionnaire findings with standard scores. The nature of the stressors and where they occur in workplaces are identified by the questionnaire so that interventions can be targeted. The questionnaire covers most relevant psychosocial domains (e.g. demand–control–social support, effort–rewards, job demands–resources, work–family conflict, social capital, socio-technical). One component of the questionnaire is shown in Table 11.3 to illustrate the type of questions asked.

The HSE Stress Indicator Tool for work-related stress

Several free tools are available to both measure stressors and analyse the findings obtained from the application of their questionnaires. Guides for the use of the tools and how to respond to findings accompany some of them. Several have algorithms embedded in them to analyse survey information and generate reports. It is advisable to discuss the suitability of specific tools with local experts as their utility will vary across countries and regions.

The Health and Safety Executive's (HSE) *Management Standards Indicator Tool* is a well-established tool (www.hse.gov.uk/stress/standards/downloads.htm).

The indicator tool is a free 35-item questionnaire, available in PDF format, based on the HSE's management standards on work-related stress. It is designed to be scored by the complementary HSE Management Standards Analysis Tool (Excel spreadsheet) to allow either stand-alone stress assessments or to form part of a larger company-wide survey. The HSE emphasises that the indicator tool should not be used as the only measure of stress within organisations. Some examples of items in the tool are shown in Table 11.4. In 2013, Canada produced the *National Standard of Canada for Psychological Health and Safety in the Workplace* to guide organisations in promoting mental health and preventing psychological harm at work, providing guidelines, tools and resources (https://www.mentalhealthcom-mission.ca/English/what-we-do/workplace/national-standard).

11.6 Bullying, mobbing and harassment at work

The total cost of bullying-related absenteeism, lost turnover and lost productivity for organisations in the UK was estimated at £13.75 billion in 2007. This reflected a 1.5% reduction in the overall productivity within the UK; when considered more widely,

TABLE 11.3

A section of the Copenhagen Psychosocial Questionnaire (COPSOQ).

Scale	Dimension name	Item name	Level	Question	Response options[a]
Quantitative demands	QD	QD1	MIDDLE	Is your workload unevenly distributed so it piles up?	1
		QD2	CORE	How often do you not have time to complete all your work tasks?	1
		QD3	CORE	Do you get behind with your work?	1
		QD4	LONG	Do you have enough time for your work tasks?	1R
Work pace	WP	WP1	CORE	Do you have to work very fast?	1
		WP2	CORE	Do you work at a high pace throughout the day?	2
		WP3	LONG	Is it necessary to keep working at a high pace?	2
Cognitive demands	CD	CD1	LONG	Do you have to keep your eyes on lots of things while you work?	1
		CD2	LONG	Does your work demand that you remember a lot of things?	1
		CD3	LONG	Does your work require that you are good at coming up with new ideas?	1
		CD4	LONG	Does your work require you to make difficult decisions?	1
Emotional demands	ED	ED1	MIDDLE	Does your work put you in an emotionally disturbing situation?	1
		ED2	CORE	Do you have to deal with other people's personal problems as part of your work?	1
		ED3	CORE	Is your work emotionally demanding?	2

(Continued)

TABLE 11.3 (Continued)

A section of the Copenhagen Psychosocial Questionnaire (COPSOQ).

Scale	Dimension name	Item name	Level	Question	Response options[a]
Demands for hiding emotions	HE	HE1	LONG	Are you required to treat everyone equally, even if you do not feel like it?	1
		HE2	MIDDLE	Does your work require that you hide your feelings?	2
		HE3	MIDDLE	Are you required to be kind and open towards everyone – regardless of how they behave towards you?	2
		HE4	MIDDLE	Does your work require that you do not state your opinion?	1
Influence at work	IN	IN1	CORE	Do you have a large degree of influence on the decisions concerning your work?	1
		IN2	LONG	Do you have a say in choosing who you work with?	1
		IN3	MIDDLE	Can you influence the amount of work assigned to you?	1
		IN4	MIDDLE	Do you have any influence on what you do at work?	1
		IN5	LONG	Can you influence how quickly you work?	1
		IN6	MIDDLE	Do you have any influence on how you do your work?	1
Possibilities for development	PD	PD1	CORE	Do you have the possibility of learning new things through your work?	2

[a] Response options: 1: always (100); often (75); sometimes (50); seldom (25); never/hardly ever (0). 1R: always (0); often (25); sometimes (50); seldom (75); never/hardly ever (100) (reversed scoring). 2: to a very large extent (100); to a large extent (75); somewhat (50); to a small extent (25); to a very small extent (0).

TABLE 11.4

Some items from the Health and Safety Executive's (HSE) Management Standards Indicator Tool for work-related stress.

Item	Responses (five-point Likert scale)				
I am clear what is expected of me at work.	Never	Seldom	Sometimes	Often	Always
I can decide when to take a break.	Never	Seldom	Sometimes	Often	Always
I know how to go about getting my job done.	Never	Seldom	Sometimes	Often	Always
If work gets difficult, my colleagues will help me.	Never	Seldom	Sometimes	Often	Always

it equated to a financial impact on GDP of close to £17.65 billion. Moreover, up to 20% of the over half a million annual work-related stress cases can be attributed to bullying behaviours. The UK Advisory, Conciliation and Arbitration Service (ACAS) published research in 2021 that shows that the cost of conflict to UK organisations was £28.5 billion, which amounts to a cost of more than £1000 for each employee. The research reflected that 9.7 million employees experienced conflict in 2018/2019.

What is workplace bullying?

Workplace bullying is harmful and targeted behaviour that happens at work. It might be spiteful, offensive, mocking or intimidating. It usually forms a pattern and tends to be directed at just one person or a limited few.

A few examples of bullying include:

- targeted practical jokes
- being purposely misled about work duties, such as incorrect deadlines or unclear directions
- continued denial of requests for time off without an appropriate or valid reason
- threats, humiliation and other verbal abuse
- excessive performance monitoring
- picking on an individual or individuals with overly harsh or unjust criticism
- spreading malicious rumours.

Criticism or monitoring is not always bullying; for example, objective and constructive criticism and disciplinary action directly related to workplace behaviour and/or job performance are not considered bullying. However, criticism meant to intimidate, humiliate or single someone out without reason would be considered bullying. Bullying and harassment can happen face to face or by letter, email or phone.

Since bullying is often verbal or psychological in nature, it may not always be visible to others.

Identifying workplace bullying

Bullying can be subtle. One helpful way to identify bullying is to consider how others might view what is happening. This can depend, at least partially, on the circumstances. But if most people would see a specific behaviour as unreasonable, it is generally bullying.

To constitute bullying behaviour it must be repeated over time. This sets it apart from harassment, which is often limited to a single instance. In most countries, bullying itself is not against the law, but harassment is. This is when the unwanted behaviour is related to one of the following:

- age
- sex
- disability
- gender reassignment
- marriage and civil partnership
- pregnancy and maternity
- race
- religion or belief
- sexual orientation.

Persistent harassment can become bullying, but since harassment refers to actions towards a protected group of people it is illegal, unlike bullying.

Early warning signs of bullying can vary:

- Co-workers might become quiet or leave the room when the individual in question walks in or they might simply ignore the individual.
- The individual might be left out of office culture, such as chitchat, parties or team lunches.
- The individual's supervisor or manager might check on the individual often or ask the individual to meet multiple times a week without a clear reason.
- The individual may be asked to do new tasks or tasks outside their typical duties without training or help, even when the individual requests it.
- It may seem like the individual's work is monitored frequently, to the point where the individual begins to doubt themselves and have difficulty with their regular tasks.
- The individual might be asked to do difficult or seemingly pointless tasks and be ridiculed or criticised when they cannot get them done.

Who gets bullied and who does the bullying?

Anyone can be a bully according to 2017 research from the US Workplace Bullying Institute:

- About 70% of bullies are male, and about 30% are female.
- Both male and female bullies are more likely to target women.
- Approximately 60% of bullying comes from bosses or supervisors, with 33% coming from co-workers; the remaining 7% occurs when people at lower employment levels bully their supervisors or others above them.

- Protected (legally) groups are bullied more frequently, e.g. only 19% of people bullied were white.

The 2021 survey, as discussed below, does not show great changes from the 2017 survey. The main changes were that male bullies were slightly less likely to target female workers and the bullying of white workers had increased to 30%. The group least likely to be bullied were Asian workers at 12%. Interestingly, the 2021 survey highlighted that remote workers were more likely to be bullied than those who used a hybrid model of working (part remote, part on site) and those who worked solely on site.

It is believed that targets of bullying were more likely to be kind, compassionate, cooperative and agreeable.

Bullying may occur more frequently in work environments that:

- are stressful or change frequently
- have heavy workloads
- have unclear policies about employee behaviour
- have poor employee communication and relationships
- have more employees who are bored or worried about job security.

How can bullying affect your health?

The physical health effects of bullying may cause the victim to:

- feel sick or anxious before work or when thinking about work
- have physical symptoms, such as digestive issues or high blood pressure
- have a higher risk of type 2 diabetes
- have trouble waking up or getting quality sleep
- have somatic symptoms, such as headaches and decreased appetite.

Mental health effects of bullying

Psychological effects of bullying may include:

- thinking and worrying about work constantly, even during time off
- dreading work and wanting to stay at home
- needing time off to recover from stress
- losing interest in things that the individual usually likes to do
- increased risk for depression and anxiety
- low self-esteem and suicidal thoughts.

11.7 Gender at work

Recognising diversity, including gender differences, in the workforce is vital in ensuring the safety and health of men, women and non-binary workers. A gender-sensitive approach recognises that – because of the general distribution of gender by jobs, their different societal roles, the expectations and responsibilities they have – women and men may be exposed to different physical and psychological risks in the workplace, thus requiring differing control approaches and measures. This approach also improves the understanding that the sexual division of labour, biological differences, employment patterns, social roles and social structures all contribute to gender-specific patterns of occupational hazards and risks. For OSH policies and prevention strategies to be effective for all workers, this dimension needs to be taken into account and policies must be based on more accurate information about the relationship between health and gender roles.

The ILO has written a useful document – *10 Keys for Gender Sensitive OSH Practice – Guidelines for Gender Mainstreaming in Occupational Safety and Health*. This is paraphrased below.

Gender-sensitive OSH practice

Guideline 1: Taking a gender mainstreaming approach to reviewing and developing occupational safety and health legislation Traditionally, men are more likely than women to work in hazardous industries such as mining, forestry, fishing and construction. In light of the above, men are more likely than women to be exposed to risks that, if not adequately controlled, can result in serious or fatal accidents. As a consequence, OSH laws have traditionally focused on visibly dangerous work largely carried out by men; while the focus in the case of women (especially pregnant women) has been on protective laws prohibiting certain types of hazardous work and exposures, such as working in mines, at night, with lead or ionising radiations or carrying heavy loads. Work undertaken by women is generally regarded as safe, because it is less hazardous, and women's occupational injuries as well as illnesses such as work-related stress, MSDs or dermatitis have been under-diagnosed, under-reported and under-compensated compared with those of men. Commensurately, men's reproductive health hazards have been considered less relevant in the context of OSH legislation.

With the introduction of equality legislation in industrialised countries, protective regulations that were considered a restriction to women's opportunities for participation in paid employment have been removed, and modern laws to protect workers' health and safety aimed at being 'gender neutral' (being neither advantageous nor disadvantageous to either sex) were enacted. However, two considerations need to be made:

1. In developing countries the restrictions to women's night work and other hazardous sectors such as mining still provide for women's protection from extreme working conditions and violence.
2. Gender-blind legislation may overlook gender differences in exposure to hazards and risks.

Most OSH legislation throughout the world still hides gender differences instead of assessing risks with a gender perspective and managing preventive measures taking into account the needs of both sexes. This gender-neutral legislation is often based on the assumption that it will apply equally to all workers as it does not explicitly recognise gender differences and therefore may not ensure equity in protecting male and female workers.

Legislation on violence and harassment
Many studies show that women are at particular risk of physical and psychological violence, both in and outside the workplace. Women are concentrated in many of the occupations with a high risk of violence: working in contact with the public and in solitary settings, particularly as teachers, social workers, healthcare workers and as clerks in banks and shops. Women also tend to work in low-paid and low-status jobs, where violence is more common; men predominate in better paid, higher status jobs and supervisory positions. Men tend to be at greater risk of physical assault, while women are particularly vulnerable to incidents of a sexual nature.

Globally, psychological violence at work and especially bullying, mobbing and harassment are reported to be a major concern. In response to the changing workplace and the increase in psychosocial hazards and risks, many countries are increasingly regulating workplace bullying, violence, discrimination and harassment (including sexual harassment) by introducing new legislation or incorporating new provisions in existing legislation to specifically address these risks. Other countries have opted for non-regulatory instruments, such as codes of practice and provisions in collective agreements. Several court rulings in different countries have recognised psychological violence as an occupational risk, equal in importance to other hazards in the work environment.

Guideline 2: Developing OSH policies to address gender inequalities in OSH practice

Gender-neutral policies are supposed to use the knowledge of gender differences in a given context to overcome biases in delivery, to ensure that they target and benefit both women and men irrespective of their sex.

Some policies that appear gender neutral may be shown, after a close assessment, to be gender blind, meaning that they do not specifically recognise gender differences. Not acknowledging gender differences may mean that apparently neutral policies impact differently on women and men and reinforce existing inequalities. A lack of distinction between male and female needs and characteristics provides for assumptions that incorporate biases in favour of existing gender relations by not reflecting the substantial differences in the lives of women and men.

Guideline 3: Ensuring consideration of gender differences in risk management

Risk assessment and management emphasises the need to adapt the work to the individual worker and to identify the risks to which workers may be exposed and protect workers against them.

The management of diversity in the workplace requires inclusive risk management measures that pay attention to the specific risks faced by women and men, young workers, older workers, migrants or persons with disabilities;

and necessitates the design of specific preventive and protective measures according to the requirements of those groups of workers.

Gender differences in exposure to musculoskeletal disorder risks

MSDs are the most common health impairments in the workplace. Women tend to suffer more from pain in the upper back and upper limbs as a result of repetitive work in both manufacturing and office work; this is accentuated during pregnancy. They also often have jobs that require prolonged standing, while men tend to suffer more from lower back pain from exerting high force at work.

Psychosocial risks: stress, violence and sexual harassment at work

Owing to the type of work that many women carry out and because of societal roles and social structures, they are generally at a higher risk of psychosocial hazards and risks that can cause work-related stress, burnout, violence, discrimination and harassment. Women entering non-traditional occupations are particularly at risk of discrimination and sexual harassment. Research has found that women's stress levels remain high after work, particularly if they have children living at home. Men, however, generally unwind rapidly at the end of the working day.

Reproductive health

Although, in general, men's OSH has received more attention than women's, this is not true for reproductive health. Occupational research and measures to protect workers' reproductive health at work have focused primarily on protecting pregnant women – and particularly the fetus.

There are many workplace hazards that can affect the reproductive health of both sexes and their offspring. These include chemical, biological and physical hazards, including pesticides, metals, dyes and solvents; noise and vibration; radiation; and infectious diseases. In addition, heavy lifting, standing or sitting for long periods of time have all been identified as occupational risks for pregnant women. Certain hazards can also affect men's fertility, sex drive or sexual performance as well as their ability to father healthy children, and some can cause cancer of male reproductive organs. They can also affect the woman, the child and the pregnancy, even if they have not been directly exposed to harmful agents themselves if they are carried in sperm or seminal fluid.

Guideline 4: OSH research should properly take into account gender differences

Research on OSH is of vital importance in stimulating and informing action to improve safety and health in the workplace. However, research tools and methods on OSH that were originally developed in relation to predominantly male-dominated sectors may not be relevant to analysing women's jobs to achieve this desired improvement.

Most studies looking at women's occupational health have concentrated on sectors where they predominate, such as healthcare, as well as on psychosocial stressors. Very few toxicological and physiological studies have been carried out. Researchers have often not considered gender- and sex-specific factors when designing studies and analysing data, rendering the study 'gender blind'. This is demonstrated by the use of gender-neutral expressions such as 'worker', 'employee' or 'driver', making it impossible to tell whether men or women or both sexes were included.

This situation has been improving. Research has found that even where men and women have the same job they may carry out different tasks and have different perceptions of the risks generated by the work involved and different health outcomes. For example, 'light' tasks assigned to female hospital cleaners actually included high workloads with postural constraints, repeated movements, a constant work pace, very little rest time, with frequent static postures and bent or stretched positions. 'Heavy' tasks assigned to male hospital cleaners, such as sweeping, were carried out in less tiring, upright positions.

Guideline 5: Developing gender-sensitive OSH indicators based on sex--disaggregated data

OSH indicators provide the framework for assessing the extent to which workers are protected from work-related hazards and risks. They are used by enterprises, governments and other stakeholders to formulate policies and programmes for the prevention of occupational injuries, diseases and fatalities, as well as to monitor the implementation of these policies and programmes and to signal particular areas of increasing risk such as a specific industry, occupation or location. They include the following:

- indicators of outcome, such as the number of occupational injuries and diseases, number of workers involved and workdays lost;
- indicators of capacity and capability, such as the number of inspectors or health professionals dealing with OSH; and
- indicators of activities, such as the number of trainee days or number of inspections.

Guideline 6: Promoting equal access to occupational health services and healthcare for all workers

WHO estimates that in developing countries only 5–10% of the working population has access to occupational health services. Some occupational health service providers have multidisciplinary teams including occupational hygienists, ergonomists, psychologists, safety and health specialists and counsellors. Across the world there are different models for the provision of occupational health services. In Europe these vary from the French system, grounded in occupational medicine and mandatory medical examinations, to the multidisciplinary models of Scandinavia.

Guideline 7: Ensuring the participation of both men and women workers and their representatives in OSH measures, health promotion and decision-making

Across the world, there is a general lack of gender balance in decision-making. The same is true with regard to decision-making concerning OSH. Women are in a minority in OSH decision-making bodies, such as national safety councils, occupational health services and enterprise-level safety and health committees.

Guideline 8: Developing gender-sensitive OSH information, education and training

The provision of information, education and training is crucial in ensuring that gender is mainstreamed into OSH policy and practice. As stated earlier, there is a general lack of awareness about the differences in the way that men and women may be exposed to risks at work. This applies to female-dominated occupations and sectors; to female workers moving into traditionally male-dominated occupations and sectors; to the extra responsibilities that women face as paid workers and unpaid carers for their families; and to the psychosocial risks, such as a threat of violence, of harassment and of discrimination, that many women face in their work roles.

Guideline 9: Designing work equipment, tools and personal protective equipment for both men and women

Across the world, work equipment, tools and personal protective equipment (PPE) have been traditionally designed for the male body size and shape. Moreover, the design of most PPE is based on the sizes and characteristics of male populations from certain countries in Europe, from Canada and from the USA. As a result, not only women but also many men experience problems finding suitable and comfortable PPE because they do not conform to this standard male worker model. With global migration this situation has become more evident in multiethnic workplaces. Poor fit to work equipment and tools can lead to poor working posture, leading to an increased risk of MSDs, while poor fit to PPE will lead to reduced protection. Hand tools and workstation heights are often uncomfortable for workers who are smaller or indeed taller and larger than the 'standard' worker. While the use of work equipment, machinery and tools designed for men contributes to women's work accident rates, men are also involved in accidents because of a poor match between equipment, tools, PPE and the worker. Women entering traditionally male jobs in areas like construction, engineering and the emergency services are particularly at risk from inappropriately designed equipment, tools and PPE.

Guideline 10: Working time arrangements and work–life balance

As a consequence of a world increasingly working around the clock, there are now millions of shift workers, including night workers. Nearly 20% of the working population in Europe and North America now work shifts, most commonly in the healthcare, manufacturing, industrial, transport, communications and hospitality sectors. As has already been described in this chapter, shift work is associated with high levels of stress, particularly where work schedules are inflexible and workers do not have control over their work. Family life and social life are often disrupted, with workers becoming isolated from friends and family. Additionally, female workers working shifts can face an increased risk of violence when, late at night, relying on public transport. Other health effects in both men and women include reliance on sleeping pills or stimulants, drug and alcohol misuse and disruption of the hormonal system. There is a clear gender gap in working time. Part-time employment is much more common among women than men. More than twice the number of women than men work part-time across the world, although part-time working is increasing almost everywhere for women and men alike. Part-time workers may not always receive equal safety and health protection and, although they spend less time at work, their injury rate per hour worked is higher than that for those working full-time. At the other end of the scale, an estimated 22% of the global workforce now works more than 48 hours a week. Men tend to work longer average hours than women worldwide. The effect of unpaid work outside normal employment (working at home) must not be forgotten, as this work affects the total hours worked by those undertaking it, normally female workers. As with shift work, fatigue associated with working long hours (wherever the work is carried out) can lead to an increase in the risk of accidents.

A continuing focus on gender mainstreaming

Despite gender mainstreaming gaining prominence as a concept through policy, practices and initiatives within countries and organisations, with the realisation that it helps in redressing the inequalities that continue to exist between the genders in terms of their OSH, it remains a practice that is ad hoc rather than the norm. This facilitates a continuation of the 'gender-neutral' approach to OSH. This has to change to ensure that all workers are assessed correctly to allow the appropriate preventative measures to be put in place, as well as to ensure that these are evaluated consistently to guarantee their continued effectiveness. Research by the European Agency for Safety and Health at Work resulted in case studies and overviews (*Mainstreaming gender into occupational safety and health practice*; *New Risks and Trends in the Safety and Health of Women at Work*), which provide examples on how this essential practice could be implemented in organisations.

11.8 Role of occupational health practitioners in managing occupational stress

As mentioned earlier, occupational stress needs to be managed across the three levels, the organisational, the workgroup and the individual. The occupational health practitioner's role spans the three facets.

Unsurprisingly, management may choose to deal with occupational stress through interventions aimed at employees rather than at organisational reforms. There may be a focus therefore on providing training in individual stress management techniques, rather than improving workplace communication and providing a timely and relevant response to any queries on what was communicated. The more holistic, and successful, reforms require greater management commitment and time, deeper analysis of stressors and to be dealt with promptly, without disrupting production. The occupational health practitioner needs to encourage a more comprehensive approach in the enterprise that emphasises the potential benefits, such as protecting product quality, lower absenteeism and loyalty to the company. Additionally, the occupational health service can promote and conduct workplace surveys of potential stressors, locate the workplace departments with the stressors and obtain employees' suggestions for remedial actions. Employer and employee commitment to addressing the stressors is necessary to make their identification useful, and occupational health services can contribute to achieving this.

For several reasons, workers suffering the adverse effects of occupational stress may receive little support from colleagues and management. Their co-workers may be dealing with the same stressors adequately and thus feel that individual weakness is responsible for poor work performance and absenteeism; they may have to work harder to fill in for work not done; and they may perceive employees with anxiety and depression induced by occupational stress as more difficult to work with, rather than acknowledging their ill health. Management has to deal with production issues and co-workers' unhappiness with their colleagues' performance, and sometimes an unfounded sense of favouritism, if usual disciplinary procedures are waived to support the troubled employee. Industrial relations are thus often strained. A fundamental role of the occupational health practitioner in this situation is to contextualise the deficits in the person's work and to present a management plan aimed at remedying the problems that takes the matter out of a strictly Human Resources Department response. The management plan should cover the primary, secondary and tertiary interventions described in Section 11.2. Communication about the aims of the plan to colleagues, with consent from the affected employee, can help reduce tensions. Once animosity is established it may be difficult to overcome. Early intervention is thus encouraged.

Additionally, practitioners may be required to identify workplace stressors of individual workers and comment on the diagnoses, anxiety and depression commonly found, and their relation to work and prognosis. Consultation with psychologists or psychiatrists is recommended.

Further Reading

Arends, I. (2015). (Mental Health and Work)). *Fit Mind, Fit Job: From Evidence to Practice in Mental Health and Work*. OECD/ODCE https://doi.org/10.1787/9789264228283-en.

Gervais, R.L. (2021). Gender-sensitive interventions in the workplace: examples from practice. In: *Aligning Perspectives in Gender Mainstreaming: Gender, Health, Safety & Well-Being* (eds. J. Hassard and L.D. Torres), 117–132. Cham: Springer https://doi.org/10.1007/978-3-030-53269-7_7.

Health and Safety Executive. (n.d.). *What are the Management Standards?* https://www.hse.gov.uk/stress/standards (accessed 14 May 2021).

Namie, G. (2021). *2021 WBI U.S. Workplace Bullying Survey*. https://workplacebullying.org/wp--content/uploads/2021/04/2021-Full-Report.pdf (accessed 14 May 2021).

Norman, S.B. and Maguen, S. (2021). *Moral Injury*. US Department of Veterans Affairs. https://www.ptsd.va.gov/professional/treat/cooccurring/moral_injury.asp (accessed 14 May 2021).

Saundry, R. (2021). *Estimating the Costs of Workplace Conflict*. ACAS. https://www.acas.org.uk/estimating-the-costs-of-workplace-conflict-report#technical-appendix (accessed 14 May 2021).

European Commission (2000). *Guidance on Work-Related Stress. Spice of Life or Kiss of Death? Employment & Social affairs. Health and safety at work. European Commission. Directorate--General for Employment and Social Affairs. Unit D.6.* Luxembourg: Office for Official Publications of the European Communities.

CHAPTER 12

Risk Assessment

Pocket Consultant: Occupational Health, Sixth Edition. Kerry Gardiner, David Rees, Anil Adisesh, David Zalk, and Malcolm Harrington.
© 2022 John Wiley & Sons Ltd. Published 2022 by John Wiley & Sons Ltd.

12.1 Introduction to risk assessment

In the UK's Health and Safety at Work, etc. Act 1974, the concept of risk assessment was introduced (but, unfortunately, only by implication) by the phrase 'so far as is reasonably practicable'. A number of subsequent pieces of UK legislation, such as the Control of Lead at Work Regulations 2002 and the Ionising Radiations Regulations 1999, required the risks to health from specific hazards to be 'assessed'. However, it was probably the Control of Substances Hazardous to Health (Amendment) Regulations 2004 that formalised the need for risk assessments in environments other than those for which specific legislation existed.

The approach of risk assessment in Europe is now much more common because of the 'Framework' Directive (89/391/EEC), which the UK has implemented predominantly by means of the Management of Health and Safety at Work Regulations (MHSWR) 1999 and other related regulations. The fundamentals of all of these regulations are the three tenets of occupational hygiene/health:

- anticipation/recognise
- evaluate
- control.

Since these various pieces of legislation have come into force, there has been some confusion about the terms used in risk assessment, specifically 'hazard' and 'risk'. These terms are defined elsewhere in this book (see Chapter 6), but also here for the purpose of emphasis and clarity.

A *hazard* is something with the potential to cause harm, such as a substance, a piece of equipment, a form of energy, a way of working or a feature of the environment. *Harm* (in terms of occupational health) includes death and major injury and any form of physical or mental ill health. *Risk* is a measure of the likelihood that the hazard (defined previously) will manifest some degree of harm. It follows, therefore, that the highest risk is where something very hazardous is almost certainly going to result in severe harm.

Other than for simple legislative compliance, the only real reason for determining risk is to decide what to do with the level of risk ascertained (Figure 12.1) – remember the adage 'never ask a question if you don't know what to do with the answer'! Organisations have a very wide variance in what they choose to do with risk and also differing hierarchies; to supplement those given in Figure 12.1, two more lists are given below:

- Accept the risk
- Avoid the risk
- Transfer the risk
- Mitigate the risk
- Exploit the risk

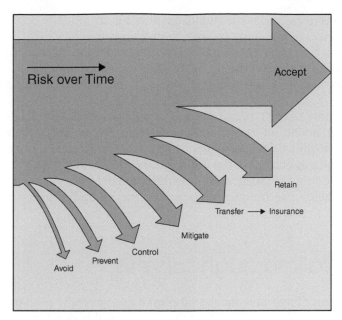

FIGURE 12.1 What to do with identified risk.

. . . and

- Avoidance
- Retention
- Sharing
- Transferring
- Loss prevention.

The current culture for these more esoteric aspects of occupational health risk, risk assessment and risk management is for them to be integrated and also form a central pillar of enterprise risk management, etc. (which will be addressed in more detail in Chapter 13).

The basic steps for risk assessment include the following elements:

- Consider all activities and situations, both routine and non-routine, including foreseeable emergencies and loss of control.
- Identify the hazards, both intrinsic and those generated by all of the activities discussed above.
- Identify which individuals or groups of workers may be exposed to the hazards (include non-employees and those identified to be at extra risk by virtue of susceptibility, illness and other medical conditions).
- Determine and assess the risks to health from the hazards.
- Determine the degree of control of these risks, and whether this is adequate and easily sustainable.

- Can this (these) risk(s) be eliminated or reduced?
- Implement new or improved risk control measures.
- Monitor the effectiveness of these controls and, if necessary or appropriate, the health of those at risk.
- Review and, if necessary, implement any appropriate corrective action.

The purpose of the structure of this chapter is to lead the reader through the basic elements of risk assessment, from the perspective both of an occupational/industrial hygienist (i.e. the environment) and of an occupational physician (i.e. the individual). This chapter does not attempt to describe the more sophisticated probabilistic risk assessment or epidemiological modelling techniques (e.g. failure modes and effects analysis and fault tree analysis).

12.2 Walk-through surveys

One of the most important and yet simplest acts – generally as an occupational health professional but, critically, in the context of this chapter – is actually to venture into the workplace and 'see for oneself' what people do and how they do it (and not just for a few minutes – longer if the outcome is chronic or if individuals are mandated to wearing personal protective equipment [PPE]/respiratory protective equipment). In order to maximise the benefit of the visit, it is common for people to use a walk-through checklist, both as an aide-memoire and to try to ensure objectivity.

The suggested pro forma below will contain elements that are not always necessary and may even be difficult to complete (technically or politically). However, it is the authors' attempt at being comprehensive, in order that the reader can extract the relevant aspects for their needs. It is also acknowledged that most workplaces contain a multitude of processes, all with their own hazards; it will therefore be necessary for the person undertaking the walk-through survey to determine whether separate sheets need to be completed for each process or section.

General site information

Name of company/factory
Address of site
Site contact (name/tel. no.)
- Managing director
- Human resources manager
- Union representative

Site details

- Site engineer
- Past activities (brief)
- Current activities
- Employee details
  - No. of employees
    - Management
    - Workforce
    - Maintenance/cleaners
- Subcontracted activities
- Age profile
- Sex ratio
- Ethnicity
- Shift patterns
- Staff turnover
- Shower/changing rooms
- Canteen

Occupational health department (no. + qualifications)

Staff

- Occupational hygienist
- Occupational physician
- Occupational health nurse
- Safety officer
- Ergonomist/acoustician/etc.

Facilities

- Equipment
  - Type
  - Quantity/quality/appropriateness
  - Deficiencies

Activities

- Executive or advisory role
- Pre-purchase review of substances/equipment
- Statutory measurements
- Non-statutory measurements
- Specification/design of control measures
- Pre-employment
- Periodic health surveillance
- Post-sickness review/rehabilitation
- Disability employment procedure
- Immunisation
- Health promotion
- Counselling
- Training
- Disaster planning

Hazard	Comment	Type and adequacy of control	Action required	Person at risk				Harm					Likelihood					Risk ranking
				EMP	CON	VIS	PUB	NO	MIN	MOD	MAJ	FAT	IMP	REM	POS	PROB	DEF	
Use of equipment																		
Rotating/moving parts																		
Free movement																		
Machine/vehi-cle movement																		
Fire explosion																		
Work practices and premises layout																		
Hazardous surfaces																		
Working at height																		
Awkward posture/movement																		
Confined space																		
Slips/trips																		
Electrical																		
Electrical switchgear																		
Electrical installations																		
Electrically operated equipment																		
Portable electric tools																		
Physical agents																		
Electromagnetic radiation																		
Noise																		
Vibration																		
Heat																		
Light																		

Ionising radiation
Non-ionising radiation
Biological agents
Viruses
Bacteria
Fungi
Protozoa
Algae
Parasites
Naked genetic material
Agents of transmissible spongiform encephalopathy
Cell lines
Genetically modified organisms

Chemical agents

Dust
Fibre
Smoke
Fume
Mist
Liquid
Gas
Vapour

Person at risk. EMP, employee; CON, contractor; VIS, visitor; PUB, public.

Harm. NO, no injury; MIN, minimal (cuts, bruises, etc.); MOD, moderate (prolonged but not permanent damage or effect); MAJ, major (permanent ill health or disability); FAT, fatality.

Likelihood. IMP, improbable; REM, remote (possible, but highly unlikely); POS, possible; PROB, probably (is likely to occur); DEF, definite (will occur at some point in time).

	Comments	Action required

Psychological factors
Intensity/monotony of work
Role ambiguity and/or conflict
High demand/low control
Workplace dimensions
Contribution to decision-making
General
Safety policy (adequacy)
Written work procedures (followed?)
Housekeeping
Suitability of personal protection equipment (PPE)
Supervision of PPE usage
Interaction of workplace and human factors
  • Dependence of safety systems, a need to receive and process information accurately
  • Dependence on knowledge and capabilities of staff
  • Dependence on norms of behaviour
  • Dependence on good communication
  • Impact of reasonably foreseeable departures from safe working procedures
Perception of company commitment to health and safety
Perception of local site commitment to health and safety
Perception of workforce motivation to work safely
Dangers caused by other people
Public (violence)
Workforce (bullying)
Proximity, suitability and speed of access for emergency services		

Comments

It is worth drawing the reader's attention to a number of points before this walk-through survey pro forma is used. Despite the fact that a crude means of assessing risk has been included, the primary function of such an aid will always remain the *identification* of hazards. Therefore, the most important part of the form is the 'comments' section, furnished by the reviewer's senses (sight, smell, sound, taste and touch). So much can be achieved without the need for the formal measurement of contaminants, i.e. many organic chemicals have distinctive smells, with some having their odour threshold around their workplace exposure limit (WEL) (perchloroethylene, 50 parts per million [ppm]), fine particles are made visible by shafts of light (Tyndall beam) and the ear can determine the intensity and frequency of industrial sounds.

In order to be systematic about reviewing all parts of a process, it is often best to observe the process from beginning to end, with, for example, chemicals being looked at from raw materials through to the final product. Included along the way should be an evaluation of the intermediates, by-products and waste/excess material.

For most of the hazard types listed above, it is also important to be aware of the route of entry into the body. For example, a volatile liquid can be ingested, inoculated, absorbed via the skin or, most commonly, inhaled (vapour).

On the pro forma, the means of separating harm and likelihood into one of the five groups is crude but is designed to assist in the process of assessing and ranking risk. There may be some situations in which anomalous risk rankings arise, but the individual is advised to review these with care.

12.3 Sampling strategies

The previous section on walk-through surveys provided some information on the questions to be asked and the observations made to make a qualified judgement about the risks to health in an environment. When decisions cannot be reached by these means, or when an estimate of the level of exposure is required (e.g. odourless and/or lethal gases, compliance with WELs, design of ventilation system, litigation), measurements taken as part of a coherent sampling strategy are necessary.

Most occupational measurements are taken for comparison with WELs or relevant standards (noise, ionising radiation, etc.). Occasionally, more enlightened companies are taking measurements for epidemiological purposes. For some time, the perception has been that the sampling strategies for the two are markedly different, but current thinking is suggesting that a well-constructed strategy should provide adequate data for both. However, regardless of this, all sampling strategies should contain the same basic elements, having answered or at least considered the following simple questions (and they will look very similar to those presented in Chapter 14):

- Why sample?
- Level of approach?
- What to measure?
- How to sample?
- Whose exposure should be measured?
- Where to collect the sample?
- When to measure?
- How long to sample for?
- How many measurements?
- How often to sample?
- What to do with the data?
- What to record?

Why sample?

A number of reasons for taking measurements have been alluded to above, but it is critical that the individual undertaking any sampling is very clear exactly what the purpose is of the collection of such data and what they are going to do with the results. The reason that more than one sample needs to be taken is that real-world exposure varies massively – from moment to moment, person to person, place to place, etc. This variability is dependent upon many factors such as the nature, density and intensity of activity/process people, the contaminant(s) of interest and environmental components, including temperature, wind speed and direction and humidity. Examples of the influence of these factors are shown in Figure 12.2.

Level of approach?

Having determined the reason for sampling, it is then necessary to determine the need or importance of the answer, thereby prioritising which contaminants and/or processes are associated with the highest degree of risk. Some risk determinants include: the number of potentially exposed individuals; the toxicity of the substance(s); the quantities used over some arbitrary reference period; the likely duration and concentration of exposure (plus exposure via routes other than inhalation), i.e. dose; the existence of and confidence in control measures; the likelihood and magnitude of change to the process and its control; and the presence of substances that may be potentiators or act synergistically or antagonistically with contaminants.

Occupational/industrial hygiene surveys can be broken down into four levels relative to the level of priority assigned: an initial assessment, a preliminary survey, a detailed survey and routine monitoring. The level of survey is obviously related to the importance associated with the answer (as described above), and the magnitude of the survey is related to the factors involved (e.g. numbers of people, expected/known 'within and between person' variability). Figure 12.3 shows a self-explanatory flow diagram to aid in the visualisation and understanding of this process.

What to measure?

Rarely, in industrial situations, is only one substance used (usually this is not a problem for other contaminants, such as ionising radiation and noise, where the sampling instrumentation is designed to be contaminant specific); therefore, a decision must be made as to which, of potentially many substances, should be measured. Reference to the original aim of sampling will assist (i.e. compliance or health risk). There are three main options, which involve the assessment of: (i) all, or many, of the contaminants; (ii) the 'mixture' as a whole; or (iii) reference/surrogate substance(s).

i.   The increasing availability of techniques able to identify and quantify large numbers of contaminants has improved the possibility of measuring multi-contaminant mixtures; however, this process will certainly be expensive. For compliance purposes, there may be a number of substances in the mixture with WELs and with the same site of action, thereby necessitating this approach, together with the use of the additive equation

$$C_1 / L_1 + C_2 / L_2 + C_3 / L_3 \ldots < 1$$

where C is concentration and L is limit.

This approach may also be necessary when the components in the mixture and their relative ratios are constantly changing.

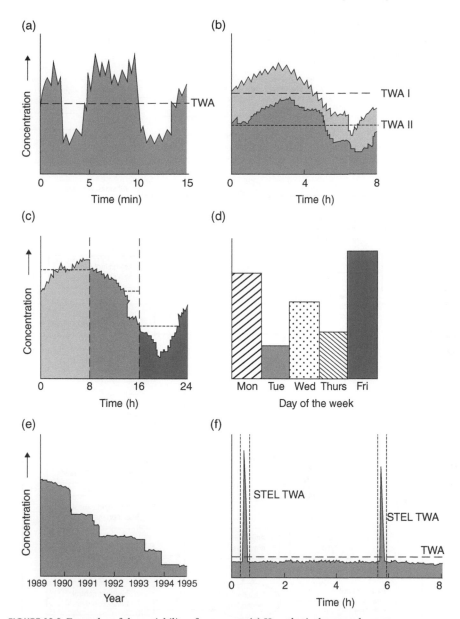

FIGURE 12.2 Examples of the variability of exposure. (a) Hypothetical personal exposure as measured by continuous monitoring and the integrated 15-minute time-weighted average (TWA) exposure. (b) Hypothetical continuous trace and integrated TWA personal exposure for two individuals undertaking the same work over an eight-hour period. (c) Hypothetical continuous trace and integrated TWA personal exposure for three individuals undertaking the same work on different shifts over a 24-hour period. (d) Hypothetical eight-hour TWA personal exposures for an individual undertaking the same work over a period of one week. (e) Hypothetical trace of weekly TWA personal exposures for an individual undertaking the same work over a number of years. (f) Hypothetical trace of personal exposure and eight-hour and 15-minute TWAs of a contained process with occasional fugitive emissions. STEL, short-term exposure limit.

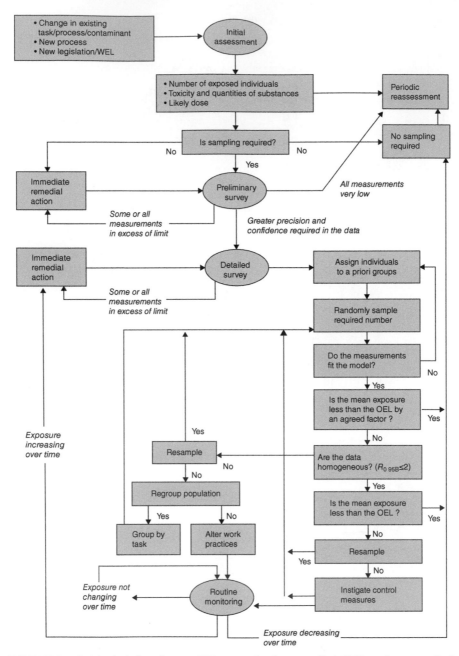

FIGURE 12.3 A decision logic flow diagram. OEL, occupational exposure limit; WEL, work exposure limit.

ii.   Instead of breaking down a mixture into its component parts (as in (i) above), the contaminant of interest is, by definition, a mixture (e.g. rubber, foundry or welding fume). The WEL is therefore set and assessed on this basis. Again, this approach may satisfy the needs of compliance testing but not those of health risk assessment; for example, with welding, issues such as the proportion of hexavalent chromium may be important for both compliance and health risk assessment. Another example is the measurement of non-specific dusts (either respirable or total inhalable), whose values are compared with the respirable and inhalable dust standards of 4 and $10\,mg\,m^{-3}$, respectively.

iii.   Where a mixture has been well characterised in terms of constituents and relative ratios throughout a process, it is possible to measure one or a limited number of these as a surrogate for the whole. The choice of which one(s) may be dictated by the difficulty/ease of measurement/analysis and/or the state of toxicological knowledge and existence of WELs.

If approach (iii) is to be undertaken, then the basis on which the WELs have been set, the toxicity of the various components (i.e. carcinogen), the proportion of each component in the bulk material and the volatility (and, thereby, the likely airborne concentrations of each component) should be addressed. It is believed that, using method (iii), if the concentration of the most volatile and/or toxic substance is under control, then, by default, so should everything else be.

A useful means of combining both the WEL (ppm) and the volatility of a substance (which is temperature dependent) is the vapour hazard index or ratio (VHR):

$$\text{VHR} = \frac{\text{concentration of saturated vapour} \left(\text{SC} \right)}{\text{WEL}}$$

where WEL is the relevant WEL for the material in question (in ppm by volume) and SC is the saturation concentration (also in ppm), given by:

$$\text{SC} = \frac{\text{VP}_{\text{STP}} \times 10^{6}}{\text{BP}}$$

in which the barometric pressure (BP) is 760 mmHg and VP_{STP} is the vapour pressure in millimetres of mercury at standard temperature (20 °C) and pressure (760 mmHg).

Applying the above to the examples of hydrazine and hexane, we obtain the following:

Hydrazine	SC = 13 158 ppm
	WEL = 0.01 ppm
	VHR = 1 315 800
Hexane	SC = 163 158 ppm
	WEL = 20 ppm
	VHR = 8157.9

From these values we can see that hydrazine is potentially much more hazardous to health, despite its lower vapour pressure and, hence, lower magnitude of exposure.

In some cases, it is also important to consider the extent to which a material, when it is airborne, can exist as a vapour or an aerosol. To quantify this, SC – as defined above – is first converted into a mass concentration $(mg\,m^{-3})$. This is then compared with the WEL (also expressed in $mg\,m^{-3}$). Thus, we have the following possible scenarios.

1. If SC/WEL < 1, the airborne material will appear mostly as an aerosol.
2. If 1 < SC/WEL < 100, the airborne material will contain some aerosol.
3. If SC/WEL > 100, the airborne material will appear as vapour.

For example, mercury has a WEL listed as $0.025\,mg\,m^{-3}$ under the assumption that the material is present as vapour and that there is no aerosol exposure. Mercury has a vapour pressure of $1.8 \times 10^{-3}\,mmHg$, leading to $SC = 19.6\,mg\,m^{-3}$. Therefore, SC/WEL = 19.6/0.02 = 980. This, therefore, confirms that the setting of a WEL for mercury based on the assumption of a vapour is correct.

How to sample?

Depending on the question being addressed and the level of approach required, it is not always necessary to use the technique with the greatest accuracy, precision, sensitivity and specificity. Not forsaking practical issues, such as the intrinsic safety, user acceptability (i.e. weight and size) and performance (i.e. flow rate range and battery longevity) of the equipment, the sampling and analytical methods chosen should meet the requirements of the sampling strategy and not vice versa.

All measuring techniques are subject to error, certainly random and perhaps systematic. A knowledge of the potential errors for all parts of the sampling train and subsequent analyses is necessary to ensure that it is minimised and that comparability is maximised; it may include the contaminant stability, sampling device (i.e. dust head), sampling medium and its stability (i.e. absorber/absorber or filter), tubing, pump (i.e. flow rate fluctuations) and analytical technique. The potential and magnitude of the error vary within a sampling train and between the sampling trains required for different contaminants. For example, the flow rate can easily be set incorrectly relative to the requirements of the instrument (i.e. cyclones) or in absolute terms (i.e. the rotameter may read $2.2\,l\,min^{-1}$, but, in reality, it is $1.8\,l\,min^{-1}$, thereby oversampling disproportionately).

Whose exposure should be measured?

In all sampling strategies, the decision of who to sample is vital. In the past, compliance testing strategies have focused on 'worst-case scenarios', whereby people undertaking the jobs likely to give rise to the highest exposure, or intrinsically 'dirty workers', are sampled. The philosophy behind this was that, if the exposure was less than the WEL, then, by default, so would the exposure be in all other situations. Unfortunately, this biased selection process was driven by legislative requirements to ascertain the probability that a person would exceed the WEL on a particular day; however, these data are profoundly limited for other purposes.

The current promulgated technique is for groups of workers with common exposure to be formed either prospectively or retrospectively, and for a subset of these to be sampled randomly. Common exposure means that the group should be exposed to the same substances and that each of the exposure distributions for the individual workers should have the same means and standard deviations. This is often referred to as homogeneity.

Prospective grouping

The grouping of prospective employees relies on the ability of the occupational hygienist to assign individual workers to a group on the basis of observations, such as the similarity of tasks, contaminants and environment (process equipment and controls). A proportion of workers from within each group should be selected randomly and sampled, with the data assessed for homogeneity. Environments in which populations generate data that meet this definition of homogeneity are almost unheard of, and therefore a more 'workable' definition is required. In the UK, for example, the Health and Safety Executive (HSE) has suggested a crude but useful rule, i.e. if a worker's exposure is less than half, or greater than twice, the group mean, he or she should be reassigned to another group. Another definition of a homogeneous or monomorphic group is described below in the retrospective grouping of employees.

Retrospective grouping of employees

It is not always possible to assign workers to the correct groups simply on the basis of observation, especially those involved in maintenance or non-routine tasks where it may be preferable to sample everyone randomly. This procedure gains in significance if it is possible to undertake at least two sets of repeat measurements on those sampled and helps to identify the components of variability of exposure, i.e. total distribution and distributions within and between workers. The groups of workers can then be calculated on the basis of the exposure data (concentration and variability). A grouping is deemed to be monomorphic if 95% of the individual mean exposures lie within a factor of 2. This implies that the ratio of the 97.5th percentile to the 2.5th percentile ($R_{0.95B}$) is not greater than 2, which equates to a between-worker geometric standard deviation (GSD) ($\sigma g\beta$) of 1.2 or less. If the groups used in an epidemiological study are not homogeneous, then the distribution of each group may overlap (i.e. lack contrast) and hence non-differential misclassification exposure may occur. This tends to attenuate the exposure–response relation – although it is more important for the occupational/industrial hygienist to ensure that, even if the groups are not homogeneous, they do not overlap – wherein the estimate of the relative risk at a certain exposure level will be unbiased but lacking precision.

Where to collect the sample?

The occupational/industrial hygienist has two main choices with regard to the location of the sampling device: to place the equipment on the individual (personal) or to fix it to a tripod, in which case it will be static over the duration of sampling (static or area). If an assessment of compliance or health risk is being undertaken, the preferred location is personal, as this is most likely to reflect the individual's exposure. In fact, for all but a few substances (e.g. cotton dust and subtilisins [proteolytic enzymes]), the WELs are specific to personal exposure.

It is conventional to call the micro-environment to which an individual will be exposed the 'breathing zone', and this is defined as approximately 20–30 cm from the nose/mouth (Figure 12.4a). Typically, the sampling device is located on one lapel, however marked spatial variation between the two lapels is possible; hence, the hygienist should be aware of this. It is also known that substances with a high degree of thermal buoyancy, such as welding fume and colophony, generate a reasonably well-defined plume that rises sharply owing to its own natural thermal buoyancy. A significant proportion of this may miss the lapel-located sampler, but,

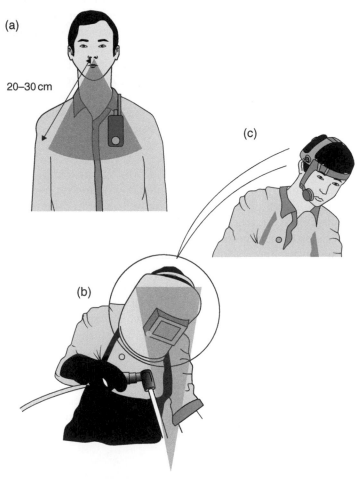

FIGURE 12.4 Location of a sampler. (a) Breathing zone highlighted with the sampler located in its classic 'lapel' position. (b) Well-defined plume missing the normal 'lapel' position (a), and (c) sampler located underneath a welding helmet next to the nose/mouth. Source: Health and Safety Executive (HSE), 1990. Licensed under OGL (crown copyright).

as a result of the nature of the work and therefore the required body position, will generate significant exposure. The welding head sampler is therefore mounted on a cranial cap or on the inside of airstream welding helmets (Figure 12.4b). Clearly, consideration of the work activity must be given before placement of the equipment, and discussion with the worker with regard to 'wearability' may be necessary.

As there is a poor relationship between static samples and real personal exposure, their use is less prevalent; however, they do have specific roles. The main one is in the assessment of the requirements and performance of control measures. The fixed location of the sampler strengthens the validity of comparing concentrations pre- and post-control intervention, without the additional variability inherent in an individual moving around the workplace. Some measuring devices are large and barely portable. This is especially true for continuous monitoring devices, or where very large volumes of air need to be sampled owing to the low ambient concentrations. Occasionally, static samples can be used as a surrogate for personal exposure, especially where the nature of the work may make the wearing of additional sampling equipment more hazardous or where a clear relationship between static measurements and personal exposure has been defined (e.g. on return roadways in coalmines).

When to measure?

Processes can be split into three main types: continuous, cyclic or random, with most major processes being made up of different proportions of all three – for example, in a chemical factory, the production is continuous, the packaging is cyclic and the reactive maintenance is random. If a worker's job involves just one of these types of process, both cyclic and random exposures will vary considerably, but will be more stable for a continuous process. This exposure variability will be even greater if a worker is involved in two or more types of process. Clearly, there is a need to be aware of this variability, and to sample at such times as to reflect this most accurately. If a random sampling programme is used, care must be taken to ensure that sufficient samples are obtained so that rare tasks are likely to be included.

How long to sample for?

This is an area of great potential divergence between the requirements of compliance and epidemiology. Compliance testing requires the comparison of exposure with legislative airborne standards, of which there are, in the main, two time-weighted average (TWA) reference periods – eight hours and 15 minutes. However, it is not necessary to sample for these exact durations because, within the reference time, there may be periods of known exposure (zero or some other value). This thereby facilitates greater precision and accuracy to be gained for the periods that are evaluated. It is then possible to calculate the TWA exposure relative to the control periods.

Epidemiological evaluation poses greater problems because it is necessary to have some knowledge of the rate at which the contaminant causes a biological effect. Thus, if the substances have an acute effect (seconds to hours) the duration of sampling must be able to reflect this variability within a shift, whereas if the effect is chronic a more appropriate duration may be a weekly, monthly, annual, average or lifetime dose.

For substances known to cause an immediate effect on, for example, mucous membranes, such as sulphur dioxide, ceiling values are quoted in some countries. The instantaneous measurement of these contaminants is difficult as instrumentation only exists for a small number of substances, and the accuracy, precision and specificity are often limited. Epidemiologically, the problem may be compounded further by issues of the exposure profile. It has been postulated that it is in some way the 'peakiness' of the exposure (profile) to sensitisers that causes the sensitisation rather than the dose.

Periods of work greater than eight hours The ever-changing requirements of employers, in terms of the duration of work or shifts, may mean that potential difficulties arise when comparing exposures with WELs devised for five 8-hour days per week. Clearly, the longer the day over which the contaminant is absorbed, the shorter the period of recovery before the next insult. For substances with very short half-lives this may not be a problem, but for those whose half-lives approach or exceed 16 hours (the period of recovery for an eight-hour working day) the body burden may rise over the week/shift period. A number of sophisticated models utilising pharmacokinetics have been put forward, but, unfortunately, they require a great deal of substance-specific information, which is very rarely available. A more simplistic yet elegant model by which WELs can be adjusted was postulated by Brief and Scala (1975) for longer working periods:

$$\text{WEL multiplication factor} = \frac{8}{H} \times \left(\frac{24 - H}{16} \right)$$

where H is the number of hours worked per day.

How many measurements?

The only way to ensure that an absolute measure of an individual's exposure has been achieved is to measure them on every day of their working life for every contaminant. Clearly, this is not possible, but equally foolish is the perception that one can take a few measurements and, by so doing, characterise an individual's exposure. Therefore, it is usually a balance between the scientific (statistical) needs of multiple samples and the logistical/political/financial aspects of reality. Obviously, the further towards the scientific needs one is able to go the better. Fortunately, there are some crude guides that assist us in the process of selecting the number of samples.

The US National Institute for Occupational Safety and Health (NIOSH) promulgated a method by which one could decide that one wanted at least one measurement from the sampled population to be in the top $T\%$ with $C\%$ confidence. This was designed specifically as a compliance tool but has been used in epidemiological studies. Tables exist wherein one specifies the upper fraction of exposure (i.e. top 10%) and the confidence with which one wants to find an exposure measurement in that fraction (i.e. 95% confidence). The total number of individuals in the defined homogeneous group is determined (group size), and the required number of samples to be taken in that day is read off (Table 12.1). These values are not dependent upon knowledge of the distributional form.

Knowledge of the geometric mean (GM) and GSD from previous surveys can be used to calculate the required number of samples. If no data are available, mean exposures and their standard deviations can be either estimated or extracted from published data for comparable industries. It is preferable to overestimate rather than underestimate the GSD, as this will maximise the sample size (i.e. $n > 2$). Therefore, the number of samples required (n) can be calculated from these data using the formula:

$$n = \left(\frac{t\text{CV}}{E} \right)^2$$

where CV is the coefficient of variation (standard deviation divided by mean), E is the acceptable or chosen level of error and t is the t-distribution value for the chosen confidence level ($n_0 - 1$) degrees of freedom.

For example, for normally distributed amorphous silica data, with an arithmetic mean of $6.0\,\text{mgm}^{-3}$, standard deviation of $2.0\,\text{mgm}^{-3}$, chosen error limit of 5%, a 95% confidence level and $t = 1.960$ (degrees of freedom):

$$n = \left(\frac{1.960 \times 2.0 / 6.0}{0.05} \right)^2$$

$$n = 171 \text{ samples}$$

Therefore, to estimate the mean concentration of the population within 5% of the 'true' mean with 95% confidence, 171 samples from the same group would be needed! Clearly, the greater the homogeneity and acceptable/allowable error and the less the confidence required, the smaller the number of samples needed.

Much more sophisticated techniques exist for the calculation of the required number of samples, especially for epidemiological use, but it is suggested that the reader refers elsewhere for these – particularly Kromhout et al. (2005).

How often to sample?

As with the number of samples, the answer to this question is reliant upon the variability – specifically, the day-to-day variance. The greater the day-to-day variance, the greater the frequency of required sampling. In addition, if certain events happen on an infrequent basis, and a random sampling schedule is being

TABLE 12.1

Sample size selection (US National Institute for Occupational Safety and Health (NIOSH)).

Top 20% with 90% confidence (use $n = N$ if $N \leq 5$)		Top 20% with 95% confidence (use $n = N$ if $N \leq 6$)		Top 10% with 90% confidence (use $n = N$ if $N \leq 7$)		Top 10% with 95% confidence (use $n = N$ if $N \leq 11$)	
Size of group (N)	No. of samples required (n)	Size of group (N)	No. of samples required (n)	Size of group (N)	No. of samples required (n)	Size of group (N)	No. of samples required (N)
6	5	7–8	6	8	7	12	11
7–9	6	9–11	7	9	8	13–14	12
10–14	7	12–14	8	10	9	15–16	13
15–26	8	15–18	9	11–12	10	17–18	14
27–50	9	19–26	10	13–14	11	19–21	15
51–∞	11	27–43	11	15–17	12	22–24	16
		44–50	12	18–20	13	25–27	17
		51–∞	14	21–24	14	28–31	18
				25–29	15	32–35	19
				30–37	16	36–41	20
				38–49	17	42–50	21
				50	18	∞	29
				∞	22		

used, it is necessary to sample often in order that at least one estimate will include this rare occurrence. Again, esoteric techniques exist to calculate accurately the frequency, but are outside the remit of this text.

What to do with the data?

It is prudent to know exactly what you are going to do with whatever data are collected; this is the least the individuals who supplied the data deserve. Unfortunately, this is not always the case and one is reminded of the adage 'Don't ask a question if you don't know what to do with the answer.' A number of statistical packages are now available, but care needs to be taken because most of these are significantly more sophisticated than the user's ability to interpret the plethora of inappropriate analyses performed.

The belief exists that almost all personal exposure data are log-normally distributed; however, this assumption is rarely tested. It is possible to test the skewness and kurtosis of a distribution, but this is complex and not always informative. More readily interpretable and certainly less complex is the cumulative probability plot. This is a plot of the individual data points as a cumulative frequency curve, where the percentage scale has been adjusted so that log-normally distributed exposure data will produce a straight line. The drawn line will summarise the characteristics of the population from which the samples were taken and enables generalisations and predictions to be made (Figure 12.5).

To draw a log-probability plot, the data should be ranked in ascending order, the number of results counted, the appropriate plotting points taken from Table 12.2

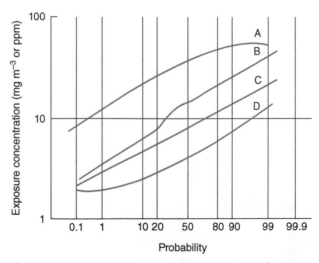

FIGURE 12.5 Four hypothetical probability plots: A, probability plot of a right-truncated distribution; B, probability plot of a mixture of two distributions; C, probability plot of a log-normal distribution; D, probability plot of a left-truncated distribution.

TABLE 12.2

Log-probability plotting points.

Rank order	Sample size (n)																Rank order
	5	6	7	8	9	10	11	12	13	14	15	16	17	18	19	20	
1	12.9	10.9	9.4	8.3	7.4	6.7	6.1	5.6	5.2	4.8	4.5	4.2	4.0	3.8	3.6	3.4	1
2	31.5	26.6	23.0	20.2	18.1	16.3	14.9	13.7	12.7	11.8	11.0	10.3	9.8	9.2	8.7	8.3	2
3	50.0	42.2	36.5	32.1	28.7	25.9	23.7	21.8	20.1	18.7	17.5	16.4	15.5	14.7	13.9	13.2	3
4	68.5	57.8	50.0	44.0	39.4	35.6	32.4	29.8	27.6	25.7	24.0	22.5	21.3	20.1	19.1	18.1	4
5	87.1	73.5	63.5	56.0	50.0	45.2	41.2	37.8	35.1	32.6	30.5	28.7	27.0	25.5	24.2	23.0	5
6		89.1	77.1	67.9	60.7	54.8	50.0	46.0	42.5	39.6	37.0	34.8	32.8	31.0	29.4	27.9	6
7			90.6	79.8	71.3	64.4	58.8	54.0	50.0	46.5	43.5	40.9	38.5	36.4	34.5	32.8	7
8				91.7	81.9	74.1	67.6	62.1	57.5	53.4	50.0	47.0	44.3	41.8	39.7	37.7	8
9					92.6	83.7	76.3	70.2	64.9	60.4	56.5	53.1	50.0	47.3	44.8	42.6	9
10						93.3	85.1	78.3	72.4	67.4	63.0	59.2	55.8	52.7	50.0	47.6	10
11							93.9	86.3	79.9	74.3	69.5	65.3	61.5	58.2	55.2	52.5	11
12								94.4	87.3	81.3	76.0	71.4	67.3	63.6	60.3	57.4	12
13									94.8	88.2	82.5	77.5	73.0	69.1	65.0	62.3	13
14										95.2	89.0	83.6	78.8	74.5	70.6	67.2	14
15											95.5	89.7	84.5	79.9	75.8	72.1	15
16												95.8	90.3	85.4	81.0	77.0	16
17													96.0	90.8	86.1	81.9	17
18														96.2	91.3	86.8	18
19															96.4	91.7	19
20																96.6	20

12.4 The Control of Substances Hazardous to Health (Amendment) Regulations 2004

This section provides a brief synopsis of the requirements of the Control of Substances Hazardous to Health (Amendment) Regulations 2004 (COSHH). The reason for their inclusion is that they provide an excellent example of legislation that dictates a structured process, wherein the employer must review the workplace to identify hazards (as highlighted in Section 12.2) and, if necessary, to collect exposure data in a rigorous and reliable way, and reveal the structure and style of modern risk assessment legislation. Although the exposition of this legislation is in this chapter about risk assessment it is worth emphasising that the absolute fundamental intent of COSHH is 'control' – the risk assessment element is but the first part of the journey. This is worth stating as so many believe that, once the risk assessment is complete, it is 'job done'.

The following is a summary of the essential sections of COSHH. It should be noted that the wording below is that of the authors and not that of the regulations as published.

Regulation 6 – Assessment of the risk to health created by work involving substances hazardous to health

An employer shall make a suitable and sufficient assessment of the risks to the health of workers exposed to substances hazardous to health with a view to controlling those hazards.

Regulation 7 – Prevention or control of exposure to substances hazardous to health

Every employer shall ensure that the exposure of employees is prevented or adequately controlled. Where a WEL exists, exposure should be reduced 'as far as reasonably practicable' (AFARP) below that limit. Where a WEL exists, exposure should be: (i) not exceeded, or (ii) if exceeded, the reasons identified and appropriate action taken to remedy the situation as soon as reasonably practicable (ARP). Control should not be achieved by resorting to respiratory protective equipment, but, if it has to be used, it shall be suitable for the purpose and HSE approved. The principles of good practice for the control of exposure to substances hazardous to health are specified as:

a. design and operate processes and activities to minimise emission, release and spread of substances hazardous to health
b. take into account all relevant routes of exposure – inhalation, skin adsorption and ingestion – when developing control measures

c. control exposure by measures that are proportionate to the health risk
d. choose the most effective and reliable control options which minimise the escape and spread of substances hazardous to health
e. where adequate control of exposure cannot be achieved by other means, provide, in combination with other control measures, suitable personal protective equipment (PPE)
f. check and review regularly all elements of control measures and their continuing effectiveness
g. inform and train all employees on the hazards and risks from the substances with which they work and the use of control measures developed to minimise the risks
h. ensure that the introduction of control measures does not increase the overall risk to health and safety.

Regulation 8 – Use of control measures

Every employer shall ensure that the control measures or protective equipment are properly used, and every employee shall make full and proper use of the control measures and equipment provided and report any defects.

Regulation 9 – Maintenance of control measures, etc.

Every employer shall ensure that the control measures provided are maintained in an efficient state and working order and are in good repair.

Where local exhaust ventilation is provided, its performance shall be examined and tested at least every 14 months, except for certain specified processes and where respiratory protective equipment is provided, then it shall be examined and tested at suitable intervals. Records of any test made under this regulation shall be kept for five years.

Regulation 10 – Monitoring exposure at the workplace

Whenever necessary to maintain adequate control of exposure, to protect the health of employees or for substances listed in schedule 5, regular monitoring is required, the records shall be kept for at least five years or, if required to be kept with medical records as described in Section 11, records shall be kept for 30 years.

Regulation 11 – Health surveillance

- Where appropriate for their protection, employees exposed to substances hazardous to health shall have regular and suitable health surveillance if exposed to a substance or if engaged in a process listed in schedule 6, or if an identifiable disease or ill effect may occur, or if there are valid techniques for the early detection of disease or ill effect.

- The employer is to keep an approved health record of those employees for 40 years.
- Where an employee is exposed to a substance listed in schedule 6, art II, health surveillance shall include medical surveillance by an Appointed Doctor.
- The frequency of medical surveillance is specified in schedule 6, part II, and can continue for a specified period after exposure has ceased.
- An EMA or appointed doctor may inspect any workplace in order to carry out his/her functions under this regulation.
- An EMA or appointed doctor can prevent an employee from working with that substance or he/she can lay down conditions under which that employee shall work.
- An employee shall present himself/herself for medical examinations which shall be during working hours and at the employer's expense and, if on the employer's premises, shall be in suitable accommodation.
- An employee may see his/her own medical record and if aggrieved by what it contains may apply for a review.
- Medical records shall be made available to an EMA or appointed doctor as he/she may reasonably require.

Regulation 12 – Information, instruction and training for employees who may be exposed to substances hazardous to health

- An employer who undertakes work that may expose an employee to substances hazardous to health shall provide such information, instruction and training as is adequate for him or her to know: the nature of the substance and the risks to health created, the precautions that should be taken, the results of any monitoring and whether the WEL has been exceeded, and the collective results of any health surveillance undertaken under Regulation 11.
- Every employer shall ensure that any person who carries out work in connection with duties under these regulations is given such information, instruction and training as will enable him or her to carry out that work effectively.

COSHH assessments

It could be suggested that the section on chemical/biological agents of the walk-through survey, described in Section 12.2, could be supplemented by the assessment required under these regulations. A pro forma approach is again necessary for these assessments, and one is given below.

ASSESSMENT FORM
Company name
Works address
Location of workplace
Single workstation/process assessment   One substance/more than one
Number of workers exposed
List of substances used
Name (trade and IUPAC)
Physical state (dust, fibre, gas, etc.)
Mode of exposure (inhalation, skin)
Toxicity class (very toxic, etc.)
WEL
Known occupational exposure
Toxic effects of each substance (brief description of chronic and acute effects on target organs)
Sketch and/or flow chart of process if relevant (use separate sheet if necessary)

SOURCE OF EXPOSURE
(In the descriptions below outline how the substance(s) come into contact with the worker(s))

Storage (description to include type of container, location, method of opening, also how stores issues are controlled) ....
....
....
Are leaks possible?   Yes/No   If yes, give method of prevention if any
....

Packaging and labelling
Is suitable packaging and labelling provided?   Yes/No
If no, state what improvements should be made ....
....
Transport and transfer (describe how substances are moved from store to point of use)...
....
Is inhalation or skin contact possible?   Yes/No
If yes, state which and describe the method of control if any ....
....
Are spills possible?   Yes/No   If yes, state how and the method of control if any ....
Use (describe how substance is used; refer to the sketch where necessary)
....
Is inhalation or skin contact possible?   Yes/No
If yes, state how and method of control if any ....
....

Disposal of excess material (describe how disposal is achieved) ....
....
Is inhalation or skin contact possible?   Yes/No
If yes, state how and method of control if any ....
....
Emissions to atmosphere (describe what is likely to be present in any
emission to outside atmosphere from within the building) ....
....
Are these emissions likely to cause any environmental problems?   Yes/No
If yes, state how they can be minimised ....
....
Waste products (describe what products and how they are disposed of;
include these products in the list of substances above) ....
....
Is inhalation or skin contact possible?   Yes/No
If yes, state how and method of control if any ....
....
Intermediate products (list any intermediate products that might occur
and state where they could be inadvertently emitted into the workroom;
also include these products in the list of substances above) ....
....
....
Is inhalation or skin contact possible from these fugitive emis-
sions?   Yes/No
If yes, state how their effects could be minimised ....
....

MONITORING
Workplace monitoring
Are airborne concentrations monitored?   Yes/No   If yes, state frequency
....
....
If no, state whether measurements should be taken; give details ....
....
Give results with dates; if frequently or routinely, give the results of the last
three surveys (where appropriate with summary results) and state reference number of the appropriate reports or result sheets (append extra
sheets if necessary) ....
....
....
....
Do the results above show that a hazard to health exists?   Yes/No   If yes,
give details
....

Are surface contamination measurements necessary?   Yes/No
If yes, give details ....
....
....

Health/medical surveillance
Is health/medical surveillance undertaken?   Yes/No
If yes, give or append collective results ....
....
....
If no, state whether surveillance should be undertaken and give details ....
....
....

Biological monitoring
Are biological measurements taken?   Yes/No
If yes, state what and give reference numbers of records and summary of
results; do not mention individuals ....
....
....
Do results of health/medical surveillance or biological monitoring show
any risk to health? Yes/No   If yes, give details ....
....

CONTROL
Ventilation methods of control
If ventilation methods of control are used, state frequency of routine
measurement and give reference number of record sheet ....
....
Do the results show any malfunctioning of the ventilation systems?   Yes/No
If yes, give details ....
....

Protective equipment
If protective equipment is used, describe the type used and method of
selection, inspection and maintenance ....
....
Is protective equipment suitable and in good order?   Yes/No   If no, give
details ....
Is decontamination of protective equipment necessary?   Yes/No
If yes, is it undertaken?   Yes/No   If yes, give details ....
....
If no, what is required? ....
....

Other methods of control not mentioned above
Give details of any methods of control ....
....
Are these methods operating satisfactorily?   Yes/No   If no, state what
improvements could be made ....
....

Training
Do any of the work methods described involve special training?   Yes/No
If yes, give details ....
....
....
Is any training given with regard to the health and safety aspects of the
work?   Yes/No
If yes, give further details ....
....
....
Is this training adequate to minimise the health risk?   Yes/No
If no, give details of extra training required ....
....
....

Welfare and personal hygiene
List the provisions for welfare and personal hygiene ....
....
....
Are these provisions satisfactory?   Yes/No   If no, state what improve-
ments are required...
....

Health and safety work sheets
Are any health and safety work sheets issued?   Yes/No
If yes, append a copy
If no, give details of what should appear on such a sheet; append a draft
if possible ....
....
....

THE ASSESSMENT
Having considered the information provided on the previous pages, I
am/we are of the opinion that (tick as appropriate):
- risks to health are unlikely
- risk is significant but adequate controls are in operation
- risk is significant and controls need to be applied as follows ....
....

- risk is unknown; the following actions are recommended ....
....
....

This assessment should be reviewed (tick as appropriate):
- when the above actions are implemented
- when circumstances change
- .... months from the date given below

Assessor(s)
Name .... Qualifications ....
Position ....
Signature .... Date ....

Initial assessment procedures

In order to make a start on the assessment, it is useful to have a sequence of actions to follow.

1. *List the substances in the area to be assessed.* This important first stage helps to define the size of the task. If the list becomes very large, the areas to be assessed should be reduced and subdivided into manageable packages. A decision is required on whether a complete production process is to be assessed or whether a subprocess within it is more manageable. The number of individual substances appearing in any one operation will probably be the deciding factor. It is also important to determine the volume of storage and use of the substances under review.

2. *Determine which of those substances are actually used.* This important consideration has proved to be a useful economic exercise in itself, as many companies are finding their storerooms and cupboards well stocked with chemicals no longer used but not yet discarded. They are also finding that different sections of the plant are using different chemicals for the same or similar processes, and that some rationalisation of their purchasing policy is required which will benefit the company financially. The COSHH assessment has provided the ideal opportunity to remove all the old substances from the site, some of which may be in an unstable condition and others in containers that are deteriorating rapidly and may soon become an occupational or environmental danger.

3. *Determine the true chemical names and/or Chemical Abstracts Service (CAS) numbers.* Most substances appear in the workplace under a trade name or code number. If the toxic nature of the substance is to be determined from the standard texts, a precise identification is required. All chemicals are issued with a unique name by the International Union of Pure and Applied Chemistry (IUPAC) and a unique number known as the CAS number.

4. *Obtain suppliers' data sheets.* There is a duty under Section 6 of the Health and Safety at Work, etc. Act 1974 for suppliers to provide adequate information on substances supplied, and this is reinforced by The Consumer Protection (Enforcement) (Amendment etc.) (EU Exit) Regulations 2019. This information is usually provided by the supplier in the form of a safety data sheet (SDS). The quality of the information supplied is very variable – the best giving all the information required to appraise the toxicity of the substance, the worst giving information that is misleading and sometimes dangerous. It is advisable to have standard letters available to request this information and more strongly worded back-up letters in the event of default.

5. *Evaluate data sheets.* It is wise to check the validity of the information supplied on the data sheets. For example, the IUPAC name of the substance or substances may not be given, making it difficult to check the toxicity information provided. Alternatively, if the substance is a mixture of chemicals, such as a proprietary solvent, not all the ingredients may be shown. It is understandable if the exact formulation of a mixture is not given, because the supplier has 'trade secrets' to protect, but a list of substances present without the exact proportions can be given without running the risk of industrial espionage!

6. *Check the toxicological data given and rewrite the data sheet.* Once the name of the substance is known, a simple check on the accuracy of the toxicological data given should be made before writing the data sheet to suit the way the substance is used in the situation being assessed. The data sheet will need to be rewritten or supplemented to take into account the way in which the substance is to be used. The suppliers cannot be expected to anticipate the way their substance is to be stored, transported or handled in the workplace under review, but the employees will require some guidance. This is a requirement of Regulation 12 of COSHH.

7. *Inspect the places where the substances are handled.* Now is the moment to inspect the way the substance is being handled to establish the modes of exposure and the possible risk to those employed. The ways in which the material is stored, transferred to the point of use, dispensed into the process and disposed of after use all pose a potential risk to those involved. It is in this way that it is possible to establish whether the exposure is to the skin or via inhalation, the two most common modes. At the same time, on-site observations can be made of the eating, drinking and smoking activities in the workplace, all of which can be a potential means of causing systemic absorption.

8. *Inhalation route – check airborne monitoring.* If the substances are dusty or volatile, and there are open containers providing surfaces for evaporation, there is a likelihood of inhalation being the main route of entry. If it is not possible to assess/quantify by other means, it may be necessary to measure the airborne concentration of the substances in the 'breathing zone' of the worker and to compare the results with published standards. Occupational/industrial hygiene surveys may need to be arranged.

9. *Skin contact route.* Observations on the method of handling will reveal whether skin contact is likely. When liquids are being transferred from one receptacle to another, even if mechanically handled, splashing could occur, and, with any open surface of liquid, accidental contact is possible. In addition, the handling of wet materials with unprotected hands is an obvious source of exposure. Measurements of airborne exposure may not be adequate to establish the degree of exposure, but the wary eye, backed-up with a knowledge of the material's potential dangers, may be what is needed to assess this hazard. If not, biological monitoring should be considered.

10. *Look at the method of control.* The performance of control methods (Chapter 15) needs to be assessed. In some cases, this can be performed by observation, whereas, for others, it will involve some technical measurements. If airborne substances are being controlled, the ultimate test is the airborne concentration in the breathing zone of the workers involved. If the levels are substantially below an applicable WEL, usually it is not unreasonable to assume that control has been achieved. More subtle methods of control involving working procedures and good supervision will have to be checked and seen to be working satisfactorily before accepting that the process is free from risk.

11. *Implement improvements before the final assessment.* If, as a result of this initial assessment procedure, some obvious faults are seen, they should be rectified speedily before completion of the final assessment. If the improvements appear to require time to implement, an interim assessment should be made with a view to reassessment later.

12.5 Control Banding

Occupational health and safety professionals require a systematic process for risk assessment and control that is based on science. Traditionally, that has been anchored in the quantitative methods described above, but there is a complementary qualitative process known as 'control banding' that also provides a solid scientific foundation. Control banding is a complementary approach to protecting worker health that arose in the mid- to late 1990s and has become more mainstream in professional practice over the past decades. These strategies offer simplified solutions for controlling workers' exposures to constituents that are found in the workplace in the absence of firm toxicological and exposure data. It is with this absence of information, especially when work is performed with chemicals that do not have established WELs, that control banding utility in the occupational/industrial hygiene profession is becoming a more mainstream practice.

Control banding can be considered a qualitative or semi-quantitative approach to risk assessment and risk management that groups occupational risk *control* strategies into *bands* based on their level of rigour. For example, the HSE developed a COSHH Essentials control banding strategy to assist the vast majority of small- and medium-sized industries (SMEs) in the UK that may not have the finances for professional occupational/industrial hygienist specialist assistance to perform the required chemical risk assessments. This outcome came with HSE's realisation that there were many substances for which WELs would never be developed and that the majority of SMEs did not understand and did not have the resources to meet the COSHH requirements to conduct risk assessments for chemicals used in the workplace. In response, the HSE established a working group of key stakeholders to develop a simple system for generic risk assessment. This approach, which leads to selection of appropriate controls, was first published as *COSHH Essentials: Easy Steps to Control Health Risks from Chemicals* and is now available as an online application (https://www.hse.gov.uk/coshh/essentials/coshh-tool.htm). This COSHH Essentials approach includes four levels for controlling exposures to chemicals:

    1.1   good occupational/industrial hygiene practices, including PPE
    1.2   engineering controls, including local exhaust ventilation
    1.3   containment, and
    1.4   the need to seek specialist advice.

Control banding is the stratification of work-related risks into 'bands' that have each been assigned controls based on the potential hazard and, in some cases, the potential for exposure. Most control banding strategies focus resources on the prevention of workers' exposure to chemical substances purchased and used in bulk form, either liquids or powders used in larger quantities. Control banding has grown well beyond these bulk chemical origins and is now applied into the broader occupational safety, health and hygiene realm. These newer applications provide utility for a wider variety of workplace hazards, including nanomaterials, safety, ergonomics and comprehensive occupational risk management, although the focus here is primarily on chemicals. It should be noted that there are similar strategies, such as hazard banding or occupational exposure banding, that seek to offer only the stratification of chemical risks and do not utilise commensurate controls as an outcome. Hazard and control banding provide a process for evaluating hazards and risks in situations where WELs may or may not exist. Some experts see this as a benefit as decoupling hazard banding from control banding allows assessment of hazards to be used in hazard communication to promote greater understanding after a substance has been introduced into a workplace. Hazard banding and occupational exposure banding, although not a substitute for WELs, yield insight into the relative toxicity of substances and can be used to aid in substitution and design of controls coupled with the knowledge of the physical state of the substance.

Various qualitative risk-ranking and banding concepts and principles have been developing since the 1970s within pharmaceutical, insurance, biological and radiological industries. These combined in the late 1990s to result in a simple but powerful concept:

Health hazard + Exposure potential → Generic risk assessment → Control strategy

The UK HSE played a pivotal role in developing a regulatory approach based on these concepts. The key components of control banding models include the hazard banding, exposure potential and control approaches. It is important to point out, however, that COSHH Essentials is limited to substances classified under the historic British The Chemicals (Hazard Information and Packaging for Supply) Regulations 2009 (CHIP), thereby excluding, for example, pesticides and pharmaceuticals, which are outside the scope of those regulations, and also process-generated hazards such as wood dust, silica dust and welding fumes (tending now to be covered by task-specific control guidance sheets [CGSs]). Exposure potential, when used as a component of control banding applications like COSHH Essentials, may be based on quantity in use, volatility or dustiness, and frequency and duration of exposure. The volatility of a liquid chemical can be obtained from SDSs and the other factors can be estimated for a given task by non-experts based on simplified guidance and easily selected input parameters. A given chemical's hazard may be captured by hazard statements (formerly known as risk phrases or R-phrases) commonly found in SDSs or other indicators of toxicity or hazardous properties.

The adoption of the Globally Harmonized System (GHS) of classification and labelling of chemicals has been an important concept for expanding the reach of control banding in a standardised format within national regulations. The GHS is a common and coherent approach to classifying the health, physical and environmental hazards of chemicals, and to communicating the hazards through labels and SDSs. GHS includes the core set of label elements that has aided in the harmonisation of hazard statements (H-statements) for each category and class of chemicals covered. It also has a harmonised approach to classifying mixtures of these chemicals. Adopted by the United Nations in 2003, the GHS is now aligned within legislation in over 60 countries. Global implementation of the GHS would thus provide an international system upon which to base control banding. This standardisation of H-statements for expanding the reach of control banding has already been implemented by regulation in the European Union (EU) and the USA's Occupational Safety and Health Administration (OSHA) is now aligned with the Hazard Communication Standard with the latest edition of GHS. The World Health Organization's International Programme for Chemical Safety is now modified to follow the GHS criteria for classification and the harmonised H-statements and is updating these periodically to account for the latest scientific developments, providing a source of information on many of the most commonly used chemicals.

The COSHH Essentials adds two significant developments to the generic risk assessment process: it is specifically developed for SMEs and it includes control advice in the form of CGSs. This former element is a significant difference as most earlier control banding approaches, such as those for the pharmaceutical industry, were intended for use by experts like toxicologists. The latter component of CGSs build on this simplification as they are designed for both common and specialised tasks and form a key component of COSHH Essentials. Additional control banding strategies focus on the dynamics of the task performed to directly assign PPE and control options without the interim step of assessing potential exposure (thus providing 'direct advice'). Over 300 CGSs have been published; in addition, there are over 200 additional direct advice sheets (DASs) covering many industries, including microelectronic chip manufacturing, offshore oil, printing, welding and construction work. Each CGS and DAS is structured according to a standard format and contains sections on access, design and equipment, maintenance, examination and testing, cleaning and housekeeping, PPE, training, supervision, a short list of references, a sample schematic of an engineering control and an employee checklist for proper utilisation of controls. The Asbestos Essentials series is a good example of the applications of the control banding strategy where direct advice can be given in the form of CGSs, based on good control practice reached by consensus of industry experts. These DASs and CGSs require no detailed data input. They can be downloaded (https://www.hse.gov.uk/coshh/essentials/direct-advice/index. htm) by selecting task sheets on equipment and methods and activities, such as non-licensed work with asbestos cement, textured coatings, insulating board and other asbestos-containing materials.

It is widely agreed that the COSHH Essentials approach should not be adopted uncritically by other countries as the approach must be seen in the context of personal protection, training and health surveillance as appropriate. An additional and substantial point is that this approach is not intended to replace exposure measurement, interpretation, substance and chemical control. Before control banding strategies can be accepted, adapted and implemented on a wide scale, a few issues must be addressed regarding validation and verification. As presented here, validation refers to the many components related to accuracy of the model itself, and verification refers to the correct installation, operation and maintenance of controls. With a qualitative risk assessment process, it is expected that outcomes may skew towards recommending more conservative control options; therefore, there is the potential for an over-prescription of controls that may lead to unnecessary expense. However, this an accepted approach as leaning towards the conservative is far more acceptable than outcomes with an under--prescription of control that could lead to a false sense of worker safety, serious injury and even death. There are multiple decision points in the application of control banding that may contribute to error; each step of the control banding strategy should be validated independently of the others, including issues related to the creation of the model, application of the model and failure analyses at each step of the control banding process (e.g. assignment, reporting and understanding of H-statements). Verification would include evaluating the installation/operation/use of controls to reduce exposures in specific workroom situations through follow-up surveys.

Beyond bulk chemicals

In expanding control banding concepts beyond management of bulk chemicals, it is recognised that, while hazards vary, two criteria remain constant: (i) hazard, exposure, and risk levels must be derived using rigorous scientific principles and (ii) less acceptable risks must be linked to increasingly stringent controls, using increasingly conservative decision criteria where knowledge is limited. While many questions about the specifics of this process remain unanswered, the basic premise of banding hazards, exposures and controls holds continued promise for applications beyond bulk chemicals and for further refinement as screening tools for use by health and safety experts and non-experts. On the control guidance side of the control banding tool applications, there has been development of banding strategies for ventilation requirements in laboratories. The Laboratory Ventilation Management Program uses American National Standards Institute (ANSI) Z10, ANSI Z9.5 and control banding strategies to create a tool to establish institutional target ventilation rates. A comparable methodology was also inspired by control banding strategies to provide health and safety staff with limited resources with the ability to conduct laboratory assessments using a hazard mapping methodology to assist in risk ranking to make informed decision recommendations to upper-level management. In addition, respiratory protection selection tools have been developed in the UK for effective use with H-statements and process-generated substance scenarios. Canada has developed a Web-based respiratory protection guide for bioaerosols that can also be used in the healthcare, agricultural and business sectors and the US OSHA has created an Advisor Genius eTool to assist users in the selection of an appropriate respirator based on the NIOSH Respirator Decision Logic and the OSHA Respirator Protection Standard regulations. Control banding has also become an essential component internationally for assessing and controlling exposures in the nanotechnology industries and for addressing work-related communicable diseases, as it is now considered a logical and proven approach to utilise in the absence of toxicological research, WELs and regulations (see Chapter 18 for more on both topics).

In the last decade, multidisciplinary control banding strategies have been designed for integration within standardised occupational health and safety management systems such as the ISO 45001 and OSHAS 18001 standards and environmental management systems such as ISO 14001 standard with the goal of providing a unified environmental and occupational risk management approach. For this expansion of control banding applications currently available, the art of qualitative risk assessment is quite basic. A hazard is defined and considered, the level of risk is stratified to a minimal number of components and the commensurate controls necessary to reduce each risk level to an acceptable outcome becomes the output. Determining the number of risk levels, which fits the concept of bands or binning, is a result of balancing the intricacy or complexity of the hazard with the needs of the worker. This simplified approach can provide solid benefits for interdisciplinary health, safety and environmental control banding efforts can be seen as these applications are tending towards using common models, strategies and outcomes. This commonality of information presented in more simplified formats creates an opportunity for improved communication both within and between health and safety professionals and can thereby create beneficial risk communication improvements with workers and their managers. An example of this generic approach can be seen in the 4×4 risk matrix model that applies the control outcomes previously described for occupational/industrial hygiene applications in Figure 12.7.

Control banding strategies and applications have also been developed outside of the occupational/industrial hygiene realm. The European Framework for Psychosocial Risk Management (PRIMA-EF) incorporates control banding concepts to

Probability

		Extremely unlikely (0–25)	Less likely (26–50)	Likely (51–75)	Probable (76–100)
Severity	Very high (76–100)	RL 3	RL 3	RL 4	RL 4
	High (51–75)	RL 2	RL 2	RL 3	RL 4
	Medium (26–50)	RL 1	RL 1	RL 2	RL 3
	Low (0–25)	RL 1	RL 1	RL 1	RL 2

Control bands:
RL 1: General ventilation
RL 2: Fume hoods or local exhaust ventilation
RL 3: Containment
RL 4: Seek specialist advice

FIGURE 12.7 Risk level (RL) matrix as a function of severity and probability. Source: Paik et al. (2008).

integrate the hazards of chemical and physical stressors such as solvents, noise or stress into the realm of the mental wellbeing of employees and total worker health applications. This framework acknowledges that the hazards of these stressors, in a social and organisation context, can contribute to different sorts of harm such as the systemic stress that is manifested from fear of exposure to harmful solvents. A control banding framework has also been incorporated into the International Labour Organization's (ILO) Ergonomic Checkpoint materials – publications that aim to reduce work-related accidents and injuries by suggesting proven and inexpensive ergonomic solutions such as better designed tools, use of carts, materials-handling techniques and workstation arrangements. The original checkpoints manual presents 132 realistic and flexible interventions that are aimed at reducing injury in the workplace without the expense of hiring consultants. The efforts of the ILO checkpoints programme have resulted in a series of three mobile 'apps' that address ergonomics (general and agriculture) and stress prevention at work. Users can access detailed checkpoints with illustrations, create custom checklists and prioritise and export notes in the workplace right from the app.

Occupational safety strategies have also been developed as, in line with the banding of chemicals by toxicity, classifications already exist for various variables of accident causation. Banding safety risks for selection of appropriate barriers for injury prevention is similar to selecting appropriate engineering controls based on chemical hazard bands in control banding. Barriers to injury, including management factors, are strongly related to the quality of safety management systems and are important parameters for risk prevention. This approach for safety has been called a barrier banding model that considers the application of safety phrases to accident scenarios or related situations and guides the user to the type of precautions needed to prevent traumatic injuries. Similarly, a comparable risk management system has been developed for industrial safety field practitioners to assist in performing risk assessments of accidents based on expert evaluation data to assist in the development of guidelines to develop preventative barriers and their maintenance. The implementation of this risk-level assessment protocol assists in providing the right information to management to prioritise decisions necessary to achieve emergency prevention, the ongoing assessment of safety barrier maintenance proactively and accident prevention measure effectiveness overall. Additionally, a qualitative, risk-based control banding strategy for the assessment and control of potential environmental contaminants using the same 4×4 risk matrix approach based on severity and probability that is presented above has also been developed. Using this same graded approach provides not only a simplified risk assessment and control format that is easy for environmental analysts to use but also a standardised and beneficial approach to risk communication for working with health and safety professionals, management and workers alike. This control banding model provides an effective means for determining standardised responses and controls for common environmental issues based on the level of risk. The model is designed for integration within occupational health and safety management systems, like ISO 45001, to provide a multidisciplinary environmental and occupational risk management approach. Qualitative environmental control banding strategies are now available to identify controls for tasks based on US and EU regulations that are also intended for addressing other local, regional and national regulations for construction, research activities, facility maintenance and spill remediation that affect air, water, soil and waste disposal.

With these multidisciplinary applications now available, a framework and protocol designed for an industry can also be developed utilising comparable control banding strategies. The construction industry presents a pervasive and consistent set of tasks performed globally that is ripe for a comprehensive, systematic approach to assess and control occupational risks holistically. There is a construction toolbox design that is based on these same control banding strategies that includes international input on multidisciplinary approaches for performing a qualitative risk assessment on the severity and probability of a construction project within the same 4×4 risk matrix scoring framework Figure 12.7. The outcome of this scoring determines a risk 'band' for a given project that is used to identify the appropriate level of training to oversee construction work. Identifying a graded risk banding of projects is extremely important for planning and budgeting construction efforts; however, as this risk banding can be performed before the project begins, the input parameters for severity and probability can be adjusted in planning by modifying task parameters to ensure that the right level of oversight expertise is available in advance and fits the projected costs. Construction project tasks are also given a graded risk control level (CL1–CL4) commensurate to risk that assists in identifying the appropriate control methods to perform the work safely. This format harnesses multiple solutions-based national programmes and publications for controlling construction-related risks with simplified approaches across the health and safety professions. A more comprehensive occupational risk model based on control banding is the Risk Level Based Management System (RLBMS) that is designed to focus environmental, health and safety resources on the highest risk procedures at a given workplace. The model utilises control banding's qualitative risk assessments performed in advance of work being performed. The model uses the same risk matrix presented above; however, the control outcomes present a gradient of increasing rigour of documentation required to ensure regulatory requirements. RLBMS creates an auditable tracking of activities, maximises health and safety staff time in the field and standardises a graded approach to documentation as a control outcome commensurate with a given task's risk level. Quantitative validation of risk levels and their exposure control effectiveness is prioritised at the higher levels of risk and is collected in a traditional personnel exposure monitoring regime for regulatory auditing.

As can be seen by this growing collection of control banding applications, the topic remains a subject of much enthusiastic praise as well as objective criticism. With all the growth and regulatory acceptance of the banding strategies, there remains a lack of understanding that control banding strategies are intended for applications in specific situations, primarily in cases of inadequate data to assess toxicity and/or exposure, or in situations in which health and safety professional expertise is not available, affordable or accessible. Control banding strategies are not intended to replace traditional industrial approaches, specifically WELs and monitoring of air contaminant levels, and, in fact, many proponents of these approaches have made clear statements about the need to continue to monitor workers' exposures. Perhaps the greatest strength of control banding is as a potentially powerful tool for knowledge management. Knowledge management is an emerging field focusing on assessing the creation, transfer and utilisation of knowledge to address specific challenges. The development of hazard control guidance materials, CGSs and the application of control banding strategies provides the means for effective occupational health and safety knowledge management. The global explosion in electronic communications has shown itself to be well suited to facilitating management and transfer of this knowledge. Realistically, many of the several billion workers throughout the world, and even many millions in the USA and UK, will never benefit from direct health and safety expertise; they may, however, benefit from the non-expert advice transferred via control banding strategies. The obvious goal of any control banding strategy is to reduce the burden of occupational injury and illness. Wider application of control banding should increase public understanding of the need to control occupational exposures to chemicals and other hazards, leading to an increased recognition of the need for professional expertise and useful solution-based databases. There are undoubtedly situations in which control banding cannot provide the precision and accuracy necessary to protect worker health; alternatively, there are undoubtedly situations in which control banding will provide a higher level of control than is necessary. Despite these limitations, control banding strategies have the potential to be excellent screening tools in the hands of both experts and non-experts to assist in providing necessary controls to reduce workplace exposures.

12.6 Biological monitoring and biological effect monitoring

Biological monitoring (biomonitoring) in occupational health and safety is the detection of substances (biomarkers) in biological media of workers and the comparison of their concentrations with reference or limit values. It has several applications but this section is limited to chemical exposures. The fundamental aim of biomonitoring is to obtain data on the efficacy of exposure control and to correct deficiencies, either due to systematic failures (inadequate extraction ventilation or poorly selected PPE are illustrative) or because of an individual's poor adherence to good practices. Additionally, employees with evidence of excessive uptake of a toxicant may need individual attention, either medical or administrative, such as relocation to a lower exposed workstation or worksite. Biomonitoring can help in exposure assessment of specific chemicals, characterisation of exposure pathways and identification of potential risks. Biomarkers can detect the exposure or a biological effect of the exposure (biological effect monitoring) or reveal susceptibility. Within the occupational context, biomonitoring is a key tool for assessing overall systemic exposure. It is of particular importance when assessing actual worker risk, as air monitoring alone may either over- or under-estimate the total uptake of certain substances. Biological monitoring may thus help in the interpretation of a worker's airborne exposure and also identify those substances where skin and gastrointestinal uptake are relevant. Biomonitoring may be interpreted at group or individual levels. The media most commonly used are urine and blood (with saliva, hair, semen and faeces also being used); although a multitude of substances can be measured, there are still only limited numbers of validated methods and limit values with proven value, meaning they are indicators of failures in exposure controls or predictive of health consequences.

Classification of biomarkers

A biomarker can be any substance that can be monitored in tissues or fluids and that correlates with exposure or predicts or influences health. Biomarkers are signs of exposure, (reversible) effect or susceptibility with possible adverse health outcomes. Biomarkers are classified into three categories depending on their use or the specific testing context.

A **biomarker of exposure** is the substance, or its metabolite, or the product of an interaction that is measured in a compartment or a body fluid. For example, lead in blood may fairly represent lead exposure of an individual.

A **biomarker of effect** in occupational health is a measurable physiological alteration that can be associated with exposure to a workplace agent. The effect is usually reversible but may indicate the potential for disease occurrence. For example, the change in concentration of red blood cell cholinesterase resultant from application of organophosphate pesticides.

Biomarkers of genotoxicity (chromosomal aberrations, micronuclei, Comet test) are used to identify exposure to genotoxic chemicals, usually at group level. They are sensitive but not specific indicators and are generally inadequate for routine occupational risk assessment purposes.

A biomarker of susceptibility is the marker of an ability to respond adversely to the challenge of exposure to a chemical. Genes can make certain individuals more vulnerable to toxins. Atopy is an example of susceptibility to become sensitised to some allergens. Biomarkers of susceptibility are generally not recommended for occupational biomonitoring.

Exposure and biotransformation

The three main exposure pathways to chemicals are inhalation (lungs), dermal (skin) and gastrointestinal (ingestion), with inoculation being more rare. Biological monitoring considers the overall systemic exposure regardless of the source or pathway. Biomarkers may also reflect circumstances such as a change in atmospheric pressure, co-exposures and respiratory rate (e.g. heavy work-load), which may all lead to a higher (or lower) uptake of the substance.

Once it enters the body the chemical (and its metabolites) can:

- be distributed among body compartments (e.g. blood, soft tissues, bone)
- undergo various modifications (biotransformation)
- cause functional changes and diseases
- get excreted.

All these pathways are particular to the chemical substance concerned and may be specific to the individual. They may be influenced by internal or external non-occupational factors (Figure 12.8).

In the process of biotransformation, the external chemical substances are transformed in the body (metabolised). Enzyme activities are the fundamentals of individual variability and susceptibility, including determining metabolic pathways and speeds of metabolism, absorption and excretion. There are many modifiers in biotransformation: sex, age, body mass, co-exposures (workplace, non-occupational, e.g. diet, including fat, alcohol and medication). Compared with the original substance, its degradation products may be less or more harmful (the latter = activation). These metabolites may be used as biomarkers (of exposure or effect) as well.

Toxicokinetic features explain that many substances (although identifiable in the metabolic process) cannot be used for biomonitoring because of short half-life and/or disappearance from the accessible matrix, e.g. from the blood or the urine.

Sampling strategy and chemical analysis

Planning a biomonitoring programme for a specific purpose starts with the selection of an adequate sampling strategy (see Section 12.3). The number of workers selected and their location in the workplace should be determined with the objective of the programme in mind. If dermal exposure is the concern, then workers with

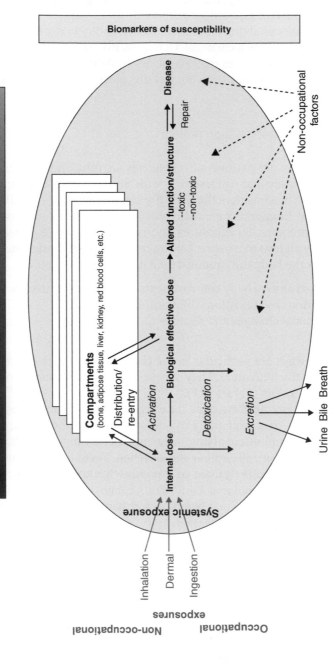

FIGURE 12.8 Overview of the process of exposure and biotransformation and possibilities of biomonitoring. Source: Adapted from Manini et al. (2007), complemented by Náray & Kudász (2015).

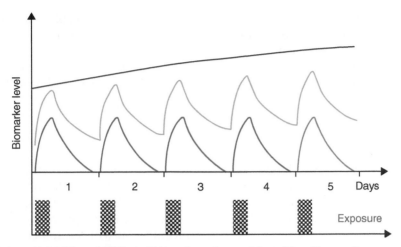

FIGURE 12.9 Different half-lives of biomarkers. Source: Adapted from Fiserova-Bergerova et al. (1997), complemented by Náray & Kudász (2015).

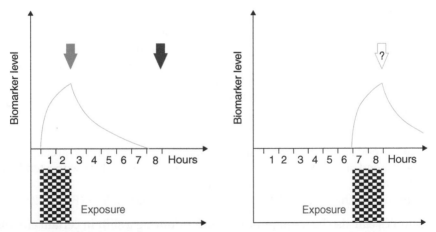

FIGURE 12.10   Possible pitfalls in biomonitoring of irregular exposures and short-half lives of biomarkers. Source: Miklós Náray and Ferenc Kudász - Authors own construct.

potential skin contact should be the core group. Ideally, a biomarker of exposure is specific for the exposure concerned (single chemical substance or a group) and reliably detectable, using non-invasive sampling. Periodical examinations are set either at fixed intervals or according to the previous biomonitoring results.

The analytical method is critical for the validity/reliability of a biomarker: accuracy, precision, reproducibility, recovery, sensitivity and specificity all influence the consistency with the limit and reference values concerned. Several factors may affect the quality of the samples and the measurement of biomarkers: type of matrix (see Biological matrices), point in time of collection, containers and preservatives and other additives used to stabilise the sample, storage temperature, exposure to ultraviolet light (i.e. sunlight) and transport time. Reliable and validated analytical methods must be used supported by internal quality control and preferably external quality assurance schemes.

The success of a biomonitoring programme highly depends on good cooperation of partners: workers, the employer, the occupational physician/hygienist and the laboratory.

Biomarker half-lives and timing of sampling

In the different matrices, biomarkers have different half-lives, which is the time it takes for the concentration to drop to half in whatever form being measured. Knowledge of half-lives of biomarkers then determines the appropriate sampling strategy: the timing and the frequency of sample collection. For substances with long half-lives their concentration will reach a certain value that remains stable (equilibrium) and reflects long-term intake during continuous exposure. In such cases, the timing of sample collection during a working day or even working week is not important. However, enough time must be given from exposure onset or stabilisation to reach equilibrium (e.g. lead, cadmium).

When the half-life is short (e.g. a few hours) the concentration varies remarkably during the working day or week; thus, the timing of sampling is critical. Such a concentration reflects exposure over a short time and may not be representative of average long-term exposure. A meaningful picture of the average exposure may be obtained only from several samples.

Examples of different half-lives are given in Figure 12.9. Usually sampling takes place

- at the end of a shift for short half-life biomarkers (Figure 12.9, green)
- at the end of the working week for short half-life biomarkers with a tendency to cumulate (Figure 12.9, orange); and
- any time for highly cumulating biomarkers with long half-lives (Figure 12.9, red).

Samples can also be taken prior to a shift or during a shift in certain circumstances. Generally, sampling is to be undertaken at a time when the inner and the external exposures are in a state of equilibrium, which is not to be expected in cases where exposures/activities are short (maintenance, etc.). In such cases, sampling shall be performed at the end of the relevant activity.

Figure 12.10 illustrates the challenge of biomonitoring for different exposures to substances with short half-lives:

- If exposure takes place in the first two hours of the shift, subsequent sampling (Figure 12.10, green arrow) assesses peak exposure, while end-of-shift sampling (Figure 12.10, red arrow) misses detection of the substance.
- If exposure takes place in the last two hours of the shift, sampling at the end of the shift (Figure 12.10, orange arrow) detects peak exposure. If exposure is erroneously reckoned as all day, the total daily exposure will be over-estimated.

Biological matrices

The most important routine biological samples are urine, blood and occasionally exhaled air. Hair and nails may provide information on long-term exposure, but analytical difficulties and uncertain reference values limit their use.

Urine collection is more readily accepted by workers (not invasive), but contamination of the sample, e.g. from particles on overalls, must be avoided. In routine urinary biomonitoring spot samples may be adjusted for dilution (by creatinine or specific gravity). Whether or not to adjust should be determined by the reference value: is it adjusted or not? Highly diluted or very concentrated urine samples (creatinine: <0.3, >3.0 g/l; specific gravity: <1.010, >1.030) are not suitable for such adjustment; thus, new specimens should be collected. The acceptable range should be confirmed with the testing laboratory.

Blood is the second most common biological matrix used in routine biomonitoring. Unlike urine, the composition of blood is regulated within narrow limits, thus it seldom needs adjustment. Blood sampling is useful for inorganic chemicals (e.g. metals) and for organic chemicals that are poorly metabolised and have a sufficiently long half-life.

Exhaled air analysis is non-invasive and most appropriate to estimate exposure to volatile organic substances (e.g. solvents), although it is used much less frequently.

Setting of biological limit values

Exposure concentrations equivalent to the biological limit values (BLVs) generally do not affect the health of the employee adversely, except in cases of hypersensitivity. A BLV can be either health based or exposure based. A health-based BLV is derived directly from human studies. Thus, the BLV may not necessarily have a relationship with the occupational exposure limit (OEL) but rather with the levels at which the potential adverse health effects are observed in studies. A more common practice is to derive the BLV from the OEL based on established correlations between air levels and biomarker level. In this case the BLV is obtained from the corresponding OELs by matching the 'mean' level of a biomarker in workers with the corresponding OEL. BLVs are named differently around the world. Probably the best known BLVs are the biological exposure indices (BEI values) of the American Conference of Governmental Industrial Hygienists (ACGIH) and the biological tolerance values (BAT values) used in Germany.

There may be a substantial variation among values obtained from different workers on the same day and also from day to day for a single worker; this may make dose–response relationships harder to assess and is a reason for repeat testing if concentrations are close to the BLV.

BLVs in occupational medicine are set for healthy adults. There is no general rule for setting BLVs for workers with certain health impairments. The disease may influence the biomarker level directly (e.g. biomarkers of effect), or the disease may alter the uptake, metabolism or excretion of the chemical. For these workers biomonitoring needs to be reconsidered and an individual approach may be necessary.

Certain vulnerable groups may require stricter limit values, e.g. blood lead in fertile women and young workers.

Use of biological monitoring

Whether or not biological monitoring is desirable in a workplace is influenced by many considerations. Generally, it is needed when workplace air levels of a chemical may not describe the potential uptake by employees of a substance adequately. Biological monitoring may be a statutory obligation, such as in lead-using workplaces in many countries. Good practice may underpin its utility: the law does not require it in a particular jurisdiction, but it is widely practised. Importantly, skin exposure may contribute substantially to internal concentrations, and ingestion also, although less commonly. Non-occupational environmental exposures may add to the workers' intake of an agent: arsenic in drinking water, for instance. OELs are generally set for moderate manual work: hard work (increased air intake over a shift) may render these OELs inadequate to assess uptake of a chemical (for some workers, moderate work for their colleagues can be heavy work for them because of differences in strength). The functionality of workplace hazard control measures and PPE, especially newly introduced or modified, can be determined using concentrations of biomarkers. Biomonitoring may add information for risk assessments, for example in identifying highly exposed tasks. Exposures outside formal working hours (e.g. at home to earn extra money) or prolonged shifts may increase concentrations above those expected from eight-hour levels (with commensurately less time for metabolism and excretion between shifts). Determining dose–response relations in epidemiological studies has benefited significantly from the use of individuals' concentrations of biomarkers.

Putting aside the issues around exposure determination, a primary question in deciding whether biological monitoring should be undertaken is 'Would the money spent on biological monitoring be better used to control workplace exposures, thus making biological monitoring unnecessary?' For example, if skin exposure can be eliminated, biological monitoring may become unnecessary.

Interpretation of biological monitoring results

Biomarker concentration is compared with appropriate reference values, but the user should be aware of all the uncertainty of the results and how the reference is defined; for example, contributions to the concentration of the biomarker from non-occupational sources. A biomarker above the reference value does not necessarily mean increased health risk for the individual but may rather show potentially higher exposure than the reference population.

Ethical considerations

Individual biomonitoring results are seen in some jurisdictions as medical data, thus should be handled accordingly as applicable. Interpretation of the results is the task of the occupational health team, not just a physician trained in the field of occupational health, because the data are primarily for identification of areas of over-exposure and their remediation, even if individuals with excessive uptake may need individual attention, e.g. temporary relocation to lower exposed jobs while exposure controls are improved. Individual workers should be informed of their biomonitoring results. Group data should be communicated to the employer and workers' representatives as well as health and safety committees if established. The ethical considerations must be regarded during the process of a biomonitoring study.

The International Commission on Occupational Health's code of ethics (see Chapter 20) states that 'Biomarkers must be chosen for their validity and relevance for protection of the health of the worker concerned, with due regard to their sensitivity, their specificity and their predictive value.' The principles of this internationally agreed document are:

- Biomonitoring should not be used as screening tests or for insurance purposes.
- Current knowledge in biomonitoring of susceptibility does not justify job opportunity discrimination of affected workers.
- Priority should be given to non-invasive (urine) and easily collected sampling (spot). In these cases, informed consent is usually not required for routine procedures using validated biomarkers.
- Invasive tests or tests posing a health risk call for a risk–benefit analysis, and informed consent of the worker.

References

https://oshwiki.eu/wiki/Biological_monitoring_(biomonitoring). *Accessed 8 March 2021.*

Kromhout, H., van Tongeren, M., and Burstyn, I. (2005). Design of exposure measurement surveys and their statistical analyses. In: *Occupational Hygiene*, 3e (eds. K. Gardiner and J.M. Harrington). Oxford: Blackwell Publishing.

Paik, S.Y., Zalk, D.M., and Swuste, P. (2008). Application of a pilot control banding tool for risk level assessment and control of nanoparticle exposures. *The Annals of Occupational Hygiene* 52 (6): 419–428.

Further Reading

Zalk, D.M., West, E., and Nelson, D.I. (2021). Control banding: background, evolution, and application. In: *Patty's Industrial Hygiene*, 7e (ed. B. Cohrssen). Hoboken, NJ: Wiley Publishers.

Risk Management

13.1 Introduction

Addressing occupational health risks and ensuring that they are managed should be addressed in the manner that one approaches all potential safety issues. Utilising the construction trades as an example, ill-health statistics indicate a prevalence of respiratory risks (asbestos, silica dust, inhalation of hazardous chemicals), skin exposures (chemicals, cement, sunlight), noise, hand–arm vibration and physical strains that lead to musculoskeletal disorders. An appropriate first step is to identify whether any of these risks may present themselves in the workplace. Next is to observe the work performed, the behaviours and actions workers utilise to undertake their work, the controls that they use and whether all available controls are utilised appropriately. Therefore, the same approach for avoiding accidents or infection control is also applied in the prevention of work-related illness and disease. Wherever there may be an opportunity for work-related risks to health and safety, then there is also a legal obligation to identify, control, prevent and manage these exposures to hazards and their risk. Even when all feasible and practical steps have been taken to reduce these work-related risks, residual risks to workers' health and safety may still be present. If this is the case, then it may also be necessary to ensure that there is an occupational health surveillance system in place as this may further aid in ensuring that the controls that have been identified and put into practice are actually succeeding as intended. Further, the implementation of a mechanism for feedback and improvement should also be put in place to manage the assessed risks and aid continuous improvement over time.

Pocket Consultant: Occupational Health, Sixth Edition. Kerry Gardiner, David Rees, Anil Adisesh, David Zalk, and Malcolm Harrington.
© 2022 John Wiley & Sons Ltd. Published 2022 by John Wiley & Sons Ltd.

Organisations have a responsibility to minimise workplace risks not only for their workers and their management, but also for contractors and visitors that may either participate in the tasks performed directly or be present intermittently in the workplace. The International Labour Organization estimates that there were 2.78 million deaths worldwide attributable to workplace risks in 2020. The World Health Organization estimates that the vast majority of these deaths are attributable to occupational health issues, with safety-related injuries and accidents constituting a much smaller component of these deaths than many may assume. The Institute of Occupational Safety and Health estimates that there are 660 000 deaths a year in the UK as a result of cancers arising from work activities. Taken collectively, it becomes apparent that an organisation's activities can indeed present work-related risks that can lead to disease, illness, injury, accident and serious health effects to its workers and the greater envelope of potential staffing. Therefore, there is sufficient reasoning for organisations to realise and accept the responsibility that an appropriate level of identification, control and management of these workplace risks be implemented to ensure that preventative measures are in place and to act sufficiently over time to minimise or eliminate these risks. An occupational health and safety management system (OHSMS) provides the process and programmes to assist an organisation with addressing these obligations formally and professionally.

An OHSMS can assist an organisation by translating its intention of preventing or minimising work-related risks into a systematic approach that can identify a series of ongoing processes as well as associated tools and methods that clearly and transparently present an organisational commitment to improving its health and safety performance. Worker participation in the building of an OHSMS and its processes is an essential component towards its overall success, especially when workers are also involved in its implementation, maintenance and feedback towards improvement. Workers not only are the most knowledgeable of their tasks but also can offer keen insight to their work-related hazards and afford invaluable feedback on what control strategies may be the most practical and enduring. The historical development of OHSMS standardised expectations began with the British Standards Institution's (BSI) development of BS 8800. The BS 8800 guidelines then became the OHSAS 18000 series of standards that, up until recently, has served as the preferred and accepted OHSMS around the world. This then became the model for the development of ISO 45001:2018, a global standard with the goal of enabling organisations to manage work-related risks optimally and provide measurable objectives towards improving their health and safety programme's performance. ISO 45001:2018 also includes an emphasis on employees' competency in understanding how to undertake their work safely as well as workers' participation and its importance for achieving a fully functional and successful overall programme. Taken overall, implementing an OHSMS can also address organisational strategic objectives while ensuring both that workers are healthy and safe while preserving, if not enhancing, its economic objectives.

13.2 Process

As with all risk management, the concepts of hazard and risk are inherent components and should be understood. Hazards are a particular exposure to a situation that has the potential to cause injury, illness or both. All things in a workplace that have this potential can therefore cause an accident or a work-related disease. Hazards can be physical, chemical or biological and include everything from working at heights, vehicular traffic, slips, trips and falls, as well as chemical substances or communicable diseases. Psychosocial hazards can also be considered as they can affect workers' health as a result of their perceptions and personal experiences that cover a broad range of situations that can vary from job insecurity and stress to workplace bullying or harassment. However, risk considers both the severity of the potential injury or illness and the probability that exposure to a given hazard or situation will occur. Just as exposure to risk is a given in all daily activities, workplace risk requires decisions on what is considered acceptable and what is not. This acceptable risk concept is also ingrained in risk management as organisations will need to make decisions on this based on input factors that also include legal obligations and internal policies.

As risk management should include a feedback and improvement component as part of its cycle, organisations should strive for a systematic process that includes the commonly applied Plan–Do–Check–Act method. This comprehensive examination ensures a review and assessment of tasks and how they are performed, who performs tasks and their level of expertise, work areas and materials, job processes, work-related equipment and its maintenance, and overall examination of the work environment. With this systematic process in place, the goal of identifying what adverse outcomes might occur in the workplace and offering the organisation an informed decision on risk acceptability can be achieved. In general, workplace risks should be kept to a level that is As Low As Reasonably Achievable, also known as the ALARA principle. Taken as a whole, this is the essence of risk management as the decision to ensure controls are put in place and maintained effectively over time is integral to preventing work-related injuries and illnesses and maintaining both profitability and a confident workforce that knows that its workplace prioritises the prevention of work-related risks and values its health and safety.

The risk management process includes a number of standardised steps; a good summation is:

- identification of exposed workers, which also includes vulnerable workers, workers with disabilities, maintenance, cleaners, contractors and visitors
- descriptions and characteristics of work procedures, tasks, equipment and materials
- identifying control measures, safety barriers and protective processes already in place

- historical assessments of workplace accidents, injuries and illnesses, and
- documentation on national/federal and local regulations, internal policies and existing standards.

This process can be achieved by applying a number of different techniques, including:

- workplace walk-throughs (see Section 12.2) to provide direct observations of the work being performed
- reviewing logs and records for workplace accidents, injuries and illnesses
- documentation of the equipment in use and its maintenance cycles
- compiling a list of chemical substances used and their safety data sheets
- conducting interviews with workers as well as management; consider surveys as well
- worker participation in the process, while compiling workplace information, and
- assessing all applicable regulations, legislation, standards and policies that are available.

The risk analysis process should involve:

- hazard identification based on what is currently present in the workplace
- historical records of hazard identification that may have occurred previously, and
- consideration and documentation of potential adverse outcomes that may result from any of the identified hazards and have the potential to cause work-related injury or illness.

This evaluation process should also include conducting risk assessments relating to given hazards, existing controls and previous decisions on risk acceptability. Risk assessment processes can be both quantitative and qualitative, involving experts or utilising control banding tools (see Section 12.5), and including participatory methods. Overall, risk assessment methods help to ensure that hazard severity and probability of occurrence are included in the evaluation, ranking and stratification of workplace risks into categories ranging from low to high. Once an organisation's acceptable risk criteria have been set, these risk assessment outcomes can then be compared and considered for inclusion as part of a comprehensive risk management system.

Once the risk assessments are complete, the next step is to identify what steps are necessary to ensure that the appropriate controls and safety measures are put into place and maintained over time to reduce or eliminate these work-related risks. This is known as risk control and it is important to ensure that the working population potentially exposed to these risks be considered vulnerable workers who may require additional control considerations. Risk control includes all levels from the hierarchy of controls (see Section 15.1), so engineering design, planning and implementation of controls is as important as the administrative controls for worker training, medical surveillance and record retention. As part of the control hierarchy, the first consideration should be to eliminate risks or substitute high hazard issues for a lower hazard option. If this is not possible, then risk control processes should ensure that the ALARA principle is applied. Risk control should include prevention measures, protection measures and mitigation measures. Prevention measures reduce the likelihood of work-related injuries and illnesses and include a primary consideration of engineering controls that can help design out potential exposure to hazards, but also include the multiple administrative control options available. Protection measures seek to enclose, isolate or place barriers between the hazards and the workers; the more workers protected by each of these measures the better. Mitigation measures are put into place to ensure that, should the hazardous exposure or energy be released, the severity of the potential adverse outcome is minimised or possibly eliminated. Broad examples of this include warning systems, evacuation plans and emergency response preparedness. More task-specific examples include fire extinguishers, ground fault interrupters and fall restraint devices. Taken cumulatively, just as organisations should know the risks that are inherent to their workplace, workers must know these too. That is why there are regulatory requirements for a worker's 'right to know' of the workplace hazards they are potentially exposed to and the controls in place to minimise their risks. The risk management process documents all of this information to provide an appropriate overview of the hazards, risks and controls in place as well as which work areas and tasks have ongoing assessments; the employees most at risk; the hazards present, their severity and probability of exposure; and the levels of risk that led to ensuring that commensurate controls have been put in place and are maintained.

13.3 Programmes

Organisations can adjust the design and size of an overall risk management programme to suit their needs, according to British Standards. Risk outcomes informed by the risk evaluation process afford an opportunity to sort and rank risk in line with the level of severity. Acceptable risk decisions can be obtained by comparing the value of risk outcomes with the value of risk as reflected in legislation as that can be seen as a baseline requirement. Organisations can certainly make decisions that surpass legislation requirements; however, legislation is not always available to inform decisions. There are additional occupational safety and health guidelines and various international standards that can add necessary decision-related information. As mentioned above, the internationally accepted framework of ISO 45001:2018 provides a global standard guide for the OHSMS process. This standard enables organisations to optimise their available work-related risk information to provide safe and healthy workplaces by preventing work-related injury and illness, and improve their health and safety performance in a proactive process. ISO 45001:2018 is designed to assist organisations by offering a standardised mechanism for continuous improvement, fulfilling legal requirements and achieving overall occupational health and safety (OHS) objectives in line with achieving an international benchmark.

The seven primary sections of the 11 overall elements of ISO 45001:2018 are listed below, with the first three sections introducing the standard and its scope. The seven sections are as follows.

Section 4: Context of the organisation. This section requires the organisation to determine its context in terms of the OHSMS, including parties with vested interests, needs and expectations. The requirements are defined for determining the OHSMS and general OHSMS requirements.

Section 5: Leadership. This section outlines the expectations of top management, demonstrating leadership and OHSMS commitment as well as defining the OHS policy. Top management are also to assign process owners with established roles and responsibilities.

Section 6: Planning. This section outlines the requirements for addressing risks, identifying opportunities and defining occupational risk analysis requirements. Expectations for hazard identification and assessment, determining established requirements and defining both health and safety objectives and establishing plans for achieving them are also discussed.

Section 7: Support. This section reviews requirements for supporting processes and providing resources to ensure effective operations under the OHSMS. Requirements for staffing, infrastructure, work environment, monitoring and measuring resources, competence, awareness, communication and documented information are also defined.

Section 8: Operation. This section establishes operational controls to eliminate the OHS hazards, to enable change management and to facilitate emergency response and preparedness.

Section 9: Performance evaluation. The section provides requirements for the organisational mechanisms necessary to determine OHSMS effectiveness. Essential monitoring and measuring of established performance evaluation, compliance obligation, internal audit and management review are discussed as required components.

Section 10: Improvement. The final section defines OHSMS requirements for continuous improvement to ensure that non-conformities, incidents and corrective actions are managed.

Each of these sections is designed as part of the Plan–Do–Check–Act cycle, as these elements are essential for implanting process changes in the organisation to drive and maintain improvements. To obtain ISO 45001:2018 certification it is not sufficient to simply document and implement the OHSMS as establishing its effectiveness is also necessary for standard compliance. There are established steps that assist with this and prepare organisations for certification audits. The first step is performing an internal audit to gauge the level of OHSMS compliance in line with the standard's expectations. This would include document and record reviews and identifying processes to indicate programme weaknesses and non-conformity information. The next step is for top management to review OHSMS performance information that would include internal audits, achieving objectives and affecting organisational change. This process assists management in making decisions on how to best improve the current OHSMS. These first two steps provide the information necessary for the last step of established corrective actions to bolster the OHSMS with the necessary corrections, changes and improvements. Taking these corrective actions assists in achieving full standard compliance. The certification process comprises the documentation review stage and the main audit. Auditors will first provide a comprehensive review of existing OHSMS documentation for compliance with ISO 45001:2018, but also to achieve organisational familiarity and outline the necessary processes for the main audit. The heart of the process is the main audit when auditors will conduct multiple interviews at all organisational levels and conduct ground-floor walk-throughs to observe all established processes in the field and compare observations with all document-related expectations to ensure commensurate implementation. This comprehensive process not only follows the pathway towards achieving ISO 45001:2018 certification but also assists in establishing that all necessary OHSMS elements are in place and achieved in practice.

13.4 Risk communication

As important as establishing an OHSMS is to defining a global standard for showcasing organisational excellence in health and safety programmes, achieving the ability to communicate programme elements and related issues clearly and concisely with all workers is considered, by many, to be equally essential as OHS professionals have dedicated their careers to developing the skills, knowledge and abilities necessary to become effective specialists. Although communication of risk is an important component of their chosen discipline, little time is dedicated in the educational process to teaching effective strategies for having a constructive dialogue with anyone in the risk generation/mitigation chain. Learning how to communicate risk with the actual workers is probably the most important lesson for field practitioners to learn if the end goal is achieving recognition, control and long-term prevention of workplace hazards. Risk communication challenges faced by individual OHS disciplines can vary greatly and are further affected by the type of audience, the message delivered and how well the information is understood. In this section models and strategies are presented that assist in simplifying and standardising the language that can be used by OHS professionals for communicating risk to any audience. In addition, these risk communication strategies can also benefit discussions within and between OHS disciplines to enhance a multidisciplinary risk management programme. Clear and consistent risk communication helps to ensure that all those listening can understand the risks being communicated and comprehend what their roles and responsibilities are to ensure that workplace risks are minimised or eliminated.

Risk communication in the occupational setting is most often associated with emergency preparedness and response, communication to the public and communication within and between responders to a potential crisis situation. In the occupational/industrial hygiene profession, risk communication is most important in discussions with workers; however, communicating risks in a language that workers understand can be a difficult expectation, especially when this skillset is not an essential component within the training curriculum of field practitioners. Learning how to communicate risk to workers is probably the most important lesson for field practitioners to learn if the end goal is to achieve recognition, control and prevention of workplace hazards over the long term. It is over time that the chronic exposure-related diseases develop, so ingraining the inherent workplace risks to the workforce is an essential component of risk assessment outcomes and risk management practices as a whole. It is also important for an occupational/industrial hygienist to learn how to communicate with their OHS peers as well: if the comprehensive workplace risks and necessary preventative measures cannot be understood among safety, health and environmental professionals, then they cannot be fully understood by workers either. This is especially true for the current trend of OHS generalist professionals. OHS generalists need to understand for themselves where and how the relative risks for each of the individual OHS disciplines interact and are prioritised for a given task or process. However, this essential need for professionals to have a multidisciplinary mindset is yet another under-served component of risk communication that needs to be addressed. As the concept of risk is understood differently depending on the audience, the methods to communicate risk to managers and even into corporate boardrooms also becomes a critical, yet limited, point of discussion and teaching. Collectively, this holistic mindset can be considered as a process for directional risk communication for stakeholders: the understanding of how to communicate at the worker level, the interdisciplinary level and the upper management level. To accomplish this, it is important to develop a single, simplified form of communicating risk. By doing so, everyone who is a necessary partner for the field practitioners to accomplish their goals can speak a standardised language. This helps to ensure that all those listening can understand the risks being communicated and comprehend what their roles and responsibilities are to ensure that these workplace risks are minimised or eliminated.

Defining risk

The definition of terms that we will be working with will assist in creating a solid foundation for building a standardised language for communicating risk throughout the workplace. Risk, as defined above, reflects the common viewpoint of establishing the probability that harm may occur and that hazards are considered to be anything that may cause this harm. Risk is a term that may be applied in many different contexts within the OHS professions; however, its definition is viewed more broadly across society at large. Our values are what we might potentially lose when we are exposed to risk. Economics, societal position and emotional and physical wellbeing are all categorical values that we share. These values can be improved or lessened based on the risks we choose to take, decide not to take or are forced into accepting either actively or passively. Judgements on accepting risk, which fit well within OHS discussions, are most often based on risk as a function of severity and probability. We take on a relatively high risk of compromising physical health and potential financial loss every time we get into an vehicle, but it is apparent that society either perceives this risk–benefit decision differently or perhaps does not fully understand the relative risks in making that choice. Work-related decisions about risk are often considered a product of the severity of a given hazard and the probability that an adverse outcome will occur. It is the role of OHS professionals to identify, assess, control and manage these risks feasibly. This may be a bit more complicated for some hazards that may affect each of the OHS professions differently. For example, a chemical exposure hazard might lead to acute or chronic illnesses, be a source of pollution and may also degrade the quality of a safety system in the workplace.

Communicating risk

Just as the definition of risk can pertain to personal wealth, physical health, emotional health or even one's status in society, the methods used to communicate this information to others may also vary. The true value of risk communication is when this real-time, two-way exchange of information creates a meaningful and accurate exchange of information that enables those at risk to make informed decisions to avoid or minimise potential adverse outcomes. Risk communication becomes a valuable component of risk management, integrating the assessment of risk and potential exposure that is just as necessary for investing in the stock market as it is in the workplace. This value is maximised when the exchange of information targets the right stakeholders and where the dialogue being communicated emphasises both the importance of risk management and the need for an ongoing monitoring of the risks presented. A common issue for communicating risk lies in determining the correct method of making the risk understandable and relatable to other relative risks while retaining the respect of those receiving the information. Risk communicators must also take into account another compounding factor for this issue: those receiving the message may have their own inherent fears and understanding of the risks presented; for example, a professional may communicate specific risks to potential radiation exposures really well, but there may be audience members who have already concluded that no level of radioactive exposures can ever be safe. This may complicate the role of OHS professionals communicating risk as these potential biases need to be understood and considered but may be difficult to address. In addition, accounting for these issues may be at a local level, as in the safety culture of a workplace, or perhaps at the regional level, when implementing risk management programmes in different countries worldwide.

Emergency response

Risk communication, as it relates to occupational and environmental considerations, is primarily focused within the scientific literature and through governmental institutions on the topic of emergency response. Serious emergency response parameters such as radiological or biological terrorism, chemical plant releases or explosions or infectious disease issues are all situations where sound and practical risk communication to the right target audiences is essential to ensure that potential deleterious issues are not compounded. The offering of timely and accurate objective and impartial data provides great assistance to those managing the process and confidence to the affected communities, and can aid in achieving a coordinated and effective emergency response. One method used to better understand the risk perception of a given audience relating to potential emergency or crisis situations and improving the development of communication strategies is known as the 'deliberative decision-making process'. Creating an open dialogue between government institutions, experts and the public is an excellent strategy for initiating preventative steps towards adapting the right information for the appropriate audience in a timely and consistent fashion. In an era of immediate and broadly spread media accessibility, understanding this process and the information it provides is especially important for OHS professionals. It can assist in developing a keen understanding of how to provide consistent and clear risk communication in the workplace using methods that are just as important for terrorism responses as they are for environmental policy and nanotechnology risks. As there is no singular strategy or process for risk communication effectiveness, it is very important to understand the complexity in how delivering the necessary information can be affected by both the communicator and the receiver of information.

Multidisciplinary roles in risk communication

Emergency response can certainly be an important component of the roles and responsibilities of OHS professionals, both as an active participant and in the development of plans and programmes. However, when it comes to the day-to-day activities and interactions with the workers who professionals are morally and ethically required to protect, there is far less information available to effectively assist in communicating risk and achieving a reduction in work-related exposures to hazards. It is important for OHS disciplines to understand their own strengths and weaknesses. Most professionals spend their entire career developing the skills, knowledge and abilities necessary for their field practitioner specialties. Their level of success is often built upon performing their roles and responsibilities in an environment where normal communication skills are enough for addressing routine issues and problems. Although OHS staff may be comfortable in their professional duties conversing on more technical topics among themselves, the ability to communicate this information to the workforce and their management may need development. Communicating risks can become even more complicated when anger, criticism, fear, lack of trust and other emotionally driven issues become entangled within workplace discussions. It is important for OHS practitioners to understand their innate communication styles. Everyone has strengths and weaknesses within their natural habits for communication and understanding these is an essential component for learning how to change and improve this skillset. This process begins by under-standing the pitfalls of risk communication inherent to their discipline and other OHS professions. It is also about learning how to overcome these personal and professional hurdles while remaining competent. Questions must be answered in a language of risk understood by workers, managers and all potential stakeholders.

When it comes to effective risk communication the OHS professions are each faced with unique hurdles that are important to address individually. In so doing, a better and more efficient method for understanding one's strengths and weak-nesses is very helpful. It is necessary to understand the audience's perception of the communicator's expertise, the potential complexity of the message they are communicating and how the audience may be affected by the message. In addition, there is the growing population of OHS generalists who are self--employed, working with small consulting companies or working for multina-tional firms that are increasingly being found to have an amazingly small OHS staff. An increasing number of OHS professionals work for consulting firms that provide broad services to industry and government on a contractual basis. This includes those who work for insurance carriers that provide consulting services to the company's various clients. In some instances, these relationships are sta-ble and allow the development of industry-specific expertise. In other cases, the OHS practice is broad-based and varied, not affording professionals the opportu-nity to strengthen skillsets. Consulting practice presents considerable challenges in risk communication as well, as professionals may be required to influence internal corporate culture and intervene with stable prevention activities exter-nally from the company. Therefore, many companies are outsourcing OHS responsibilities that include occupational/industrial hygiene, occupational safety, occupational health and environmental analyst functions. Manufacturers may ask their OHS staff to monitor not only the indoor air quality but also the hazardous emissions released into the air and water of surrounding commu-nities. Public health agencies or environmental groups may hire or otherwise call upon OHS professionals to monitor pollutants in community air and water as well. Therefore, it is also essential for OHS generalists to understand the risk communication expectations of the individual OHS professions as they are em-ployed to potentially provide this information to workers, to workplace man-agers, to the public and to the environmental community.

CHAPTER 14

Principles of Occupational Epidemiology

14.1 Introduction

Definition

Epidemiology may be defined as the study of the distribution and determinants of health-related states or events in specified populations, and the application of this study to the control of health problems. Whenever consideration is given to the health of groups of people – and this is invariably so in occupational health – the principles of epidemiology must be understood. Therefore, occupational health professionals need not only to be conversant with the methods of epidemiological investigation but also to be able to incorporate some of these concepts into their work. Collecting, presenting and interpreting data for annual reports is one example of the practical application of epidemiological principles. Even if the various disciplines never wish to undertake an epidemiological study, at the very least they

Pocket Consultant: Occupational Health, Sixth Edition. Kerry Gardiner, David Rees, Anil Adisesh, David Zalk, and Malcolm Harrington.
© 2022 John Wiley & Sons Ltd. Published 2022 by John Wiley & Sons Ltd.

must be able to understand and perhaps even evaluate such studies. This chapter aims to cover these areas.

Consideration of the definition given above implies that epidemiology concerns a study of the distribution of the disease and a search for the determinants of the observed distribution. Clearly, the clinical disciplines within occupational health will concentrate on this disease/condition outcome whereas all of the specialties involved in measuring substances/agents/etc. will be concerned with the exposure assessment element with the epidemiologists relating one to the other. Epidemiological methods provide the means to relate health status to the exposure experienced by study subjects.

The process of elucidating disease causation using epidemiology involves three types of investigation:

1. a description of the current status of health of the 'at-risk' group or its exposures (descriptive epidemiology)
2. ad hoc studies to test aetiological hypotheses to get closer to the likely cause (analytical epidemiology), and
3. the design and execution of a study that aims to alter exposure to the putative risk factor to assess whether this leads to an altered disease rate (experimental epidemiology); the last type of study is frequently difficult to design and execute for ethical reasons but, in the final analysis, epidemiology is concerned with preventing ill health by establishing the causes of disease and removing them.

Uses

In occupational health, epidemiology has five main uses:

1. the study of disease causation or associations with risk factors
2. the study of the natural history of a disease
3. the description of the health status of a specified population
4. the evaluation of intervention in health-related issues
5. the development of hygiene standards from epidemiological studies of exposure and health outcome.

Sources of data

Population census and death registrations were first introduced for political and legal reasons. They have, nevertheless, been a never-ending source of data for the investigation of occupational causes of disease. Pension records, sick benefit schemes and treatment records have likewise been used. In fact, epidemiologists will use almost any source of personal health record to further their research, although few have been collected initially with such research in mind! However, the emergence of powerful personal data protection legislation in many countries threatens the very existence of some types of epidemiological research.

National or regional records (vital statistics)

During an individual's lifetime, major milestones are recorded for various purposes. Birth, marriage, divorce and death are all recorded whether on a regional or national basis. The registrations are undertaken locally and stored centrally.

Death certificates

Death marks the final event in an individual's health record. It is readily verified, and in countries where registration is complete it provides a reasonably accurate and quantifiable measure of life-threatening illness in the community. Inaccuracies in such countries apply only to the cause of death, not to the fact of death. Internationally agreed coding systems exist for death certificate information – the latest is the 10th revision of the International Statistical Classification of Diseases and Related Health Problems (ICD-10; https://icd.who.int/browse10/2010/en) but ICD 11 is due for release – and this enables death certificates to be analysed by underlying cause. It also allows for more valid between-study comparisons.

It has been established with reasonable certainty that death certificates are fairly accurate in high-income countries and, if based on broad diagnostic categories, the 'true' cause of death is correctly coded in over 80% of cases. This accuracy varies with the disease: subcategories of cardiovascular and respiratory disease can be notoriously difficult to define, whereas a disease such as leukaemia is much more accurately defined as it requires a precise pathological diagnosis prior to the institution of treatment. In fact, in many parts of the world informative death certificates are the exception – significant research has been undertaken in low- and middle-income countries where verbal autopsies (information on death circumstances collected from relatives, friends, etc.) are used because the death certificates may simply state 'natural causes' or not exist at all.

Occupation is typically recorded on the death certificate as the 'last known' or usual occupation. Although uniformly applicable, it leads to a statistic of limited value when studying retired decedents or persons whose death was actually caused by a previous or secondary occupation. For example, the occupational categories 'retired', 'housewife' and 'civil servant' are epidemiologically useless. Similar inaccuracies are noted when pneumoconiosis is seen to be the cause of death in a car park attendant: this is not due to the dust generated as cars drive in and out of the parking area past the man's booth, but to the fact that the attendant is probably a pensioned-off coal miner. Such inaccuracies can sometimes be circumvented using factory pension scheme records (see 'Local records').

Birth certificates

In the past, these records were primarily used for the establishment of denominators for the calculation of infant disease rates. The recent advent of recording congenital malformations and pregnancy complications, as well as birth weight and duration of pregnancy, has afforded an opportunity of using these records when studying the effects of the mother's as well as the father's occupation. The strictures regarding diagnostic accuracy are, however, similar to those for death certificates.

Morbidity

Nationally or regionally acquired morbidity records regarding health and safety at work are available in some countries. They may be less accurate than mortality records (albeit that Scandinavian disease registers are generally good) and for epidemiological purposes may require supplementation with ad hoc recording in order to make them acceptable. Errors in diagnosis, failure to report accidents, illness and injury, and incomplete coverage by law all militate against these sources of data as ideal epidemiological tools. Sickness absence data are particularly deficient regarding female employees and are notoriously inaccurate, except for the broadest diagnostic groupings. Nevertheless, such statistics can indicate gross secular changes and may highlight new hazards. For diseases that are not life-threatening, these are crucial measures of occurrence.

Newer surveillance schemes based on voluntary reporting of certain diseases by occupational health practitioners and hospital specialists are proving to be useful adjuncts to the national statistics.

Local records

These may be acquired through hospitals, family doctors, factories, schools, pension schemes, insurance policies, professional associations and trade unions. All such records have been used at one time or another by occupational health epidemiologists. However, they are all collected for purposes unrelated to epidemiological study, and their accuracy, completeness, comparability and relevance are always doubtful.

Ad hoc records

Some large industrial organisations now maintain continued surveillance of the 'high-risk' workers, not only as they move from job to job within the company but also if and when they leave or retire. These exposure registers can be of inestimable benefit later on in assessing the health status of workers in various exposure circumstances many years previously. At present, there are few industries in which retrospective exposure data of any worth are available.

Notification and registration of certain specific diseases have been made compulsory from time to time. Early examples include various infectious diseases such as whooping cough or measles. More recently, cancer registries have been established in a number of countries. The more efficient ones now boast a diagnostic accuracy in excess of 98%, with a high level of enumeration. Other examples include registers set up to monitor specific diseases such as mesothelioma, angiosarcoma of the liver, pneumoconioses, adverse reactions to certain drugs, specific congenital malformations and certain disabilities, such as blindness.

Despite this wealth of health records, the epidemiologist frequently has to search several sets to obtain only a portion of the information required regarding an employee's health. It may still be necessary to contact the employee or his or her next of kin for further data. Even if a total picture of that employee's health from the cradle to the grave is acquired, it may still be too imprecise about possible occupational hazards and their relationship to the worker's health owing to the paucity of exposure data at the factory or factories at which the person worked.

14.2 Measures of exposure and health outcome

Information relating to hazard exposure and health outcome acquired from the above data sources has to be expressed in terms that permit comparisons between and within populations. This section deals with some of those measures and the concepts underlying their use.

Exposure

For the foreseeable future, this will remain the least accurate measure and therefore the weakest link in the chain between cause and effect. The majority of epidemiological studies investigating occupationally related causes of disease falter when it comes to establishing, with accuracy and precision, the exposure histories of the populations of workers under study, unless it is rapid disease onset and acute exposure being assessed, e.g. allergens and asthma.

In the final analysis, the ideal epidemiological study will show a dose–response relationship between a suggested cause and the disease outcome. This adds great strength to the association being causative and also materially assists in establishing safe (or relatively safe) working conditions for future generations of employees.

At present, past exposures are frequently classified as low, medium and high or merely expressed in years of exposure of whatever degree. This is most unsatisfactory. Ideally, past exposure information should be of high quality and measured with great accuracy/precision and sensitivity/specificity, using standard, or comparable, instrumentation. It should not only provide information on, say, the concentrations of the toxic material potentially (and realistically) absorbable by the workers, but also provide accurate data on variations in that concentration during the work cycle – daily, weekly, monthly – and its duration.

In addition, data should be available on other relevant exposures, especially those associated with the disease under investigation; for example, smoking and chronic obstructive pulmonary disease (COPD). These include changes in the physical and chemical formulation of the toxic substance in the worker's immediate environment as well as an assessment of possible interactions between various noxious elements, whether they be additive, multiplicative, synergistic or even negative, as well as confounders, i.e. other causes of the disease such as smoking in lung cancer/COPD investigations.

At present such data are rarely available, and if available are virtually never complete. Thus, they furnish epidemiologists with a continuing source of major error (attenuation) in their investigations.

The range of possible exposure groupings is:

1. ever/never employed in the industry
2. length of service in the industry

3. job categories by precise division or task duties (qualitative)
4. job categories ranked ordinally by exposure intensity
5. quantitative exposure intensity categories
6. quantitative dose categories.

Health outcome

Measures of occurrence

In epidemiology, the most common measures of occurrence are the incidence and the prevalence. Incidence is commonly expressed as rates per 'person-periods' (usually person-years). The 'incidence' of a disease relates to the occurrence of new cases and the 'incidence rate' relates to the number of new cases that occur in a given population over a given period of time. (Strictly speaking, the 'incidence rate' [or incidence density] should be distinguished from the 'cumulative incidence', which relates to the proportion of persons developing the disease. Also, incidence [and prevalence] can be expressed as episodes of disease rather than persons.)

The 'prevalence' of a disease concerns the existing number of cases of the disease at one point in time or over a period of time. Prevalence is, therefore, in strict terms, a ratio of the number of existing cases to the population at risk at a given time over a given period.

Prevalence and incidence are related to each other with reference to a given disease through the duration of disease. The relationship can be expressed thus

$$\text{Prevalence} \propto \text{incidence} \times \text{duration}$$

Pictorially, this can be conceived as a reservoir (Figure 14.1) supplied with water from streams above and released through the dam below. The quantity of water in the lake (the prevalence) is dependent upon the amount flowing into it from the streams above (the incidence) and the amount of water leaving the lake below the dam (those people with the disease who cease to have the disease – they recover or die). One implication of this relationship is that, although the incidence of a condition is declining, the prevalence can be rising. This occurred with human immunodeficiency virus (HIV) infection in many countries: effective public health promotion programmes reduced incidence but at the same time the introduction of antiretrovirals meant that people with HIV infection lived longer, thus increasing the prevalence in the population. In practical terms, incidence may need a clear definition for the occurrence of chronic diseases with a vague or prolonged onset, e.g. lung cancer. Typically, the incident case is then identified at diagnosis, rather than at disease onset, which is unknown. Incidence is a more straightforward measure when the disease is acute and has a clearly defined onset.

Measures of frequency

These are rates of one sort or another. Although rates are established to allow comparability between populations, they can be confusing if a clear idea of their

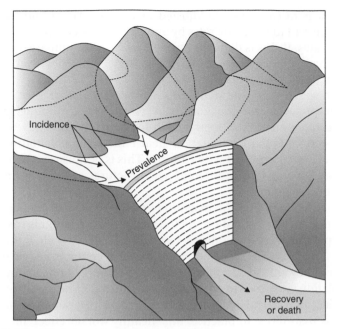

FIGURE 14.1 Relationship between incidence and prevalence.

limitations is not established. In essence, there are three measures of frequency of a given event (death, disease, accident, etc.):

1. crude
2. adjusted
3. standardised.

These and other epidemiological definitions are lucidly defined in *A Dictionary of Epidemiology* (see Further reading).

For illustration purposes, we will concentrate on measuring the frequency of death, but any health-related event can be so measured.

$$\text{Crude death rate} = \frac{\text{total deaths in the population at risk}}{\text{population at risk in person} - \text{years}}$$

Such a death rate is far from ideal as the deaths relate to both sexes, and, more importantly, to all age groups. Comparison of two crude death rates could lead to erroneous conclusions. For example, the crude death rate for town A (an industrial centre) is 12 per 10^6 per year and the rate for town B (a seaside resort) is 15 per 10^6 per year. The implication is that town B is a less healthy place than town A. This is because no account has been taken of the age breakdown of the populations. Town A has a younger population and the age-specific deaths are all higher than in town B, but town B has an older population. The way around this dilemma is to calculate an adjusted death rate. This removes the latent weighting inherent in the crude rates by another set of weights – in this case, the age-specific rates. If this is done for towns A and B, the comparison now shows town A to have higher age-specific death rates than town B and summary statistics can be calculated to reflect this.

Although widely used, the standardised mortality rates (SMRs) do have pit-falls in interpretation for the unwary. First, as the technique involves an indirect age adjustment, SMRs calculated for two or more study populations, using the same standard population death rates for calculating expected deaths, should be interpreted with caution. This is because the two index pop-ulations may have markedly different age structures and the age adjustment may thus be inadequate.

The second point is that the magnitude of the SMR is dependent upon the choice of the standard population. As the standard population is frequently the national population, it is, by definition, less healthy than a working (occupational) population. This is because the national population contains people who do not work because they are sick, disabled or dying. Therefore, if one assumes that the index population is exposed to no serious occupational hazards, the SMR for that occupational group, calculated using national data as the standard, should inva-riably be less than 100%. In practice, this 'healthy worker effect' means that an unexposed occupational group, when compared with the national population, should have an SMR of about 80–90.

The third factor is that SMRs gloss over age-specific differences in the working population. Not all workers are exposed equally to the putative hazard – it might be more severe in the youngest group, or more noticeable by its cumulative effect in the older groups. A way around this is to consider age-specific SMRs.

A fourth factor that could be relevant is socio-economic class. There are differ-ences in SMR by socio-economic class and the proportion of each in the two populations compared may not be equal. Allowances can also be made for this. Although socio-economic class is a convenient grouping, it is made up of inter-related factors that include income, education and way of life (such as housing and site of house) as well as occupation.

Finally, it is necessary to mention the proportionate mortality ratio (PMR). This statistic, although not as robust as the SMR, is useful particularly when populations at risk are not accurately known. The PMR is the proportion of deaths from a given cause in the index population divided by the proportion of deaths from that cause in the standard population.

The relevance of time, place and person

From what has gone before, the reader should, by now, have realised that num-bers, the currency in which epidemiologists deal, have to be continually reviewed in light of factors that could lead to comparison problems. In short, epidemiolo-gists strive to compare apples with apples, not apples with oranges.

Assembling the data for an epidemiological investigation is a bit like piecing together the crucial elements in a criminal investigation or occupational/industrial hygiene sampling strategy. The questions are the same:

1. To whom?
2. Where?
3. When?
4. By what? (Why?)
5. How?

The sixth question that is vital to health prevention can be added to these – **So what**?

The main characteristics affecting person, place, and time are summarised in Table 14.1.

Measures of risk Risk estimation is primarily a function of data analysis but can be conveniently considered here. Two measures are commonly used:

1. relative risk
2. attributable risk.

Relative risk is the ratio of disease rate in exposed persons to the disease rate in non-exposed persons. *Attributable risk* is the difference between disease rates in exposed persons and disease in non-exposed persons.

The magnitude of the relative risk is a measure of the strength of the association between the risk factor and the disease – the magnitude of the statistical significance is not related to this strength.

Case–control studies (see 'Case–control and follow-up studies') do not usually permit relative and attributable risk values to be obtained as described above, as such studies do not usually permit direct measurement of disease rate but measure the relative frequency of risk factor exposure.

TABLE 14.1

The Main characteristics affecting the person, place and time.

Person	Place	Time
Age	Natural boundaries	Day
Sex	Political boundaries	Month
Ethnic group	Urban/rural boundaries	Year
Social class	Place of work in factory	Season
Occupation	Environment	—
Marital status	Climate	Secular and cyclic
Family	Migrant status	—
Genes	—	—

14.3 Causation or association

Before considering specific types of epidemiological studies, one further concept needs to be emphasised: the statistical association of a risk factor with a disease does not necessarily prove causation. The association could be spurious or it may be indirect through other known or unknown variables. Epidemiological techniques can never prove that A causes B, but they can often provide considerable support (or denial) for a causal hypothesis.

Such support can be conveniently considered under nine headings (for the original exposition of these nine factors, the reader is referred to Bradford Hill [1965]):

1. Strength of association – is the disease more common in a particular group of workers; if so, by how much?
2. Consistency – has the association been described by more than one researcher and preferably using different methods of enquiry?
3. Specificity – is the disease restricted to certain groups of people and to certain sites?
4. Time – does the suspect cause always precede the disease and is the time interval reasonable?
5. Biological gradient – is there a good dose–response relationship?
6. Biological plausibility – does the association seem reasonable or is it absurd?
7. Coherence – do all aspects of the causality hang together in a logical and feasible way?
8. Experimental evidence – can the causality be tested experimentally or does experimental evidence support causality?
9. Analogy – has a similar suspect cause been shown for related causes or effects?

Rarely will all nine points be present in the proof of a hypothesis, nor do they all carry equal weight.

However, the more there are the stronger the association and the more likely it is that there is a causal relationship. But, as Bradford Hill says:

All scientific work is incomplete – whether it is observational or experimental. All scientific work is liable to be upset or modified by advancing knowledge. That does not confer upon us a freedom to ignore the knowledge we already have, or to postpone the action that it appears to demand at a given time.

Study design

Consideration of the design of an epidemiological study requires advance planning. It does not just happen. Having said that, it is usually impossible to stick rigidly to a classic study design as practical considerations will modify such an ideal situation. What is fundamental to all epidemiological studies is the need to have a question that demands an answer.

Study design consideration can be divided into two parts: (i) goals and (ii) options.

Goals
The ultimate aim of an epidemiological study is to obtain accurate information about the object of the study. Practical restrictions present before, during and after the investigation may limit the feasibility of obtaining the most accurate picture. The balance between these two opposing forces can be denoted as the efficiency of the operation as a whole (Figure 14.2).

Validity
Validity is related to the general (external) and the specific (internal). In the general sense it is concerned with how the study results could be extrapolated in a more general context. For example, if a study showed that farmers in a particular area had a higher prevalence of fractured legs than office workers, can these results be extrapolated to all farmers? Or are there specific circumstances in the study area that show that the farmers or the landscape, climate, their tractors, etc. are significantly different from the population of such workers as a whole to militate against such generalisations? (Perhaps the control group is inappropriate and therefore it is the factor that vitiates generalisation.)

In a specific sense, the study groups may be biased. Bias can take many forms and some can be controlled at the design stage. Three broad groups can be distinguished:

1. Selection bias concerns the way in which the study populations were assembled and includes the validity of choosing the chosen population, for example 'Were they volunteers?'; 'Were they lost to follow-up?'; 'Were they a survivor population?'; and 'Did they all come from the same hospital/district?'.
2. Information bias relates to the quality and accuracy of the data gathered. It includes errors by the interviewer or the interviewee in the diagnosis or the exposure measures and so on.
3. Confounding is a factor that independently influences both the exposure and the outcome and thereby suggests a spurious direct relationship between the two. The classic example is age. The older the worker, the

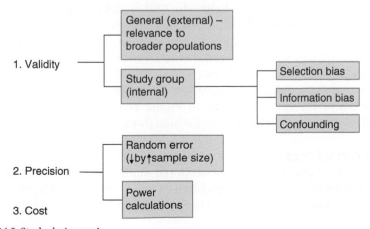

FIGURE 14.2 Study design goals.

more likely he or she is to have been significantly exposed to the occupational hazard and the more likely to have the illness in question – given that most diseases are age dependent.

Precision

Precision is another aspect to be considered. If a study plan involving a particular size of population (or measurements) were implemented repeatedly and independently an infinite number of times, the results would be grouped about a mean value. Departure from this mean value would give an estimate of random error. A small random error would indicate high precision. Information regarding the precision of the study is augmented by increasing the sample size or by increasing the number of times the measurements are made. Wherever possible, it is valuable to calculate the likelihood of discovering a real effect given the study population size. Formulae are available to undertake these so-called power calculations.

Cost

The cost of the investigation can be measured in terms of time, effort and personnel. The efficiency of the study is a measure of the value of the information gained against the cost of the study.

Options

The goals of rational study design require that certain choices are made in terms of the way the investigation is executed (Figure 14.3).

Timing

A choice of prime importance is the timing of the investigation. Figure 14.4 depicts the life history of a factory population on a calendar–time/age–time format – and can be used to illustrate these options in timing. Real-life events are, of course, more complex than in this example but the principles remain the same. The factory concerned opened in 1965 with a population of workers aged 18–40 years. The passage of time (horizontal scale) is, of course, accompanied by the ageing of the population (vertical scale). The population is assumed not to alter and therefore progresses diagonally across the figure. In 1980, a major expansion programme with the advent of new processes necessitates enlarging the workforce with predominantly men younger than those in employment. This new cohort ages *pari passu* as the extant group. (An alternative model is the introduction and cessation of a particular process in 1965 and 1980, respectively.) If we wish to investigate this process and/or the population, we have several options with regards to timing and the direction of the study. Referring to Figure 14.3, the study could be cross-sectional (vertically orientated) or longitudinal (horizontally orientated).

Cross-sectional studies

The decision to undertake a cross-sectional study generally means a quick, cheaper opportunity to study the problem in hand. These advantages are offset by the limitations imposed by having to assess the population at risk in a narrow

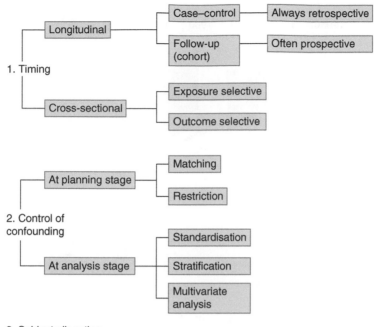

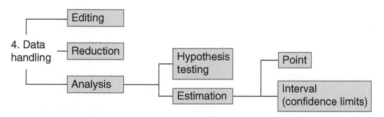

FIGURE 14.3 Study design options.

time frame. The narrowness of the time interval means that the investigators may find it difficult to look at exposure and outcome as a time-dependent relationship. But there are methods to overcome temporality between exposure and outcome. You can ascertain the outcome in, say, 2020, and then obtain exposure data from several sources: company occupational hygiene records, questionnaires, job exposure matrix (JEM), etc. Of course, the extent of bias in the exposure measures needs to be assessed as a limitation. A big issue in cross-sectional studies is the healthy worker effect. Sick/affected workers are not at work (too sick to work or made redundant) and not at the workplace to be studied, so occurrence is typically under-estimated. The cross-sectional study tends to ascertain either outcome or exposure more reliably.

Case–control and follow-up studies These investigations take longer to do and are more expensive but provide, by virtue of the study being concerned with a period of time rather than an instant, an opportunity for looking at an exposure

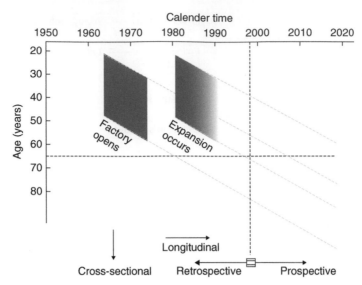

FIGURE 14.4 Some age–time factors in study design.

and its outcome as a time-related chain of events. Two types of study design are commonly employed: (i) the case–control study (or, more accurately, case–referent study) and (ii) the follow-up study (which includes cohort investigations) (Figure 14.5).

- *Case–control studies* tend to be retrospective. They begin with a definition of a group of cases with a disease and relate these and the non-cases (control subjects/referents without the disease) to the past exposure history. Case–control studies are particularly useful for rare diseases and those with long latency. In occupational epidemiology, the main drawback here is the accurate ascertainment of exposure history going back anything up to 40 years. Although longitudinal in that exposure in the past is sought, the past can be recent, and the case–control design has been successful in investigating acute-onset conditions: gastroenteritis (food poisoning) soon after a work function; Legionnaires' disease during a conference; and organophosphate poisoning are examples.
- *Follow-up studies* do not necessarily suffer such limitations if the exposure is defined and accurately known, and a group of exposed (and usually non-exposed persons) are followed up to assess the eventual outcome of such exposure. Such studies may be prospective or retrospective in directionality. A prospective study establishes a group to follow up from initiation of the study to disease onset or end-of-study date, a prolonged undertaking for diseases of long latency. A retrospective study identifies a group that existed in the past and examines records of exposure and disease up to a pre-determined later date. Good records of exposure and disease outcomes are necessary for reliable findings. (Note: a study that uses a group of workers currently in employment or in employment at a particular time and then delves into past

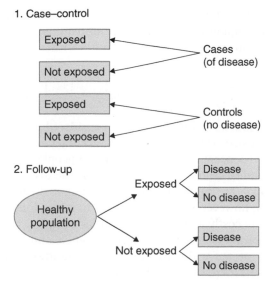

FIGURE 14.5 Longitudinal studies.

exposure and disease status so that the exposures of those with and without the disease can be compared is a cross-sectional study, not a retrospective follow-up study.) Follow-up studies are designed to observe incidence and, ideally, should span a period of time in excess of the maximum induction period for the exposure factor to produce a putative outcome.

Control of confounding factors The control of confounding factors can be undertaken at the planning stage or during data analysis. During planning, matching the cases (or exposure group) with persons without the characteristic essential for selection may reduce or eliminate such confounders. For example, age matching eliminates the problem of inadvertently comparing old with young. The alternative to matching is the restriction of the cases and their referents to narrow strata, which effectively excludes unwanted confounding. Such stratification without restriction can be carried out during data analysis, or standardisation procedures can be adopted instead. Complex inter-reactive confounders can be minimised by multivariate analysis.

Subject allocation Studies are often published in which numbers in the referent (control) group exceed the cases by a factor of 2 or more. This can strengthen the validity of the comparison and, thereby, the conclusions that are drawn. The law of diminishing returns, however, begins to operate after the case–referent ratio exceeds 1 : 3, and 1 : 5 is rarely exceeded – largely for reasons of economy.

Data handling Three main procedures are employed:

1. the editing of the collected data to a readily usable form
2. its reduction to a manageable size, and, finally,
3. the analysis.

Analytical procedures tend to test hypotheses propounded at the outset of the investigation or are employed to estimate various parameters, either to one point or, more commonly, to establish confidence limits for the calculated estimates.

14.4 Which type of study do I use?

For many years, follow-up studies have been considered to be the epidemiological study par excellence. Their reputation for accuracy is based partly on their inherently unbiased concept – a group or groups of people are chosen in terms of characteristics manifest before the appearance of the disease in question, and then these individuals are followed over time to observe the frequency of the disease. By definition, however, such studies tend to take a long time to complete and, in addition, are costly and frequently rather complex. Nevertheless, some epidemiologists nowadays feel that a well-designed and efficiently executed case–control study 'nested' within a cohort carries the advantages of both studies while minimising the disadvantages of each.

The choice between the two is dependent upon the question posed in the exposure/health outcome equation. This can be summarised as follows:

Question	Study type
A causes B?	Either
	Case–control (disease rare)
	Follow-up (exposure rare)
A causes B1, B2, B3?	Follow-up
B caused by?	Case–control
B caused by A1, A2, A3?	Case–control
B caused by A?	Case–control

Selecting cases (and control subjects) can, however, be difficult. Here are some questions that the researcher should ask before making a choice:

1. Have I collected information on the control subjects with the same zeal as the cases?
2. Are the response rates from both cases and control subjects similar?
3. How well are these referents matched to the case?
4. Have I methods to deal with all important potential confounders (matching or in adjustment in analyses)?
5. Have I 'over-matched'?
6. Do the referents come from a population similar to the cases? (For instance, if the controls had developed the disease would they have entered the study as a case?)
7. Could I choose an equally good comparison group more cheaply or more quickly?

Shortcomings in the epidemiological method

By now it will be clear to the reader that the epidemiological method is not without its difficulties! In brief, the main problems can be summarised as follows:

- a healthy worker effect – the study group is artificially healthier than the comparison group either because atypically healthy people were recruited into specific jobs at the workplace (e.g. at a pre-placement medical) or sick workers left it prior to the study
- the comparison group has a different general health status from the cases
- a poor response rate
- high turnover of study populations – selecting in (or out)
- latency between exposure and effect longer than study period
- insufficient evidence of differing effects by differing exposures
- poor quality of health effects data
- poor quality of exposure data, multiple exposures
- no effect of exposure noted – 'Does this imply a true negative result or merely a poor or small study (non-positive result)?'

14.5 Disease clusters

A cluster or outbreak occurs when the number of cases of a specific health outcome or disease exceeds what is expected in a population. In the occupational health context, a cluster may be at a workplace, in a community around it, in a group of former employees or any combination of these three. Clusters arise because of workplace exposures – a real effect of work processes – or by chance: there are millions of enterprises and groups of workers globally, and, hence, uniform distributions of health effects among them is truly an extremely remote possibility. Clusters in communities and among former workers are typically epidemiologically complex and not usually within the competency of occupational health services, so they are not considered here.

Clusters are not infrequent, and they generally cause concern among workers and their families, management and occupational health professionals. Consequently, there is usually pressure on occupational health services to investigate them. An investigation is usually appropriate, but with provisos because the cluster may be due to just chance – if this happens, then resources will be wasted if an unnecessarily comprehensive investigation is undertaken, and the findings of the investigation may be misleading if interpreted as if an a priori hypothesis is being tested. For example, if finding that the observed number of cases is statistically significantly larger than the expected number then this would be taken to mean that workplace factors necessarily account for the excess, or any real increased risk to health for that matter. There are many pitfalls in cluster investigations. (See Kreiss and Monson [2017] in Further reading.)

What then should be the approach to investigating a workplace cluster possibly related to work by occupational health professionals serving an enterprise?

Clear communication at the beginning is necessary. Anxiety and mistrust may accompany disease clusters, especially if the condition is serious, such as cancer. The methodology, interpretation of findings and steps to be taken after the investigation should be discussed.

The nature of the cluster should then be defined. In particular, the occurrence of a specific health outcome or disease needs to be confirmed. Importantly, unrelated health effects of various body systems may be misinterpreted as a cluster. At times it is necessary to actively find cases in the workforce not already documented. But one should be cautious about seeking common non-specific health effects, as false positives (conditions unrelated to work) will be found which will complicate the investigation. Once it has been established that a specific health effect is present in a group of workers, a simple appraisal of whether the numbers of cases are unexpectedly high should be undertaken. Sometimes regional disease rates are readily available, in which case increased disease occurrence can be assessed objectively. If not available, the assessment is more subjective. Consultation with local specialist health units may be helpful in reaching a conclusion. Remember that hypothesis testing is not appropriate; this appraisal is to answer a simple question: on the face of it, does it seem that there are more cases than one would expect?

Next, the location within the enterprise of the cases should be mapped; are most of them in the same factory area or on the same production line, for instance? This is to aid a thorough scrutiny of the workplace exposures of the affected workers. (If they are dispersed through the enterprise, a cluster is not excluded.) Then an assessment of whether the exposure, production process or nature of the enterprise is an established cause of the condition should be done. An established cause here is one that is well documented and described in textbooks or systematic reviews or similar sources. If an established cause is identified, usual workplace procedures for managing work-related health effects should be effected. If not, novel exposure–effect associations should not be investigated unless done so formally. For example, by extending the investigation to other enterprises with the same exposures or making the same products. This is usually best led by experienced researchers such as those in public health institutions or universities. The identification of the aetiology of 'popcorn lung', a lung disease caused by a chemical flavouring of microwave popcorn, is a good example of an investigation of a cluster due to a novel exposure. (See Kreiss and Monson [2017] in Further reading.)

14.6 Conclusions

The principles of (occupational) epidemiology should be known and understood by all occupational health professionals and these fundamentals apply equally from international studies to smaller scale, factory-based investigations undertaken by one researcher. Ideally, it should stimulate all those involved in occupational health to go back out on to the shop floor and view the workforce anew. If you find a working population in which there is an exposure–health outcome question to be answered, then the authors would advise that the occupational health professionals with a question find and collaborate with epidemiologists or experienced researchers to answer the question – as you have an epidemiological study on your hands! But it is advisable to collaborate with epidemiologists or experienced researchers when designing methods to answer the question and in analysing the data collected to answer it.

Further Reading

Bradford Hill, A. (1965). The environment and disease: association or causation? *Proceedings of the Royal Society of Medicine* 58 (5): 295–300.

Kreiss, K. and Monson, R.R. (2017). Investigating an outbreak. In: *Parkes' Occupational Lung Disorders*, 4e (eds. A.N. Taylor, P. Cullinan, P. Blanc and A. Pickering). Boca Raton, FL: CRC Press.

Lash, T.L., VanderWeele, T.J., Haneuse, S., and Rothman, K.J. (2020). *Modern Epidemiology*, 4e. Philadelphia, PA: Wolters Kluwer.

Porta, M. (2014). *A Dictionary of Epidemiology*, 6e. New York: Oxford University Press, Inc.

CHAPTER 15

Control of Airborne Contaminants

15.1 Introduction

The purpose of the application of workplace control techniques is to minimise worker exposure to the potential hazard; ideally, so that exposure levels are below those that are considered to be hazardous. The success of the selected control will be judged by its ability to reduce personal risk. The control method should remain effective and maintain the same degree of protection over the working life of the process. Potential risk should be assessed by examining the results of failure of the control system. Where chronic hazards exist, an occasional transient failure may not be too serious, but any overexposure could have grave implications in the case of sensitisers and carcinogens, and, for asphyxiants, could be fatal. Thus, the control system must be designed to match the potential risk and, when risks

Pocket Consultant: Occupational Health, Sixth Edition. Kerry Gardiner, David Rees, Anil Adisesh, David Zalk, and Malcolm Harrington.
© 2022 John Wiley & Sons Ltd. Published 2022 by John Wiley & Sons Ltd.

are great, tolerances and safety factors should be planned accordingly. Where potential failure could have serious consequences, there will be a need to build in redundancy and back-up controls to warn of over-exposure.

In accordance with good occupational hygiene practice, the control systems will take two forms – software and hardware – which can be applied together or separately.

Software consists of:

- substitution of a less hazardous material (Figure 15.1)
- methods of work to reduce worker exposure
- training of workers to adopt safer methods of work
- application of work schedules or regimes to limit the number of exposed individuals and to reduce the duration of their exposure.

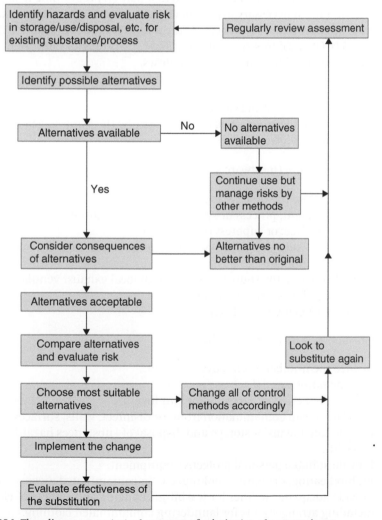

FIGURE 15.1 Flow diagram to assist in the process of substitution of a contaminant.

Hardware consists of:

- enclosure of the process
- suppression of emissions
- shielding of source or worker
- ventilation – extract at source
- ventilation – dilution to reduce concentration
- application of personal protective clothing to the worker (see Chapter 16).

As far as exposure to substances is concerned, there is a legal duty to *prevent* or *control* enshrined in many pieces of statute. For example, in the USA there is the Occupational Safety and Health Administration (OSHA) 29 CFR 1910.1450 Occupational Exposure to Hazardous Chemicals in Laboratories standard that requires employers to develop and implement a written programme to list procedures and equipment necessary to protect workers from chemical hazards. In the UK there is the Control of Substances Hazardous to Health (Amendment) Regulations 2004 (COSHH); this sets out the classic 'hierarchy of control' in which control options should be considered, as follows.

To prevent exposure (software solutions):

1. Eliminate the use of the substance.
2. Substitute by a less hazardous substance or by the same substance in a less hazardous form (Figure 15.1).

To control exposure (hardware solutions):

1. Totally enclose the process and handling systems.
2. Design the plant, process or systems of work to minimise the generation of the substance; or suppress or contain it.
3. If spills are likely, design the system/process to minimise the volume and area of contamination.
4. Partially enclose the source, together with local exhaust ventilation.
5. Provide local exhaust ventilation.
6. Provide sufficient general ventilation.

To control exposure (software solutions):

1. Reduce the number of employees present.
2. Exclude non-essential access.
3. Reduce the period of exposure for employees.
4. Regularly clean contamination from, or disinfect, walls, surfaces, etc.
5. Provide safe means of storage and disposal of substances hazardous to health.
6. Provide suitable personal protective equipment.
7. Prohibit eating, drinking, smoking, etc. in contaminated areas.
8. Provide adequate facilities for washing, changing and storage of clothing, including arrangements for laundering contaminated clothing.

When tackling a workplace health hazard with a view to reducing the risk, using engineering controls, the order in which the problem should be approached is as follows.

1. Deal with the source of emission or hazard.
2. Examine the *transmission* of the hazard between the source and the worker.
3. *Protect* the worker or the exposed population.

The hazard can be:

- an airborne pollutant, such as dust, gases and vapours; a microbiological organism; or a radioactive particle, all of which enter the body via the lungs
- a radiated emission, such as noise, heat, light or ionising and non-ionising radiation, which affects the body through the skin or other exposed organs
- a chemical in liquid or solid form, which can affect the skin or enter the body via that organ.

Source

The source can be tackled, in the case of airborne pollutants, to reduce the potential for emission as follows:

- change the process so that no hazard is created
- substitute the toxic material for one with a lower hazard potential (Figure 15.1)
- enclose the point of emission to minimise the area of outlet openings
- provide extraction ventilation to capture the material at the point of release
- suppress at source by wet methods or quenching techniques.

The emission of radiation can be approached as follows:

- reduce the intensity of the source
- change the wavelength of radiation to a safer one
- enclose the point of emission
- attenuate at the point of emission.

Transmission

With airborne pollutants, once the material is airborne and away from the source, control involves:

- shielding between the worker and the source
- application of dilution ventilation
- the use of jet ventilation to divert the contaminated air.

In the case of radiated emissions:

- increase the distance between the worker and the source
- attenuate the radiation
- deflect or divert the radiation.

Exposed population

The workers' exposure can be minimised by examining their position in relation to the hazards. In the case of air pollution:

- enclose the worker
- eliminate the need for a worker by controlling the process remotely or by automation
- wash the worker in a stream of uncontaminated conditioned (temperature and humidity controlled) air
- reduce the duration of exposure by means of job rotation
- apply a safer method of work involving less contact with the pollutant
- educate and train the worker to appreciate the hazards, so that their own behaviour will minimise the exposure
- provide respiratory protection.

With radiation and skin contact:

- enclose the worker in a protective cabin or behind shields
- remove the worker by means of remote control operation of the process or by automation
- apply a safer method of work
- educate and train the worker in the risks involved and the application of safer methods of work
- provide protective clothing for all vulnerable or exposed parts of the body.

This philosophy is represented diagrammatically in Figure 15.2.

Sources of emission

Sources of emission can be either *predictable* in time and space, being continuous or periodic, or *unpredictable* (fugitive), occurring haphazardly owing to the breakdown or wear of normal engineering items. The former can be dealt with by engineering methods, some of which are outlined below, but the latter cannot and normally involve the use of personal protective equipment (see Chapter 16). The maintenance of plant and equipment always carries a great risk of predictable and unpredictable emissions, and maintenance workers require special attention and equipment to minimise their exposure. Software should be particularly attended to because maintenance workers usually work unsupervised where access is difficult and when health and safety staff are not on site.

Control of periodic and continuous emissions

It is necessary to examine the working process carefully to establish where the sources of emission are and how an improvement can be effected. In most cases, the emission of dust and vapours can be minimised by enclosure, or by redesigning

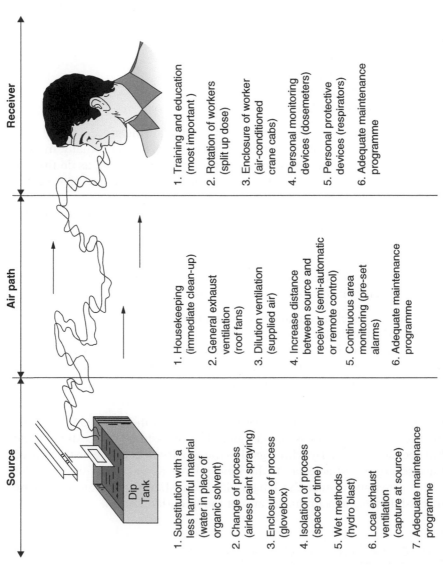

Source

1. Substitution with a less harmful material (water in place of organic solvent)

2. Change of process (airless paint spraying)

3. Enclosure of process (glovebox)

4. Isolation of process (space or time)

5. Wet methods (hydro blast)

6. Local exhaust ventilation (capture at source)

7. Adequate maintenance programme

Air path

1. Housekeeping (immediate clean-up)

2. General exhaust ventilation (roof fans)

3. Dilution ventilation (supplied air)

4. Increase distance between source and receiver (semi-automatic or remote control)

5. Continuous area monitoring (pre-set alarms)

6. Adequate maintenance programme

Receiver

1. Training and education (most important)

2. Rotation of workers (split up dose)

3. Enclosure of worker (air-conditioned crane cabs)

4. Personal monitoring devices (dosemeters)

5. Personal protective devices (respirators)

6. Adequate maintenance programme

FIGURE 15.2 Movement of a contaminant from a source to a receiver with control techniques for each component. Source: Olishifski (2002).

the process so that the escape of pollutants is reduced. The openings through which pollutants escape can be fitted with doors or covers, which remain closed most of the time and which are opened only for access. If this is impracticable, the openings for access can be fitted with extract ventilation, but it is worth remembering that the smaller the openings, the lower the air flow rate required to capture the pollutants and, hence, the cheaper the costs.

The redesign of the process can be simple, for example:

- fitting covers on containers and openings
- matching discharge ports to entry holes
- using sealed transfer systems
- using anti-splash discharge nozzles.

A more expensive solution is to enclose and automate the process completely, thus keeping the bulk of the contaminants inside; however, eventually, in most processes, the end product has to be exposed to the atmosphere, as do the raw materials at the start. With highly toxic materials, automation may be the only solution.

The provision of enclosure means that the visibility of the process is impaired; therefore, where it is necessary to observe the process, enclosure materials should be transparent. Closed-circuit video viewers could be adopted. Observation of the process is often necessary to judge whether a container is full or empty; thus, visibility is not important if an alternative means of indication is employed. This may involve one of the following:

- placing the vessel or container on a weight indicator
- using a float indicator
- using a beam of light or a stream of radioactive particles to a sensor placed on the opposite side of the vessel; the intervention of the material cuts the beam, thus indicating that it has reached that level
- using pressure switches.

Process redesign is often a cheaper expedient than the provision of extract ventilation, which requires skilful design to be successful and is costly to build and to operate, particularly with regard to the replacement of the heat removed by the discharge of extracted air to the atmosphere – as well as requirements for its maintenance and regular checking/verification. Many ventilation systems are unsuccessful owing to poor quality and/or inappropriate design.

15.2 Extract ventilation design

Where alternative solutions cannot be adopted, the pollutants can be captured before they are released into the 'general working environment' by means of extract ventilation. This can be achieved by some kind of hood, enclosure or slot, sufficiently negatively pressurised to ensure an inward current of air that will carry with it the airborne pollutants. The extract device will normally be connected to a fan via ducting, and thence to a point of discharge. An air-cleaning system in the duct may be necessary to ensure that the discharged air is sufficiently clean, either to recirculate to the workplace or to satisfy external environmental standards if released outside.

With an unrestricted suction inlet, such as a hood, air will flow from all sides, in a zone of influence that is approximately spherical, with the inlet at the centre. Thus, with unflanged hoods, air will flow in from behind the inlet as well as in front, where there may not be any pollutants, and so this air is wasted. Flanges and screens are therefore necessary to channel the air at a sufficient velocity over the point of release of the pollutant to ensure successful capture.

The *capture velocity* is defined as that velocity which will overcome the motion of the airborne pollutant to draw it into the mouth of the extract. The following factors will influence the capture velocity:

- the velocity of release of the pollutant
- the degree of turbulence of the air around the source
- in the case of particulates, their aerodynamic diameter
- the density of the materials released.

Recommended capture velocities are given in Table 15.1.

The *capture distance* is the distance between the point of release and the mouth of the inlet. The *face velocity* is the air velocity across the mouth or face of the inlet. The *aspect ratio* is the ratio of the width of the face divided by the length.

With booths, enclosures and fume cupboards, the face velocity is used rather than the capture velocity. Sufficient face velocity should be provided to prevent the pollutants released inside the enclosure from escaping back towards the worker. Recommended face velocities will depend upon the degree of toxicity of

TABLE 15.1

Recommended capture velocities.

Source conditions	Typical situations	Capture velocity (ms⁻¹)
Released into still air with no velocity	Degreasing tanks, paint dipping, still-air drying	0.25–0.5
Released at a low velocity or into a slow-moving airstream	Container filling, spray booths, screening and sieving, plating, pickling, low-speed conveyor, transfer points, debagging	0.5–1.0
Released at a moderate velocity or into turbulent air	Paint spraying, normal conveyor transfer points, crushing, barrel filling	1.0–2.5
Released at a high velocity or into a very turbulent airstream	Grinding, fettling, tumbling, abrasive blasting	2.5–10.0

the material being handled and the amount of air turbulence found at the entrance, and will vary from $0.3\,\mathrm{m\,s^{-1}}$ for an aerodynamically shaped inlet handling low-toxicity materials up to $1.5\,\mathrm{m\,s^{-1}}$ for the opposite. It must be borne in mind, however, that, with non-aerodynamically shaped entrances, the higher the air velocity, the greater the degree of turbulence created by the inlet. Turbulence often results in pollutants escaping the extract and entering the worker's breathing zone.

The shape of the extraction inlet will be dictated by the shape of the workplace and the cross-sectional area over which the pollutants are released. If the suction inlet area is too large, air distribution across the face may be uneven, allowing pollutants to escape capture over certain parts of the emission area. If the larger face dimension exceeds $1.5\,\mathrm{m}$, it is advisable to provide twin duct offtakes or split the area with two hoods. It is advisable for flow splitters to be fitted to any hood in which the velocity distribution is expected to be uneven. Table 15.2 shows the shapes and uses of different suction inlets.

Low-volume, high-velocity extract systems

This technique is useful for extraction on portable hand-held power tools, such as grinders, circular saws and sanders. The principle is to place the suction inlet as close as possible to the point of release of the particles. The capture velocity should be greater than the velocity of the particle as it leaves the tool. The closer the inlet to the point of release, the less volume flow required and the smaller the ductwork. For hand-held tools, the ducting must be light and flexible, made of plastic ribbed with reinforcing material and no larger in diameter than the hose of a domestic vacuum cleaner. The collected pollutants are usually particles of metal or wood, which are collected in an industrial type of vacuum cleaner; therefore, the whole unit is portable and self-contained.

The performance of many of the above suction inlets can be improved by the addition of a flange fitted around the periphery of the inlet. This has the effect of limiting the zone of influence to the immediate area in front of the inlet. The effect this has on the capture velocity and distance can be calculated by the utilisation of the 'Fletcher' equation (see 'Suction inlet performance').

Suction inlet performance

With straight-sided hoods and slots, centre-line velocities in the area in front of the inlet can be predicted. They are dependent upon the aspect ratio of the inlet, the mean face velocity and the distance from the hood. The relationship developed by Fletcher (1992) (see Gardiner and Harrington, 1992) is given in the expression:

$$\frac{V}{V_0} = \frac{1}{0.93 + 8.58\alpha^2}$$

TABLE 15.2		

Suction inlet shapes and uses.

Shape	Description and pressure loss calculations	Uses and features
	Canopy hood pressure loss = 0.25 × duct p_v + filter loss (if fitted)	Suitable for pollutants having a natural upward current, i.e. hot processes, cooking. Unsuitable if workers need to lean over the process. Overhead access is difficult
	Side hood (open faced) pressure loss = 0.25 × duct p_v	Suitable for bench work, but has an uneven velocity profile, i.e. the air velocity is higher at the top. Access to workplace available on three sides
	Side hood (slotted) pressure loss = 1.8 × slot p_v + 0.25 duct p_v	Suitable for bench work. The slots provide a more even face velocity profile. Access to workplace available on three sides
	Enclosure (can be open faced, but can have a sliding front as with fume cupboards) pressure loss = 0.25 × duct p_v + filter loss (if fitted)	Provides greater containment as the pollutants are released inside and should not escape if the face velocity is sufficient. Access is limited to front only. Some turbulence can be expected owing to entry of air at the edges of the enclosure, which can be minimised by aerofoil-shaped sides
	Booth with top extract and bottom supply through a perforated or gridded work surface extract pressure loss = 0.25 × duct p_v	Provides good capture of internally produced pollutants and ensures low entry velocities through opening, thus minimising turbulence. Careful design is required to balance air flow rates to ensure a 10–25% excess of extract over supply. This ensures a small inflow at the mouth
	Slot, defined as having an aspect ratio of more than 5 : 1 pressure loss = 1.8 × slot p_v + 0.25 × duct p_v	Has good access all round; suitable for surfaces of tanks or where pollutant release is spread over an area rather than from a point. Capture distance is limited
	Double slot with extraction from two sides pressure loss = 1.8 × slot p_v + 0.25 × duct p_v	Has good access all round; suitable for surfaces of tanks or where the pollutant is spread over a wide area. A double slot will always provide better capture than a single one
	Extract hood with supply slot extract pressure loss = 1 × face p_v + 0.25 × duct p_v	Suitable for control over very wide surfaces as the supply of air can sweep the pollutants into the extract. Careful design is required to balance air flow rates to ensure that more air is captured than supplied. Also, the 10° expansion of a jet of air must be borne in mind when sizing the extract hood

(Continued)

TABLE 15.2 (Continued)		

Shape	Description and pressure loss calculations	Uses and features
	Portable hood on flexible duct pressure loss = $0.25 \times$ duct p_v	Suitable for sources of pollution that are moving, such as welding on a large workpiece
	Curved slot pressure loss = $1.8 \times$ slot $p_v + 0.25 \times$ duct p_v	Suitable for extracting closely around containers
	Extract annulus pressure loss = $1.8 \times$ annular $p_v + 0.25 \times$ duct p_v	Suitable for extracting around discharge pipes and outlets
	Evacuated containers pressure loss = $0.65 \times$ duct p_v	Suitable for sources of emission that are released at very high velocities. An evacuated container is placed in the path of the particles as they are emitted. Capture velocities of about $10 \, \text{m s}^{-1}$ are required

p_v is the velocity pressure at the stated position.

where $\alpha = XA^{-1/2}(W/L)^{-\beta}$, $\beta = 0.2(XA^{-1/2})^{-1/3}$, V is the centre-line velocity at distance X from the hood mouth, V_0 is the mean velocity at the face of the hood, L is the length of the hood, W is the width of the hood and $A = LW$.

The volume flow rate through the hood can be calculated by assigning V_0 to the required capture velocity and X to the designed capture distance. The volume flow Q is then obtained from:

$$Q = V_0 A$$

This formula also applies to the relationship between the volume flow rate, cross-sectional area and air velocity in the ducts. The solution of the Fletcher equations can be simplified by using the nomogram provided in Figure 15.3.

The addition of flanges to the hoods will increase the centre-line velocities by up to 25% for hoods with a low aspect ratio, but by up to 55% with a slot of aspect ratio 16:1. The optimum flange widths are in the region of $A^{-1/2}$.

If capture distances are too great, the required face velocities to provide a suitable capture velocity can become excessive. For example, to provide a capture velocity of $1 \, \text{m s}^{-1}$ at a distance of $1 \, \text{m}$ from the mouth of a $200 \times 1000 \, \text{mm}$ slot would require a face velocity of $66 \, \text{m s}^{-1}$, which is truly unrealistic.

The prediction of velocities away from the centre line is difficult. In general, however, they will be less than the centre-line velocity on either side.

Unfortunately, the theoretical prediction of centre-line velocities assumes that the surrounding areas are free from disturbing air currents, which is often far

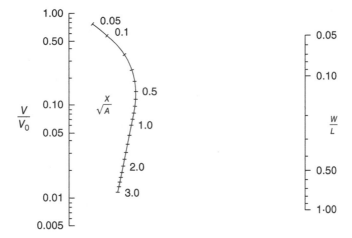

FIGURE 15.3 Nomogram for the solution of the Fletcher equations. Source: Crown copyright is reproduced with the permission of the Controller of The Stationery Office.

from the case, particularly if there is a regular movement of people and vehicles in the vicinity of the source of pollution. In addition, the edges of the hood, the workplace and the worker all contribute to local air turbulence, which can result in pollutants being drawn out of the capturing airstream and into the workplace and potentially into the breathing zone of the worker. In an ideal workplace, the entries to hoods should be of aerofoil shape to minimise turbulence.

In practice, one of the few situations in which aerofoil shapes are used is in modern fume cupboards, where they have been shown to be successful in minimising the escape of pollutants. It is possible to add aerofoils to the entrances to older fume cupboards, and they have been shown to improve capture.

Ducts and fittings

Air is conveyed from the extract inlet to the point of discharge in ducts, which take a route to suit the needs of the building in which they are housed. In order for the air to be thus conveyed, fittings, such as bends and changes of section, are required to assist in negotiating obstructions and to accommodate items of equipment, such as filters and air cleaners. The remaining parts of the system employ straight ducts. The shapes and sizes of the ducts depend upon the configuration of the workplace and the building, and the desired velocity of the air inside the ductwork. There are several factors that should be considered when deciding upon the cross-section of the ducts, and usually a compromise is made between them. For a given volume flow rate, the larger the duct, the lower the air velocity inside, and the less energy absorbed in overcoming friction. Such a duct is, however, high in capital cost. A circular cross-section is more economical in material than a rectangular one, but, in some buildings, the space available into which the duct can be placed is more suited to the rectangular shape.

If dust or larger particles are to be conveyed, it is important to ensure that they do not settle out and deposit inside the ducts to cause an obstruction or, in the case of flammable dusts, become a potential explosion hazard; therefore, the correct transport velocity is required to minimise deposition.

The *transport velocity* is the minimum air velocity within the duct necessary to maintain the particles airborne. Table 15.3 gives some recommended transport velocities. If only gases and vapours are to be carried, transport velocities are not important, and the air velocity becomes a matter of economics and/or acoustics. Optimum velocities are usually between 5 and 6 m s^{-1}, but, if noise levels are not to be obtrusive, 5 m s^{-1} should be the maximum.

In extract ventilation design, the volume flow rate (Q) is determined first by virtue of the requirements of the suction inlet. Then, having decided upon the duct velocity (V), the cross-sectional area (A) is determined from the expression:

$$Q = VA$$

Ducting is usually made of galvanised sheet steel, but a variety of other materials can be used, including brick, concrete, polyvinyl chloride, fibreglass, canvas, plastic and stainless steel. Where the air contains corrosive materials, galvanised metal is unsuitable and a corrosion-resistant material must be used.

Pressure losses

Air requires a pressure difference for it to flow, and it will always flow from the higher to the lower pressure. The source of motive power is either natural or by means of a fan. Pressure is a type of energy that appears in two forms, static (p_s) and velocity (p_v), and the sum of these is known as the total pressure (p_t). Static

---

TABLE 15.3	

Recommended transport velocities.

Pollutant	Transport velocity (m s^{-1})
Fumes, such as zinc and aluminium	7–10
Fine dust, such as lint, cotton fly, flour, fine powders	10–12.5
Dusts and powders with low moisture contents, such as cotton dust, jute lint, fine wood shavings, fine rubber dust, plastic dust	12.5–17.5
Normal industrial dust, such as sawdust, grinding dust, food powders, rock dusts, asbestos fibres, silica flour, pottery clay dust, brick and cement dust	17.5–20
Heavy and moist dust, such as lead chippings, moist cement, quicklime dust, paint spray particles	Over 22.5

pressure is exerted in all directions by a fluid that is stationary, but, if it is moving, it is measured at right angles to the direction of flow to eliminate the effects of velocity. Static pressure can be either positive or negative in relation to atmospheric pressure: on the suction side of a fan, it is usually negative, and, on the delivery side, it is normally positive. This is illustrated using the U-tube gauges shown in Figure 15.4.

Velocity pressure is the kinetic energy of a fluid in motion, and is calculated from the following expression:

$$p_v = \frac{\rho v^2}{2}$$

where ρ is the air density and v is the air velocity.

If the standard air density at $1.2\,\text{kg}\,\text{m}^{-3}$ is used, the above expression becomes:

$$p_v = 0.6 v^2$$

If v is in metres per second, p_v will be in pascals. These expressions are widely used in air flow measurement and in the calculation of pressure losses in ductwork systems.

Reynolds number

In a pipe through which fluid flows, the relationship between the energy absorbed and the rate of flow depends upon the character of the flow. At low velocities, a non-turbulent flow exists, which is termed 'laminar' or 'streamlined' flow, where the energy absorbed is proportional to the velocity of the fluid. At higher velocities, a turbulent flow exists, in which the energy absorbed is proportional to the square of the fluid velocity. The character of the flow is determined by the following variables:

- μ, the dynamic viscosity of the fluid
- ρ, the density of the fluid

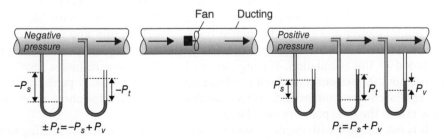

FIGURE 15.4 Examples of typical liquid-filled manometer readings on either side of a fan showing the effect of positive and negative pressure.

- v, the velocity of the fluid
- D, the diameter of the pipe.

These variables combine together to form a dimensionless number, known as the Reynolds number (Re), which may be calculated from the equation:

$$Re = \frac{vD\rho}{\mu}$$

In general, with $Re < 2000$ laminar flow exists, and with $Re > 4000$ turbulent flow exists. Between these limits, flow conditions are variable. In most engineering applications, $Re > 4000$, and it is assumed that the energy absorbed is proportional to the square of the velocity. The exception to this general statement is in air filtration, where air velocities can be very low within the filter medium, and Re approaches 2000.

The energy losses due to friction are expressed as a pressure loss, which can be calculated or obtained from charts and nomograms. With regard to straight lengths of ducting, the pressure loss can be obtained in pascals per metre, using the nomogram given in Figure 15.5. As the duct sides are parallel, there is no change in air velocity from one end to the other. The pressure losses obtained from the nomogram are therefore both total and static. The losses in most fittings are calculated by multiplying the velocity pressure at a point in the fitting by a factor determined empirically for the geometrical shape of that fitting. The resulting pressure loss is in total pressure. It is important to work in total pressure for ventilation calculations because fittings and changes of section have changes in static pressure within them, sometimes resulting in a gain of static, but a loss of total, pressure. Working in total pressure throughout avoids any confusion.

Fan required

In order to establish the duty of a fan to draw air through the system, it is necessary to sum the individual pressure losses from each of the components, starting from the suction inlet and working toward the fan (Figure 15.6). If there are components on the delivery side of the fan, it is also necessary to add the pressure losses on that side. Similarly, if a filter or dust collector is installed, the pressure loss of that component must be included. This will be obtainable from the manufacturer and should be quoted both for a clean unit and for the time when the filter needs changing or cleaning, the latter higher pressure being included in the calculation. Having summed all the pressure losses involved throughout the system (this should include the discharge velocity pressure), the fan can be chosen from manufacturers' catalogues to handle the chosen volume flow rate at the total pressure calculated.

It is not unusual with extract systems to add several branches, all feeding to a single duct and fan. When this occurs, the pressure needed to specify the fan is normally taken as that required to bring the air from the inlet furthest from the

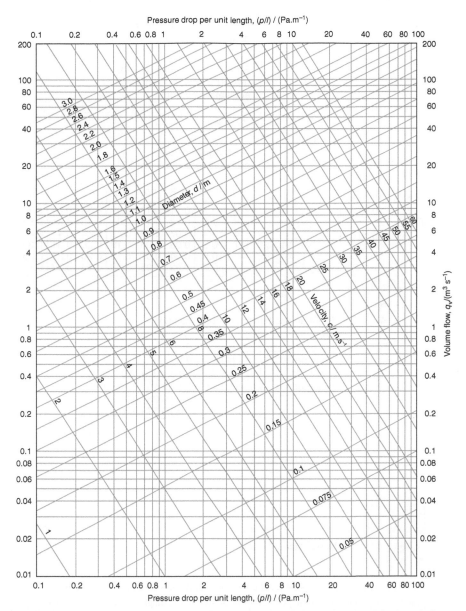

FIGURE 15.5 Nomogram for calculating air flow in round ducts (plotted on logarithmic scales). Source: CIBSE Guide C: Reference data, published by the Chartered Institution of Building Services Engineers, London.

fan through the system to the discharge point. Sufficient pressure will be available to overcome the resistance of the intermediate branches, i.e. those nearer the fan. Indeed, there may be an excess of pressure, making it necessary to restrict the intermediate branches in order to prevent an excess of air flow from

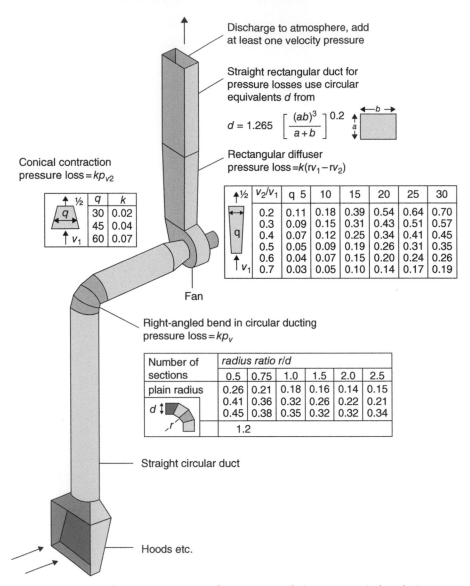

Discharge to atmosphere, add at least one velocity pressure

Straight rectangular duct for pressure losses use circular equivalents d from

$$d = 1.265 \left[\frac{(ab)^3}{a+b} \right]^{0.2}$$

Conical contraction pressure loss $= kp_{v2}$

Rectangular diffuser pressure loss $= k(rv_1 - rv_2)$

$\frac{1}{2}$	q	k
	30	0.02
	45	0.04
v_1	60	0.07

$\frac{1}{2}$ v_2/v_1	q 5	10	15	20	25	30
0.2	0.11	0.18	0.39	0.54	0.64	0.70
0.3	0.09	0.15	0.31	0.43	0.51	0.57
0.4	0.07	0.12	0.25	0.34	0.41	0.45
0.5	0.05	0.09	0.19	0.26	0.31	0.35
0.6	0.04	0.07	0.15	0.20	0.24	0.26
0.7	0.03	0.05	0.10	0.14	0.17	0.19

Fan

Right-angled bend in circular ducting pressure loss $= kp_v$

Number of sections	radius ratio r/d					
	0.5	0.75	1.0	1.5	2.0	2.5
plain radius	0.26	0.21	0.18	0.16	0.14	0.15
	0.41	0.36	0.32	0.26	0.22	0.21
d	0.45	0.38	0.35	0.32	0.32	0.34
	1.2					

Straight circular duct

Hoods etc.

FIGURE 15.6 Pressure losses in components of an extract ventilation system. p_v is the velocity pressure, the subscript referring to the position as indicated in the diagram accompanying each fitting. For a fan, see Figure 15.5; for pressure losses for hoods etc., see Table 15.2.

passing through them to the detriment of the furthest branch. This results in the multibranched system being out of balance, a common fault with many industrial systems that have been in use for some time. Balancing can be achieved by installing adjustable dampers in the intermediate branches or by making those branches higher in resistance by design. The damper method has the disadvantage of being thrown out of balance by injudicious tampering unless the damper handles are locked in the balance position. In addition, if dust is to be carried in the duct, the dampers can act as a depository, such that unwanted accumulations of dust can build up, making the damper unworkable and causing an unnecessary obstruction in the duct. Inherent balancing by design is therefore preferred. When designing a system, it is useful to draw a sketch of the layout, labelling each junction at which the air changes speed or direction, or at which two airstreams meet, by assigning the change point with a number or letter of the alphabet. In this way, each section can be identified as, for example, 3–4 or E–F. A table should be drawn up with headings as shown in Table 15.4.

The table should be filled in section by section, starting from the inlet furthest from the fan, using the design information selected as appropriate to the requirements of each section. It is not necessary to complete every column for each section, as they do not all apply, and it may be necessary to leave some sections until after the following section has been designed. The last column on the right of the table is the sum of the pressure losses accumulated from the beginning, and this provides a statement of the pressure inside the duct at that point in relation to the atmosphere. Thus, if a connection was to be made to the atmosphere at that point, the pressure difference available to overcome the resistance of the connecting branch is known.

15.3 Dilution ventilation

There are many situations in industry where it is impracticable to extract at source by means of a hood or enclosure. Typical situations include:

- where the source of emission is very large, e.g. the manufacture of boats in glass-reinforced plastic (GRP)
- where the source is moving, e.g. in a production line where products are hanging from a moving conveyor
- where the presence of a hood or enclosure would impair the transfer of products.

Control can be achieved by passing large quantities of air over the source to dilute it to a safe level or to divert it into an unoccupied space.

It is necessary to decide on the volume flow rate of air to dilute the emission to a chosen concentration, and for this the following equation should be used:

$$Q = \frac{R}{C}$$

where Q is the required diluting volume flow rate in cubic metres per second, R is the rate of emission of the pollutant in milligrams per second and C is the chosen concentration in milligrams per cubic metre. This equation assumes that the diluting airstream and the pollutants are evenly mixed.

TABLE 15.4

Headings for a table to be used in designing an extract system.

Section	Length (m)	Volume flow ($m^3\,s^{-1}$)	Duct dimension (mm)	Duct area (mm)	Air velocity (ms^{-1})	Velocity pressure (Pa)	Loss factor (k)	Pressure loss per metre (Pam^{-1})	Section pressure loss (Pa)	Cumulative pressure loss (Pa)

The chosen concentration can be the published occupational exposure limit or a certain fraction of it. For example, it would be good practice if the pollutant has a workplace exposure limit (WEL) that the chosen concentration should be as low as reasonably practicable, for example less than 25% of the published value. The rate of emission is more difficult to determine, and may be related to the rate of usage during a working period and how much of the pollutant is released into the workroom atmosphere.

For example, in the manufacture of items in GRP, the resin emits styrene; the suppliers of this resin are able to predict how much styrene is released for a given surface area during the curing process. A typical value of normal pigmented polyester resin is an emission rate of 50 g of styrene per hour per square metre of exposed surface. Thus, if 100 m^2 of GRP is emitting, the rate of emission will be 5000 g h^{-1} or approximately 1400 mg s^{-1}. Therefore, to dilute that to 25% of the published WEL for styrene (430 mg m^{-3}), i.e. 108 mg m^{-3}, a volume flow rate of $1400/108 = 13$ m^3 s^{-1} is required.

The method of introducing diluting air into the workroom needs some care. Supply grilles designed to create high velocities may provide good mixing, but would be unpopular with the workforce as cold draughts may occur. Low-velocity displacement ventilation, with the diluting air being heated to, for example, 16 °C and introduced at floor level, will gently displace the pollutant with little discomfort to the workforce.

Summary of the aims of both dilution and extraction ventilation

1. Do not draw or blow the contaminated air towards the face of the worker.
2. Place the extract as close to the source of pollution as possible.
3. Enclose as much of the source as is consistent with the work process.
4. Direct dilution ventilation so that the source of emission is entrained away from the occupied areas.
5. Discharge polluted air in such a way that it does not re-enter the building or adjacent buildings. High discharge stacks improve dispersion and minimise weather effects.
6. Make allowances for outside wind effects to prevent blowback of extracted air.
7. Make allowances for buoyancy effects of the release gases or vapours, i.e. hotter or less dense substances tend to rise when in a concentrated form, while colder, heavier substances tend to fall. There is also a tendency for a concentrated pollutant released into still or slow-moving air to form a layer on the floor or in the roof, according to its density relative to air; it can be difficult to remove this, and it can lead to dangerous accumulations if the material is toxic or flammable. This phenomenon only occurs when air is stagnant. Under normal operating circumstances, where there is movement of people and products, there is sufficient turbulence to mix the heavy vapour with room air, such that the density of the mixture is little different from that of air and no sedimentation will occur.

8. If it is important to contain the polluted air in the room in which it is released, this can be achieved by extracting 10–15% more air than supplied.
9. Do not discharge toxic or harmful substances into the atmosphere without rendering them harmless.
10. Certain gases and vapours are flammable, and their handling may come under special regulations or codes requiring flameproof equipment. Due regard must be taken of this.

15.4 Choice of fan

Having decided upon the volume flow rate to pass through the ventilation system, and the pressure or suction required to overcome friction losses through the system, it is necessary to select a fan capable of providing that duty. Fan manufacturers publish catalogues from which the correct fan can be chosen. The performance figures are often presented by means of graphs, known as characteristic curves, which show the relationship between pressure and volume flow. It is necessary to select the fan so that the duty point lies on the curve at the fan's most efficient operating condition. This will be indicated on the curve or by the manufacturer.

Most fans used in industrial ventilation are of two types: *axial flow* and *centrifugal*. Axial flow fans normally consist of a multibladed propeller-type rotor inside a cylindrical casing, often of the same diameter as the ducting. The electric motor is usually inside the casing and in the airstream being moved. These fans tend to be noisy and are limited in the amount of pressure they develop, such that they are not suited to high-resistance systems, for example those containing fabric or centrifugal filters. Some have a bifurcated arrangement, so that the motors remain outside the airstream and are suitable for systems carrying hot air or flammable vapours.

Centrifugal fans are capable of developing much higher pressures and are best suited to high-resistance systems. They can be described as having a paddle-wheel type of impeller, rotating inside a volute-shaped casing, such that air leaves the fan at right angles to the direction in which it enters. They are normally quieter than axial flow fans. Motors are normally outside the airstream, and may be directly coupled to the shaft of the impeller or connected by means of a drive, such as a V-belt or gearbox.

Many fan motors used in industry are powered by a 380–440 V three-phase electrical supply. The direction of rotation is dictated by the way in which the terminals are connected. Should they be connected wrongly, the fan will run in reverse. This could occur on installation or after routine maintenance. With axial flow fans, reversal will result in air flowing in the opposite direction, and is usually noticed and rectified. However, the flow in centrifugal fans is not reversed when the motor turns in the wrong direction, but this results in a greatly reduced air flow. As the air continues to flow in the correct direction, the error is not noticed, and may continue for long periods of time, with the consequent reduction in control efficiency. Most good fan makers indicate the correct direction of rotation on the casing, but if this is not marked, it is possible to determine the correct direction by examining the fan casing. It enlarges in the direction of rotation.

The COSHH Regulations 2004 in the UK require a thorough examination and test of ventilation systems that control substances hazardous to health to be made at regular intervals, varying between 1 and 14 months, depending upon the substance or operation that is being ventilated. US OSHA 29 CFR 1910.94 Subpart G and 1910.1450 outline requirements that include the written hazardous chemical control programme for measuring, assessing and testing industrial ventilation system adequacy that should be conducted at least once per year and after any alteration or repair to the system.

15.5 Air cleaning and discharges to the atmosphere

Air cleaning

Environmental restrictions are already placed upon employers to limit the amount and concentration of toxic substances discharged to the atmosphere, and certain registered works are required by law to do so. Therefore, attention should now be turned to limiting the emissions from ventilation systems that contain substances hazardous to health.

The removal of particles from discharged air involves various alternative principles, the choice of which is dictated by the size, nature and concentration of the particles. Large, dry particles in a high concentration from, for example, a woodworking shop are best dealt with by a centrifugal method, such as a cyclone. Small, dry particles from, for example, a lead smelter would best be removed by a fabric filter, such as those found in a bag house. Dusts that can be easily charged electrically can be removed by electrostatic means. Sticky or wet dusts will require methods involving wet scrubbing, which, although cleaning the discharged air, may lead to a secondary problem of wet sludge disposal.

The removal of gases and vapours from discharged air is generally more difficult, as the pollutant is in molecular form and does not respond to the physical forces that can capture airborne particles. Chemical adsorption and absorption are the principles employed. Wet absorption involves passing the gas-laden air through extended wetted surfaces and sprays of water or chemical solutions. Adsorption normally uses activated charcoal beds through which the gas-laden air passes, the pollutant being adsorbed onto the minute pores in the charcoal. Thermal oxidation techniques are also being developed. To achieve a high degree of cleaning, all techniques are bulky and costly to purchase and operate.

Air-cleaning techniques absorb energy from the extracted air; hence, this must be accounted for when choosing the correct fan for the job. Adding air cleaning later will invariably involve upgrading the performance of the fan to cater for the extra resistance to air flow that the device provides.

Discharges to the atmosphere

Any ventilation system that discharges air horizontally to the atmosphere will, at some time or another, encounter external wind pressures. Sometimes the direction and velocity of the outside wind will result in a reversal of the air flow in the ventilation system, and pollutants will be scattered internally rather than be extracted. Such systems require weather covers to prevent blowback, but these devices can result in polluted air remaining close to the buildings and being re-entrained into them. It is far better to discharge vertically as high as permissible with a high efflux velocity. Conical weather covers should be removed as they tend to bring pollutants down to ground level to be re-entrained into adjacent buildings. Suitable alternatives are available to prevent rain and snow from entering the discharge stack.

References

Gardiner, K. and Harrington, J.M. (eds.) (1992). *Occupational Hygiene*, 3e. Oxford: Blackwell.

Olishifski, J.B. (2002). Methods of control. In: *Fundamentals of Industrial Hygiene*, 5e (eds. B.A. Plog and P.J. Quinlan). Chicago: National Safety Council.

CHAPTER 16

Personal Protection of the Worker

16.1 Introduction

If control at source or during transmission is not possible, or if extra safeguards are required, then the worker must be protected. This can be performed in one of three ways, depending on the nature of the contaminant.

1. By washing the worker in a stream of uncontaminated air, thus displacing any airborne pollutants.
2. By segregation or separation, using a shield or air-conditioned enclosure.
3. By providing personal protective clothing.

Displacement

This depends upon the creation of a diffuse, clean air flow over the worker and towards the work, carrying away the work products, preferably towards some form of extraction system. The provision of work station supply ventilation has corresponding economies in the volume of air

Pocket Consultant: Occupational Health, Sixth Edition. Kerry Gardiner, David Rees, Anil Adisesh, David Zalk, and Malcolm Harrington.
© 2022 John Wiley & Sons Ltd. Published 2022 by John Wiley & Sons Ltd.

required in comparison with a system ventilating the whole building. Care must be taken to ensure that local turbulence is minimised, so that the effectiveness of control is maintained. This technique is most suited to well-defined work stations.

Thermal comfort of the worker must be considered, so that the combination of air temperature and velocity is such that cold draughts are not experienced at the place of work. To this end, supply diffusers must be chosen carefully, and the supply air temperature must be controlled accurately to suit the air velocity directed at the worker. This is particularly important when air is discharged from above and behind the worker, as the back, neck and back of the head are the parts of the body most sensitive to draughts. It is important to remember that even in air at a temperature above that of a normal room the individual can feel cold if the air is flowing at a sufficiently high velocity. Figure 16.1 shows the relationship between air velocity and temperature and the part of the body affected; it also shows the number of people complaining of discomfort as a percentage of the total number tested. As an example, it can be seen that a draught of $0.2\,\mathrm{m\,s^{-1}}$ at a temperature of $1\,°C$ below ambient room temperature, flowing onto the occupants' necks, will give a feeling of uncomfortable coolness to 20% of the room occupants, whereas the same draught blowing on the ankle region will cause discomfort to only 5%.

Enclosing or shielding the worker

Isolating the worker from an uncongenial or toxic environment is a technique that is often adopted when the working process is too large or too expensive to control at source or in the transmission stage. Isolation cubicles can be used to protect from noise, ionising radiation, heat and cold, as well as from airborne toxins. In most cases, the enclosure will require ventilation and, possibly, air conditioning, and the amounts of air required will need to be calculated. As a general rule, each person enclosed will require $10\,l$ of fresh air per second, but this amount can be varied, depending upon the size of the enclosure and whether or not smoking is permitted. For example, a small enclosure containing one person who smokes would require a fresh air rate of $25\,l\,s^{-1}$, whereas a spacious enclosure in which no smoking takes place could be ventilated with as little as $5\,l\,s^{-1}$ per person.

Personal protection

The organs of the human body that are vulnerable to attack from external sources are the eyes, the ears, the skin and the respiratory system. In the case of the first three, a barrier or attenuation device should be worn over the organ being protected. With regard to airborne pollutants, respiratory protection involves the wearing of a device that either cleans the polluted air to a safe level or provides a stream of uncontaminated air from a separate source.

At this juncture, it must be pointed out that Regulation 7 of the Control of Substances Hazardous to Health (Amendment) (COSHH) Regulations 2004 specifically states that employers need to ensure that their employees are not exposed to substances hazardous to health. Control of this exposure should be

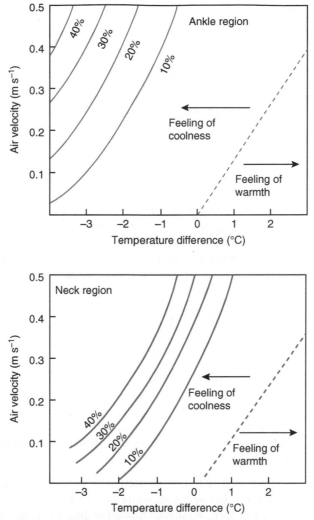

FIGURE 16.1 Percentage of room occupants objecting to draughts on the ankle and neck region.

secured by measures other than by the provision of personal protective equipment (PPE), but, where other means are not preventive or do not provide adequate control, then, in addition to those measures, suitable PPE shall be provided to control exposure adequately. The regulations require that the PPE provided must be suitable for the purpose and conform to a standard approved by the Health and Safety Executive.

Examples of situations in which the use of PPE may be necessary include the following:

• where it is not technically feasible to achieve adequate control by other measures alone, control should be achieved by other methods as far as reasonably practicable and then, in addition, PPE should be used

- where PPE is required to safeguard health until such time as adequate control is achieved by other means
- where urgent action is required, such as in a plant failure, and the only practical solution is to use PPE
- during routine maintenance operations.

In most cases, PPE appears to offer a cheap alternative solution to the provision of engineering control methods. On closer scrutiny, however, the management problems that are created by its introduction make this alternative less attractive. In order to make the decision to use personal protective devices routinely, it is necessary to hold discussions involving trade unions or workers' representatives and, once the decision to go ahead has been made, arrangements must be put in place for the education and training of the users. A complete back-up system of purchasing, storage, cleaning, repair, inspection, testing, replacement and, ultimately, detailed record keeping must also be established. Moreover, the reaction of the worker to being asked to wear the devices may involve financial inducements and changes in contract conditions before adoption, and management supervision may need to be strengthened.

16.2 Eye and face protection

Protection must be provided to guard against:

- the impact of small particles projected at a low velocity
- the impact of heavy particles at a high velocity
- the splashing of a hot or corrosive liquid
- the contact of the eyes with an irritating gas or vapour
- a beam of electromagnetic radiation of various wavelengths, including laser beams.

Each harmful agent may require a particular form of eye protection, which may be unsuitable for another agent. In some cases, the protection may need to be extended to the whole face. Whatever hazard or hazards exist, the protective device must be carefully chosen to suit.

Standards

Various standards for eye protection have been produced to assist in obtaining the correct specification to suit the harmful agent.
British Standard (BS) and British Standard European Norm (BS EN)

- *BS EN 169*. Specification for filters for personal eye-protection equipment used in welding and similar operations.
- *BS EN 170*. Specification for ultraviolet filters used in personal eye-protection equipment.
- *BS EN 171*. Specification for infrared filters used in personal eye-protection equipment.

- *BS EN 169*. Specification for filters, cover lenses and backing lenses for use during welding and similar industrial operations.
- *BS EN 166*. Specification for industrial eye protectors for general purposes.
- *BS 4110*. Specification for visors for vehicle users.

American National Standards Institute (New York)
- ANSI/ISEA Z87.1-2010, American National Standard Occupational and Educational Personal Eye and Face Protection.
- ANSI/ISEA Z87.1-2020: American National Standard For Occupational And Educational Personal Eye And Face Protection Devices; establishes the criteria for using, testing, marking, choosing and maintaining eye protection to prevent or minimise injuries from eye hazards.

General points

Eye protection takes the form of spectacles, goggles or face shields, all of which are available from a wide range of manufacturers and suppliers, in a wide range of sizes. Suitability for the hazard and comfort must be the overriding factors in choosing the particular device, as the users must have complete confidence in the protection it provides and must not be forced to remove it to relieve discomfort during the operation for which protection is required. A pre-occupation with discomfort may also distract from the task in hand and lead to errors and accidents. A good range of suitable forms of protection should therefore be made available so that the user can choose the one which suits the shape of his/her face. This may mean having products from more than one manufacturer available.

Some of the problems involved in the use of eye protectors are given below. Several can be overcome by suitable selection, but certain problems are inherent in the use of such devices.

- They may not guard against the hazard.
- They may not fit properly.
- They may be uncomfortable due to uneven pressure on the face.
- They will restrict the field of view.
- Spectacles worn for correction of vision may interfere with the wearing of eye protectors and vice versa. While safety spectacles with corrective lenses are available, their suitability is limited to minor eye hazards.
- Optical services and follow-up may be necessary to deal with problems of refraction of light.
- Eye protectors may interfere with the wearing of respiratory and/or hearing protection. Where more than one organ is to be protected, an integrated, combined protective device may therefore be more suitable.
- Owing to discomfort, the wearer may be tempted to remove the protector from time to time, with a consequent loss of protection for that period.
- Fitting, cleaning, inspecting and replacement procedures are necessary.
- Training may be required for users and for maintenance staff.

Types available

Safety spectacles are only suitable for low-energy hazards, but are available in a wide range of sizes to suit the face. Types: clear, clip-on, prescription and tinted (anti-flash).

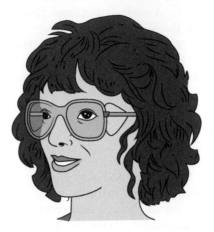

Goggles are suitable for a wide range of hazards, but are limited in fittings from any one manufacturer. Types: chemical, dust, gas, gas welding, general purpose and molten metal.

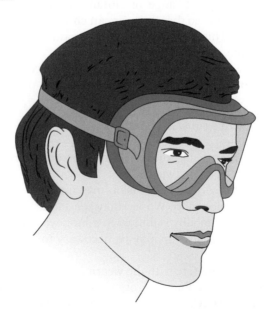

Shields are suitable to protect the eyes or the whole face; they can be attached to a helmet or a headband, but may be hand-held. Types: eye, face, furnace viewing and welding.

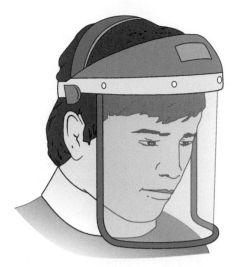

16.3 Skin and body protection

Skin protection includes guarding hands, feet and body against:

- damage from dermatitic or corrosive agents
- absorption into the body via the skin
- radiant heat
- cold
- ionising and non-ionising radiation
- physical damage.

The material as well as the thickness that is used for the gloves, apron or garment must be suited to the purpose and must be chosen carefully.

Standards and codes, BS and BS EN

Hand protection
- *BS EN 374. Part 1*. Protective gloves against chemicals and microorganisms: terminology and performance requirements.
- *BS EN 388*. Protective gloves against mechanical risks.
- *BS EN 407*. Protective gloves for thermal risks.
- *BS EN ISO 21420*. General requirements for gloves.
- *BS EN 421*. Protective gloves for ionising radiation including contamination and direct exposure to radiation.
- *BS EN 455-1*. Medical single-use gloves.
- *BS EN 511*. Protective gloves for cold.
- *BS EN 60903*. Insulating protective gloves for working with electricity.

Foot protection

- *BS EN ISO 20344*. Requirements and test methods for safety, protective and occupational footwear for professional use.
- *BS EN ISO 20345*. Specification for safety footwear for professional use.
- *BS EN ISO 20346*. Specification for protective footwear for professional use.
- *BS EN ISO 20347*. Specification for occupational footwear for professional use.
- *BS EN 15090*. Specification for firemen's leather boots.

Body protection

- *BS EN ISO 13688*. Protective clothing: general requirements.
- *BS EN ISO 11611*. Protective clothing for use in welding and allied processes: general requirements.
- *BS EN ISO 12127*. Protective clothing – protection against heat and flame; test method – determination of the contact heat transmission through protective clothing or its materials.
- *BS 7182*. Specification for air-impermeable chemical protective clothing.
- *BS 7184*. Recommendation for selection, use and maintenance of chemical protective clothing.

Types available

Hand protection

Materials	Protection	Gloves
Asbestos	Abrasion	Armoured
Cotton	Chemical	Chain mail
Leather	Electrical	Disposable
Moleskin	Fire/flame/heat resistant	Electrician's
Neoprene	General purpose engineering	Gauntlets, hand pads
Nitrile	Hygiene	Mitts
Nylon	Low temperature	Reversible
Polythene	Radiation	Surgical, X-ray
PVA		
PVC-impregnated cotton		
PVC		
Rubber		
Terrycloth		
Terylene		

PVA, polyvinyl acrylate; PVC, polyvinyl chloride.

Foot and leg protection

Anti-static footwear	Knee pads
Boots and shoes	Leggings
Chemical footwear	Moulded footwear
Clogs	Non-slip footwear
Cold-storage footwear	Overboots and overshoes
Conductive footwear	Rubber ankle boots

Foundry boots	Soles and heels
Gaiters/spats	Thigh boots
Knee boots	

Body protection

Materials	Protection	Garments
Asbestos	Buoyant	Aprons
Chain mail	Chemical	Armlets and sleeves
Cotton (denim, etc.)	Exposure	Capes
Glass fibre	Fire/flame/heat resistant	Coats and jackets
Leather	High-visibility fluorescent	Disposable gloves
Melton	Ionising radiation	Hoods and sou'westers
Moleskin	Proofed	Overalls
Neoprene	Quilted	Suits— – hot entry
Nylon, Terylene	Ventilated	Trousers
Paper and disposable		
Plastic coated		
Polyurethane		
PVC		
Wool		

PVC, polyvinyl chloride.

General points

- Protective clothing materials may be attacked and degraded by contact with chemicals. Different glove materials and their relative thicknesses have permeation rates to certain chemicals to break through intact materials, leading directly to skin contact that can vary from minutes to hours and requiring a matching of material and thickness to classes of chemicals to be used. In addition, permeation leading to degradation can also result in chemical penetration, requiring an established regimen for care, maintenance and disposal at established intervals. Protective clothing designed to withstand chemicals also comes in a variety of forms and materials, each with its own characteristics with regard to resistance to chemical permeation. Permeation rates with different manufacturers' garments may vary even with the same material. Therefore, it is important to know these breakthrough times before selection of all protective clothing materials.
- While the material may be suitable, seams and joints in garments may allow the passage of particles, liquids and/or vapours. This can be aggravated by the bellows action of body movement within a clothing assembly. In addition, continual flexing of the material allows liquids to pass through more readily.
- Protective clothing, particularly a whole-body garment, sets up a microclimate, inside which the loss of body heat may be limited, causing discomfort and leading to possible stress. Some such garments can be ventilated.
- Some garments restrict the movement of limbs, which slows the worker and increases fatigue. In addition, thicker gloves that may have been chosen

to minimise chemical breakthrough time can lead to a reduced tactile grip that can result in difficulty in handling certain items and could be deleterious for some delicate tasks.

- Provision must be made for changing, cleaning and storage of protective clothing.
- Impervious gloves must be sufficiently long to tuck under a sleeve to prevent materials from spilling inside.
- Low temperatures may make certain plastic materials too stiff to be usable.
- Caution must be exercised in the use of latex gloves, especially in those with a history of allergy.

16.4 Respiratory protection

The choice of equipment in this field is vast, ranging from the simple disposable dust mask to the full, self-contained breathing apparatus, and there is much confusion as to which device to use for a particular hazard. As the wrong choice may seriously affect the health of the wearer, and could lead to asphyxiation, advice from an expert is required. In addition, user training is essential, whatever device is chosen, and servicing and cleaning facilities must be provided.

Standards and codes, BS and BS EN

- *BS EN ISO 16972*. Respiratory protective devices – definitions.
- *BS EN 133*. Respiratory protective devices – classification.
- *BS EN 134*. Respiratory protective devices – nomenclature of components.
- *BS EN 135*. Respiratory protective devices – list of equivalent terms.
- *BS EN 136. Part 10*. Parts for full face masks for respiratory protective devices: specification for full face masks for special use.
- *BS EN 137*. Specification for respiratory protective devices – self-contained open-circuit compressed air breathing apparatus.
- *BS EN 14593*. Respiratory protective devices – compressed air-line breathing apparatus for use with full face mask, half mask or mouthpiece assembly – requirements, testing, marking.
- *BS EN 14387*. Respiratory protective devices. Gas filters and combined filters with requirements, testing, and markings.
- *BS EN 143*. Specification for particle filters used in respiratory protective devices.
- *BS EN 12941*. Respiratory protective devices: specification for powered particle filtering devices incorporating helmets or hoods.
- *BS EN 12842*. Respiratory devices: specification for power-assisted particle filtering devices incorporating full face masks, half masks or quarter masks.
- *BS EN 149*. Specification for filtering half masks to protect against particles.
- *BS EN 13794*. Respiratory protective devices for self-rescue – self-contained closed-circuit breathing apparatus – compressed oxygen escape apparatus – requirements, testing, marking.
- *BS EN 402*. Specification for respiratory protective devices for escape – self-contained open-circuit compressed air breathing apparatus with full face mask or mouthpiece assembly.

- *BS EN 403*. Specification for filtering respiratory protective devices with hood for self-rescue from fire.
- *BS EN 404*. Respiratory devices for self-rescue – filter self-rescuer.
- *BS 529*. Recommendations for the selection, use and maintenance of respiratory protective devices.
- *BS 4400*. Method for sodium chloride particulate test for respiratory filters.
- *BS EN 1146*. Specification for breathing apparatus – open-circuit escape breathing apparatus.
- *BS EN 13794*. Specification for breathing apparatus – closed-circuit escape.
- *BS EN 145*. Specification for respiratory protective devices: self-contained closed-circuit compressed oxygen breathing apparatus.
- *BS EN 136*. Specification for full face masks for respiratory protective devices.
- *BS EN 140*. Specification for half masks and quarter masks for respiratory protective devices.

Types available

The efficiency of respiratory protection in the removal of contaminants is expressed as the nominal protection factor (npf), which is defined as the ratio of the concentration of the contaminant present in the ambient atmosphere to the calculated concentration within the facepiece when the respiratory protection is being worn, that is:

$$npf = \frac{\text{concentration of contaminant in the atmosphere}}{\text{concentration of contaminant in the facepiece}}$$

The npf is used to determine the degree of protection required once one knows the concentration of pollutant in the workplace and the required concentration inhaled by the worker. However, actual protection factors, commonly referred to as effective or workplace protection factors (epf or wpf), are often much lower than the quoted npf. The reduction of protection reflected by actual protection factors may be a by-product of workers removing them when their use is necessary, due to comfort or other factors, as well as multiple issues that may affect appropriate donning and fit during tasks.

Respirators
These operate by drawing the inhaled air through a medium that will remove most of the contaminant. For dust and fibres, the medium is a filter that is replaced when dirty and these are known as particulate respirators. These can only protect against particles as they do not protect against chemicals, gases and vapours. Particulate filters are divided into three series: N, R and P; each is available at three efficiency levels: 95%, 99% and 99.97% (available as an N100, R100 or P100 for addressing any particulate). The N series filter is used in environments free of oil mists. Environments with oil mists can use either R series filters, which are good for one shift, or P filters, which may be used for longer than one work shift. Chemical cartridges or gas mask respirators are classified as air purifying for gases and vapours as they use specific mediums that adsorb chemicals to filter

or clean chemical gases out of the air as a user breathes and they are specifically designed for the gas or vapour to be removed. The medium is carried in a canister or a cartridge for ease of handling and renewal. Extreme caution must be observed to ensure that the correct medium is used for the pollutant in question; where dust and fibres are concerned, it is important to consider the size range of the particles to be removed in order to select the appropriate filter medium. Cartridges are also available for combinations of dust, gases and vapours, such as for pesticides (organic vapour canister plus a particulate filter), acid gases and ammonia, or acid gases and organic vapours. It is important to note that respirators do not provide any protection from an atmosphere deficient in oxygen.

Disposable particulate respirators (also known as an N-95) are manufactured from the filtering material; some are suitable for respirable-sized dust. The facepiece is at a negative pressure as the lung provides the motive power and can provide filtration through the material when properly fitted; npf ≈ 5.

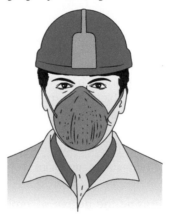

Half-mask respirators are manufactured from rubber or plastic and are designed to cover the nose and mouth; they have a replaceable filter cartridge. With the appropriate cartridge selected and respirator fitted, they are suitable for dust, gas or vapour. The facepiece is at a negative pressure as the lung provides the motive power; npf ≈ 10.

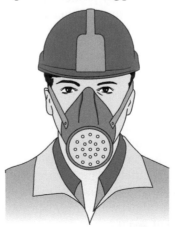

Full-facepiece respirators are manufactured from rubber or plastic and are designed to cover the mouth, nose and eyes. The filter medium is contained in a canister directly coupled or connected via a flexible tube. With the appropriate canister or cartridge selected and respirator fitted, they are suitable for dust, gas or vapour. The facepiece is at a negative pressure as the lung provides the motive power; npf ≈ 50.

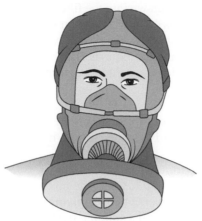

Powered respirators with a half mask or full facepiece are made of rubber or plastic and are maintained at a positive pressure as the air is drawn through an appropriately selected filter by means of a battery-powered fan. The fan, filter and battery are normally carried on the belt, with a flexible tube to supply the cleaned air to the facepiece; npf ≈ 500.

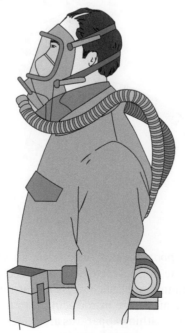

Powered visor respirators have a fan and filters carried in a helmet, with the cleaned air blown down over the wearer's face inside a hinged visor. The visor can be fitted with side shields, which can be sized to suit the wearer's face. The battery pack is normally carried on the belt. A range of filters and absorbents is available to ensure the correct one is appropriately selected, and a welder's type is also produced; $npf \approx 1–20$. It is worth noting that, for both powered respirators and powered visor respirators, because the air is drawn into the filter(s) either in the small of the back or nape of the neck, the air is often cleaner than that found in the breathing zone. Therefore, although the npf may be low, the epf or wpf may be much higher.

There are many variations in the types of the above devices, and manufacturers' catalogues and advice should be sought before a choice is made.

Breathing apparatus

This provides a supply of uncontaminated air from a source that is either drawn from fresh air or compressed air or is supplied from a high-pressure cylinder carried by the wearer.

In a *fresh air hose apparatus*, a supply of fresh air is fed to a facepiece, hood or blouse via a large-diameter flexible tube. The motive power is provided by either a manually or electrically powered blower, giving a positive pressure in the face-piece. It is important to establish a suitable fresh air base for the blower and, if manually operated, two operators should be present; $npf \approx 50$.

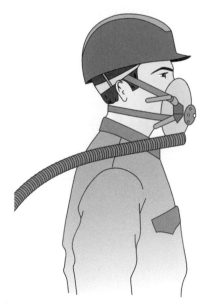

A *compressed air-line apparatus* supplies air via a reducing valve to a face-piece, hood or blouse. If the normal factory compressed air supply is used, it is necessary to filter out contaminants, such as oxides of nitrogen, carbon monoxide and oil mists, from the air before introducing it to the wearer. Specially designed air compressors for breathing apparatus are preferred, as these use special lubricating oils to minimise air contamination; $npf \approx 1000$.

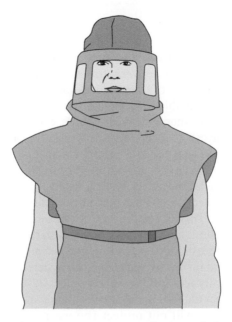

Self-contained breathing apparatus uses cylinders of air or oxygen, feeding a mouthpiece or facepiece, via a pressure-reducing valve. Open-circuit sets contain sufficient air or oxygen for a duration of use of between 10 and 30 minutes. Closed-circuit sets, which recirculate and purify exhaled breath, can last up to three hours; npf ≈ 2000.

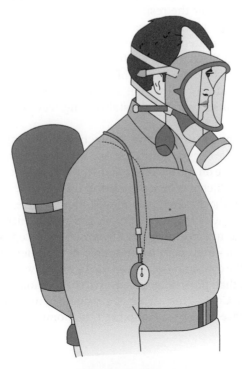

General points

With negative-pressure facepieces, the success of the device depends largely upon the adequacy of the seal between the wearer's face and the edge of the facepiece. The sizes and shapes of human faces vary so widely that it is important to have a range of sizes available to suit every wearer. Unfortunately, this type of respirator is unsuitable for men who wear beards, even with as little as two days of growth. BS 5108 suggests that the following negative-pressure test will reveal leaks both around the facepiece and elsewhere in the device. It is therefore appropriate practice for users to be given the same model and size that they were fitted with and being clean shaven as when fit tested.

To ensure proper protection, the facepiece fit should be checked by the wearer each time they put it on. This may be done in the following way. Negative pressure test: Close the inlet of the equipment. Inhale gently so that the facepiece collapses slightly, and hold the breath for 10 seconds. If the facepiece remains in its slightly collapsed condition and no inward leakage of air is detected, the tightness of the facepiece is probably satisfactory. If the wearer detects leakage, he should re-adjust the facepiece and repeat the test. If leakage is still noted, it can be concluded that this particular facepiece will not protect the wearer. The wearer should not continue to tighten the headband straps until he is uncomfortably tight simply to achieve a gas-tight face fit.

Respiratory protection is generally uncomfortable to wear, particularly those forms that use the lungs to provide the motive power and have negative-pressure facepieces. As the resistance of the filter has to be overcome by the wearer's lungs, the higher the resistance, the less comfortable the apparatus, and the greater the temptation to remove it for some temporary respite. This problem can be exacerbated when the work rate of the individual is high. It has been shown that the removal of the respirator, even for a short period of time, can seriously reduce the degree of protection given – the higher the npf, the more pronounced this reduction. These factors are related to the use of the epf or wpf discussed above for establishing true respirator effectiveness in practice.

In order to maintain an effective protection factor, all devices, with the exception of disposable ones, require cleaning and inspection after use. The manufacturer should advise on the life of the canister or cartridge, taking into account the environment in which it is being used, and this must be replaced at the interval recommended. If the mass of contaminant the cartridge/canister is capable of adsorbing is quoted, then, by combination of the average airborne concentration, duration of exposure and breathing rate, the appropriate replacement date can be calculated. However, care needs to be taken if the interval between wearing periods is long, as the concentration of the contaminant within the adsorbent will homogenise rather than progress across the cartridge/canister as a 'concentration front' (Figure 16.2). Central maintenance procedures are preferable to allowing the wearers to service their own equipment, as nominated responsible persons

(a)   Movement of concentration front over time

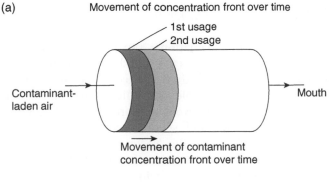

1st usage
2nd usage

Contaminant-laden air

Mouth

Movement of contaminant
concentration front over time

(b)   Homogenised concentration after being left

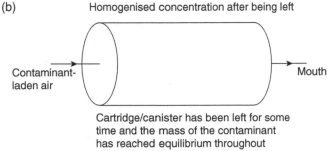

Contaminant-laden air

Mouth

Cartridge/canister has been left for some
time and the mass of the contaminant
has reached equilibrium throughout

(c)   Graphical representation of (a) and (b)

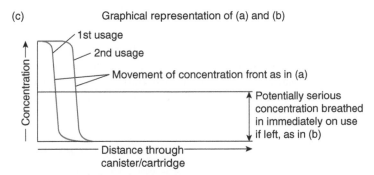

1st usage
2nd usage
Movement of concentration front as in (a)

Potentially serious
concentration breathed
in immediately on use
if left, as in (b)

Concentration →

Distance through
canister/cartridge →

FIGURE 16.2 Movement of the concentration front over time.

can build up an expertise on care and maintenance, apply routine tests and keep records on the respirators.

Wearer training and practice are essential, even with the simplest respiratory devices, but with breathing apparatus training courses must be extensive and thorough. No person should be allowed to wear a set unless he/she is seen to be fully conversant with the apparatus and knows the procedures to adopt in cases of emergency. The mines' rescue services and fire brigades have the greatest expertise and experience in the use of self-contained non-aquatic breathing apparatus in the UK.

16.5 Hearing protection

The Control of Noise at Work Regulations 2005 (Noise at Work Regulations) requires that the exposure of employees to noise should be reduced as far as reasonably practicable by means other than the use of personal ear protectors. However, it also requires that suitable and efficient personal ear protectors should be made available to all employees who are likely to be exposed to daily levels of noise between the 'first' and 'second' action levels. If employees are likely to be exposed to levels above the 'second' or 'peak' action levels, the employer shall provide suitable and efficient hearing protectors which, when worn properly, should reduce the levels to below those action levels.

Because noise is produced over a range of frequencies, the choice of hearing protection must be based upon the measured spectrum of the noise to be attenuated. Hearing protectors are either earmuffs, also known as circumaural muffs, which cover the ears, or earplugs, which are inserted into the ear canals. Within these two groups, however, there are several subdivisions. The earmuffs can have several degrees of attenuation, while the earplugs can be of a variety of materials, both disposable and reusable. Figure 16.3 shows attenuation data for four types of hearing protection, and illustrates the importance of frequency.

Types available

Earmuffs
These consist of a cup-shaped cover over each ear, held in place by a spring-loaded headband. To ensure a good seal around the ear, the cups are edged with a cushion filled with liquid or foam. The degree of attenuation is affected by the material of the cup and its lining, and the success of the device depends upon the quality of

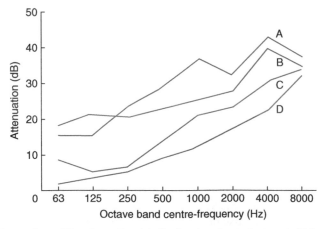

FIGURE 16.3 Comparison of the attenuation data for four hearing protectors: A, high-attenuation earmuff; B, disposable expanding polyurethane foam earplugs; C, low-attenuation earmuff; D, disposable earplugs.

the seal around the ear. Earmuffs are also available with noise-cancelling capabilities to reduce some high or peak noise exposures, such as at firearm shooting ranges. The duration for which earmuffs perform to specification can be very limited (i.e. months).

Earplugs

These can be of a variety of materials:

Disposable plugs	Reusable plugs
Glass down	Permanent moulded plastic
Plastic-coated glass down	Paste-filled rubber
Wax-impregnated cotton wool	Paste-filled plastic
Polyurethane foam	

All reusable plugs require washing after use and a sterile place for storage. Disposable plugs are available commercially in wall-mounted dispensers or in cartons containing several days' supply for one person. Manufacturers often give a noise reduction rating (NRR) for their hearing protection products. In theory, this would mean that an exposure of 100 dB(A) while wearing earplugs with a 25 dB NRR yields a true exposure to the worker of 75 dB(A); however, in practice this is not the case. The National Institute for Occupational Safety and Health (NIOSH) Occupational Noise Exposure document suggests a rough guide for derating manufacturer-generated NRRs as follows: muffs (25%), foam earplugs (50%) and moulded (flanged) plugs (70%); this will give a more appropriate exposure reduction factor in practice. A more appropriate quantitative fit testing of hearing production products has become easier to achieve and provides a true exposure reduction factor for one or more products. If noise exposure is extreme, it is possible to use earplugs in combination with earmuffs. However, there are limitations to the effectiveness of this combination. For example, combining a 26-dB NRR earplug and a 34-dB NRR earmuff will not yield an additive 60-dB noise reduction at 1000 Hz as it has been shown to be closer to 40 dB. It is thought that bone conduction is the primary reason that attenuation is limited as high-energy sound waves can be conducted via the bone to cause the wearer a direct stimulation to the middle and inner ears. A rough rule of thumb in practice is that this combination should add no more than 10 dB NRR to the earplug's effective NRR.

Theoretical protection

To calculate the degree of protection given by hearing protectors, it is necessary to measure the sound spectrum of the noise emitted at the workplace, using octave band analysis. If the result is required in dB(A), the A-weighting values at each mid-octave frequency should be from the measured sound to provide a 'corrected level'; each mid-octave level can then be added together, according to Figure 16.4.

The assumed protection of the hearing protector, also expressed in mid-octave values, should then be subtracted from the corrected level, and the result added

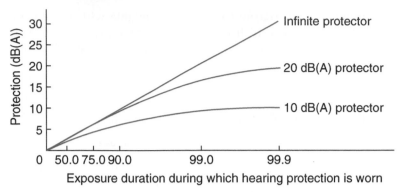

FIGURE 16.4 The effects of removing hearing protectors for short periods of time. Comparison of the protection afforded by hearing protectors that reduce the instantaneous sound level by 10 dB and 20 dB. Source: Else (1975).

as before to produce the estimated dB(A) at the wearer's ear. This can best be illustrated with an example (Table 16.1). As with respiratory protection, hearing protection can be uncomfortable, particularly if worn for long periods, as the wearer may feel enclosed and isolated and, with earmuffs, perspiration can build up around the seals. Although earmuffs provide the greatest amount of attenuation, they are easy to remove and replace. Therefore, wearers are tempted to remove them to ease discomfort. It has been shown that the removal of hearing protection, even for short periods, will reduce the overall protection substantially, the effect being increasingly more pronounced as the noise levels increase. This effect is illustrated in Figure 16.4, from which it can be seen that protection giving 20 dB(A) attenuation when worn 100% of the time will only give an effective 10 dB(A) protection when worn 90% of the time. If noise levels are much in excess of 90 dB(A), protection must therefore be worn continuously to maintain levels of below 85 dB(A) at the ear, averaged over the whole shift.

It can be seen from this that better overall protection may be provided by using a lower degree of attenuation from, for example, glass down earplugs, which may be more comfortable and more acceptable and so not be removed during the shift, than by using a higher degree of attenuation with less comfort, for example earmuffs.

Servicing and replacement facilities must be provided for earmuffs because they will deteriorate with time, in particular at the seals, which become distorted and harden with age. A range of hearing protection should also be made available so that wearers can choose the type that is most comfortable for them.

As with all forms of personal protective devices, adequate training must be given so that the wearers can understand the reasons for providing these devices. In-house training programmes should be implemented and can be aided by films and/or tape/slide presentations. Hearing protection manufacturers can assist with audiovisual aids and explanatory leaflets. As both disposable and reusable earplugs come in different sizes and are made of variable materials, newly available

TABLE 16.1

Example of calculation to find the degree of attenuation provided by a particular earmuff against a typical industrial noise.

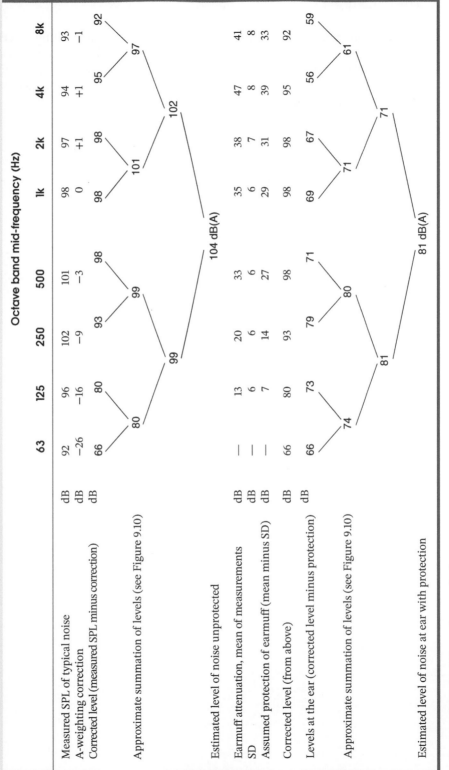

		Octave band mid-frequency (Hz)							
		63	125	250	500	1k	2k	4k	8k
Measured SPL of typical noise	dB	92	96	102	101	98	97	94	93
A-weighting correction	dB	−26	−16	−9	−3	0	+1	+1	−1
Corrected level (measured SPL minus correction)	dB	66	80	93	98	98	98	95	92

Approximate summation of levels (see Figure 9.10)

80   99   101   97 → 99   102 → **104 dB(A)**

Estimated level of noise unprotected

		63	125	250	500	1k	2k	4k	8k
Earmuff attenuation, mean of measurements	dB	—	13	20	33	35	38	47	41
SD	dB	—	6	6	6	6	7	8	8
Assumed protection of earmuff (mean minus SD)	dB	—	7	14	27	29	31	39	33
Corrected level (from above)	dB	66	80	93	98	98	98	95	92
Levels at the ear (corrected level minus protection)	dB	66	73	79	80	69	67	56	59

Approximate summation of levels (see Figure 9.10)

74   81   71   61 → 81   71 → **81 dB(A)**

Estimated level of noise at ear with protection

SD, standard deviation; SPL, sound pressure level.

computer programs can be used to assist with a quantitative fitting of certain personal protective devices in a manner comparable to respiratory fit testing. Routine audiometric measurements on workers can provide an opportunity to make contact with them and to encourage them to wear hearing protection and remind them of the basics of how to use it properly.

Reference

Else, D. (1975). A note on the protection afforded by hearing protectors implications of the energy principle. *Annals of Occupational Hygiene* 16 (1): 81–83.

CHAPTER 17

Tertiary Prevention

17.1 Introduction

The preventive approach has three stages:

- Primary prevention aims to prevent new cases of disease/injury arising.
- Secondary prevention aims to detect disease or injury at the earliest stage when the condition may be reversible or disease progression halted or slowed.
- Tertiary prevention aims to ameliorate the effects of established disease or injury.

These approaches can be applied at both a workplace population level and an individual level. In occupational health, commonly the concept of the hierarchy of controls is applied to the consideration of primary preventive measures. This chapter addresses tertiary prevention, meaning that primary and secondary measures have failed. Taking hepatitis B infection (see Section 4.2, Hepatitis B) in healthcare work as an example, primary prevention could be achieved through immunisation and safer sharps use. Secondary prevention in the same situation might include identifying healthcare workers with existing infection by screening before offering immunisation. Tertiary prevention for an individual healthcare worker with hepatitis B may involve treatment with anti-viral medication and monitoring of the viral load and markers of infectivity, which may allow a return to work – even undertaking exposure-prone procedures such as certain types of surgery.

The workplace population approach would involve adopting policies and practices that support the implementation of universal precautions, safer sharps use, immunisation programmes for workers considered at risk, appropriate hepatitis

Pocket Consultant: Occupational Health, Sixth Edition. Kerry Gardiner, David Rees, Anil Adisesh, David Zalk, and Malcolm Harrington.
© 2022 John Wiley & Sons Ltd. Published 2022 by John Wiley & Sons Ltd.

B screening and facilitating access to treatment services. Additionally, supportive employment policies should be in place including redeployment and retraining as may be required for those who are unable to return to their original work. Occupational health professionals therefore need to consider that they are not only advising individual workers and their managers but also taking account of the risks to health for the workplace population and the employing organisation.

17.2 Return to work and workplace accommodation

A common scenario for occupational health practitioners is to receive a referral from a manager of a worker on sickness absence related to a disease or workplace injury. Such a routine circumstance is actually the practical application of tertiary prevention. Workplace interventions can reduce the length of sickness absence, reduce pain and improve functional status effectively, with evidence supporting their use for musculoskeletal disorders. The type of workplace interventions considered for occupational low back pain have, for example, been a worksite assessment by an ergonomist with subsequent work adjustments, identifying barriers to return to work, agreeing solutions and involvement of an occupational physician communicating with the general medical practitioner to avoid any misunderstandings. There are guidelines giving other disease-specific recommendations, e.g. for occupational asthma and occupational contact dermatitis, to assist in the management of these conditions.

In the case of occupational contact dermatitis, once the diagnosis has been established then changes to work practices are the most effective means to allow a worker to continue in their job. Figure 17.1 illustrates the 'three peaks of occupational disease'. In this context these peaks represent that some diseases, e.g. allergic contact dermatitis, are caused by work; other diseases, e.g. atopic dermatitis, may be worsened by work; and some cases of dermatitis may be unrecognised by the healthcare professional as work related. In so much as all these cases are treated, they are subject to a level of tertiary prevention. Other preventive actions for established disease might include simple interventions, such as allowing and encouraging a worker to change any contaminated clothing quickly and to ensure the provision of disposable towels instead of using rags kept in clothing pockets. However, this may require advocacy from the occupational health professional to persuade management of the utility of such a change. On an individual basis these changes may be recognised as 'accommodations' or 'adjustments', taking into consideration all the circumstances of the case under jurisdictional human rights legislation relating to disabled persons. It is for the employer to consider the practicality of supporting the necessary changes at the request of the employee, or when it should be known to the employer, for instance, if there is information already available in an occupational health or medical report. The employer's duty to accommodate is considered to be up to 'undue hardship' or to make 'reasonable adjustments' according to the applicable legislation. In some jurisdictions, the onus on

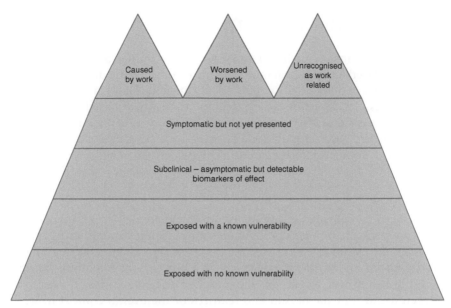

FIGURE 17.1 The three peaks of occupational disease.

companies to accommodate workers is more stringent for occupational disease and injury than for non-occupational conditions; in others it is more a moral obligation. It should be recalled that the benefits in some circumstances will not only be tertiary prevention for the individual worker, but if implemented more widely primary and secondary prevention benefits may be across the workforce, e.g. reducing skin contact with allergens and irritants that may elicit and incite contact dermatitis. Additionally, the clinical identification of skin contact allergens or irritants is helpful because their avoidance may lead to improvement or even resolution of the dermatitis. Where it is not possible to completely avoid the responsible agent, personal protective equipment may then be appropriate with monitoring of the skin condition. Where these measures fail, redeployment of the worker to alternative work may be necessary. Alongside these interventions, education of the affected worker about the occupational condition has been shown to lead to better self-management.

17.3 Workers' compensation

Supporting the affected worker through the disability management system such as with a Workers' Compensation (Industrial Injury or Disease) claim might be considered tertiary prevention as this may provide access to further employment support resources. In many jurisdictions with workers' compensation systems, an accepted claim will also lead to a different, often more rapid, treatment pathway, medical insurance provisions and additional health benefits. Conversely, a worker frustrated by the progress of their claim or engaged in acrimonious litigation may be less likely to have a positive view regarding return to work.

17.4 Disability and impairment assessment

Compensation is insurance based and often uses a framework for assessment of disability based on a medical model being a characteristic directly caused by disease, trauma or other health condition. An ancient classification system, the Barema tables, developed in the eighteenth century, was based on mediaeval laws to produce a disability percentage table. In this scheme a bodily loss or impairment, e.g. limb amputation, equates to a percentage disability and thereby to a compensation amount. The widely used *American Medical Association Guides to the Evaluation of Permanent Impairment* provide methods of deriving similar percentage disability scores often applied in various insurance schemes.

The social model views disability as a problem created by an unaccommodating physical environment brought about by attitudes and other features of the social environment. Assessment of abilities may focus on activities of daily living rather than impairments and so represents the remaining abilities. Disability is, however, a complex phenomenon and constitutes an interaction between features of the person and features of the overall context in which the person lives. A better synthesis is the biopsychosocial model; this incorporates the concepts of functionality and disability as embodied in the International Classification of Function (ICF). The ICF is the World Health Organization's framework for health and disability with a clear focus on functioning, acknowledging that anyone can experience a decrement in health and thereby experience some disability.

Tertiary prevention is of great benefit to individual workers, employing organisations and the general economy through facilitating early return to work, retention in the workforce and the avoidance of worklessness. Aside from treatment, tertiary prevention can be summarised as rehabilitation, re-education, retraining and possibly redeployment.

Further Reading

van Vilsteren, M., van Oostrom, S.H., de Vet, H.C.W. et al. (2015). Workplace interventions to prevent work disability in workers on sick leave. *Cochrane Database of Systematic Reviews* (10): CD006955. https://doi.org/10.1002/14651858.CD006955.pub3.

Adisesh, A., Robinson, E., Nicholson, P. et al. (2013). U.K. standards of care for occupational contact dermatitis and occupational contact urticaria. *The British Journal of Dermatology* 168: 1167–1175. doi:10.1111/bjd.12256.

World Health Organization (2002). Towards a Common Language for Functioning, Disability and Health: ICF – The International Classification of Functioning, Disability and Health. https://cdn.who.int/media/docs/default-source/classification/icf/icfbeginnersguide.pdf?sfvrsn=eead63d3_4 (accessed 26 August 2021).

CHAPTER 18

Special Issues in Occupational Health

Pocket Consultant: Occupational Health, Sixth Edition. Kerry Gardiner, David Rees, Anil Adisesh, David Zalk, and Malcolm Harrington.
© 2022 John Wiley & Sons Ltd. Published 2022 by John Wiley & Sons Ltd.

18.1 Introduction

In addition to the occupational health issues presented in the previous chapters, the occupational health practitioner is faced with other problems that cannot always be neatly classified under section headings. This chapter constitutes a series of short accounts of aspects of occupational health of current interest. Psychosocial aspects are now of sufficient importance to warrant a chapter of their own (see Chapter 11).

18.2 Working hours

The health issues related to working hours involve two aspects:

1. shift work
2. long hours of work.

Both of these working practices can be construed as involving 'unsociable' hours. That is, employees are, for one reason or another, required to work outside the limits considered by many people to be 'normal'. Nominally, this equates to an eight-hour 'stint' from morning to late afternoon for five days of the week. Nowadays, work patterns frequently depart from this conformity; 24-hour factories, late shopping hours, short-term ('zero-hour') contract work, demanding targets, flexible working arrangements, working from home and many other aspects of modern working life have led to extended working hours outside the 'normal' working day.

Shift work

Shift work is the 'norm' for about 20% of the workforce in most countries, but with large variations among them. The need for shift work is threefold:

1. *societal*: services and emergencies
2. *technical*: continuous process industries
3. *economic*: optimal plant utilisation.

There are various types of shift work:

- two or three shifts in a 24-hour period
- rotating or fixed shifts
- rapid or slow rotation shifts
- forward or backward rotation shifts
- 8-, 10- or 12-hour shifts.

There is no doubt that rotating shift work – particularly those systems involving night work – leads to various disruptions to normal life. These include:

- *biological*: circadian dysrhythmia, cardiovascular disorders, gastrointestinal disorders
- *psychosocial*: fatigue/sleep loss, lowered performance, mental health, increased accidents
- *individual*: perhaps greater variation than group effects; dependent on domestic/social circumstances and coping strategies. Low participation in social and family life, e.g. childcare, is a common consequence of prolonged night work requiring daytime sleep.

In Volume 124, IARC (https://publications.iarc.fr/593) reaffirmed that night shift work that disrupts circadian rhythm (meaning in light) is a probable human carcinogen (2A). The large number of women working at night (nurses for example) and the high incidence of breast cancer calls for interventions to counter the effects of circadian disruption. Prevention and compensatory measures to reduce the deleterious effects of shift work are beyond the scope of this section. Such measures have been identified, though, and occupational health practitioners should promote their adoption in the workplaces they service.

Long hours of work

Although many of the effects of rotating shift work are now well known, the effects of long working hours have received less attention in the scientific literature. Extended hours include the manager working 50–70 hours per week or the shop-floor employee working a 12-hour shift for more than four shifts a week.

Fatigue has been recognised as an effect of 12-hour shifts, but other putative effects, such as ill health, increased accident rates and poor performance, are less well documented and the issue is, as yet, unresolved. A particular problem here is that, although the 12-hour shift usually means three or four days off each week, it also allows for a second job to be undertaken – often in clandestine circumstances. This makes it difficult to assess the harm caused by just three days of 12 hours.

For the manager working long hours per week, there are virtually no studies that can answer the health effect issue. Either the studies have not been executed or the populations studied so far are rather special groups with factors that prevent any generalisation to the issue as a whole.

The European Commission has promulgated a Directive on working time (Directive 2003/88/EC), which attempts to restrict working hours in terms of both weekly total and hours to be worked in any day.

18.3 Workplace injury, incidents and management

Safety statistics

With the indulgence of the reader, data from the UK will be used in this section not because they are seen to be good but because they are readily available and clearly presented. In the UK, about 100 people are killed as a result of workplace incidents every year; in addition, about 700 000 suffer a non-fatal injury – with ~65 500 more serious injuries reported under the Reporting of Injuries, Diseases and Dangerous Occurrences Regulations 2013 (RIDDOR).

It is evident from Figure 18.1 that slips, trips and falls (on the same level) seem to dominate annually and geographically, although this may seem somewhat trivial to focus upon when juxtaposed with the data showing that in total 6.5 million working days are lost with an annual incurred cost of £5.6 billion. A cautionary note is that only about 30% of all reportable incidents to employees are reported, with the figure falling to about 5% for the self-employed.

It appears reassuring that over the past 20 years the number of workplace non-fatal injuries has fallen, although care needs to be taken in the interpretation of these data as all sorts of factors may be at play – decreasing heavy industry, a sense of futility in reporting, etc. (Figure 18.2).

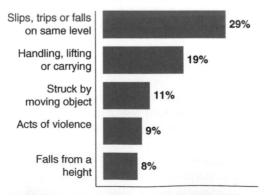

FIGURE 18.1 Non-fatal injuries to employees by most common accident kinds.

Figure 18.3 presents the rate of self-reported work-related ill health and non-fatal injury by industrial sector, demonstrating that sectors that cause injury are often not those that cause work-related ill health.

As stated above, these data are presented in a purely objective manner and to catalyse critical and insightful thought – as in, not what is the difference between the UK and France in Figure 18.4 but why?

The same is true for the stark difference between Poland and France in the data presented in Figure 18.5; and between the UK and Poland in Figure 18.6.

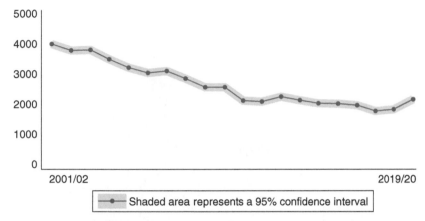

FIGURE 18.2 Estimated self-reported workplace non-fatal injury per 100 000 workers.

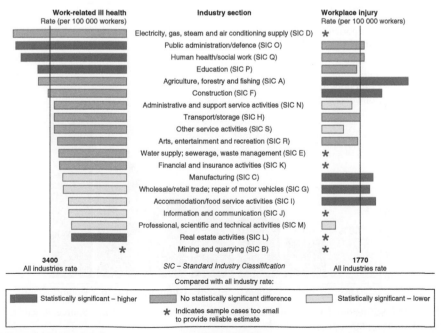

FIGURE 18.3 Rate of self-reported work-related ill health and non-fatal injury by industry.
Source: Labour Force Survey annual average estimate 2017/18–2019/20.

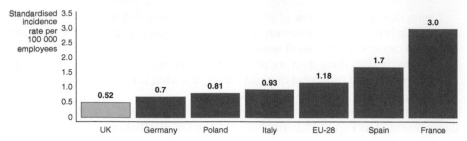

FIGURE 18.4 Fatal injuries in large European Union (EU) economies. Source: Adapted from Eurostat (2017).

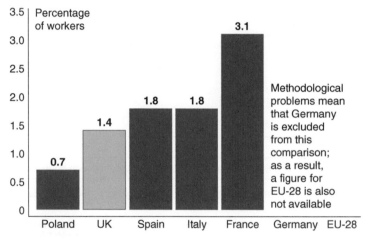

FIGURE 18.5 Self-reported work-related injuries resulting in sick leave. Source: Based on EU Labour Force Survey (2013).

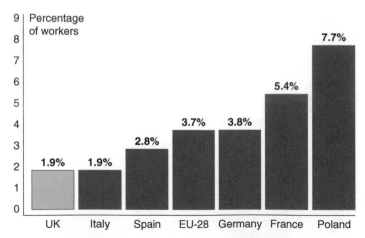

FIGURE 18.6 Self-reported work-related health problems resulting in sick leave. Source: Based on EU Labour Force Survey (2013).

Safety management

Over the last few years, there has been a shift away from the prevention of repetitions of accidents (reactive prevention), which is easier to do but unreliable, towards proactive prevention, where the probabilities of a range of unwanted outcomes are considered and an integrated control plan is implemented prior to their manifestation.

Workplace incidents are very rarely caused by a single unsafe act or condition, but more commonly by a combination of factors. An 'unsafe act' can include human actions that are unintentional, i.e. 'unintentional errors', and intentional risky behaviour, i.e. 'violations'. However, it could be said that it is unsafe acts by an individual or group, often remote in time and place from the workplace, that create conditions where unsafe acts by the workforce can lead to accidents. These remote errors by managers have been referred to as 'latent' or 'decision' failures, and those by the workforce at risk as 'active' failures.

Proactive safety management

Programmes to prevent workplace incidents must address the following four elements of the accident causation process.

1. *Multicausality*. It must be recognised that most accidents have multiple causes, and that to identify and prevent their occurrence, it is necessary to investigate all aspects of an organisation and attempt to alter its perception of occupational health and safety.
2. *Active and latent failures*. An active failure is one in which the error has an immediate adverse effect (equivalent to an unsafe act), whereas a latent failure may exist within an organisation for some time and may only manifest itself when combined with appropriate active failures (unsafe acts/conditions).
3. *Skill-, rule- and knowledge-based errors, and violations*. Skill-based errors are 'lapses' in highly practised and routine tasks. If an individual assesses a situation and makes the wrong decision, this is a rule-based error; knowledge-based errors are those in which there is no rule to cope with a situation. Violations are said to occur when an individual deliberately undertakes a task contrary to the rule.
4. *Hazard identification, risk assessment and preventive action*. The avoidance of latent failures necessitates the identification of hazards, the assessment of risk and the selection, implementation and measurement of the preventive actions taken. Clearly, it is implicit that individuals must recognise and accept responsibility and have the appropriate knowledge and skills to recognise, evaluate and control hazards.

The Management of Health and Safety at Work Regulations 1999 and the Health and Safety Executive's (HSE) publication *Successful Health and Safety*

Management (HS(G) 65, 2013) (https://www.hse.gov.uk/pubns/books/hsg65.htm) state four key functions for the management of health and safety.

1. *Policy and planning.* Determine goals, quantifiable objectives/priorities and a programme of work capable of achieving the objectives. The relative success of this programme must then be measured and, if appropriate, revised.
2. *Organisation and communication.* Clearly defined responsibility and lines of two-way communication must be determined.
3. *Hazard management.* Hazards must be identified and their risks assessed. Appropriate control measures must be determined, implemented and reviewed over time.
4. *Monitoring and review.* It is essential that steps 1, 2 and 3 are not only in place but also in use and are seen to work in the conflicting world of commerce.

Safety culture

It is possible that an organisation may have all of the relevant parts of a safety programme in place, but that the culture associated with safety may be inappropriate or even poor. Organisations with a positive safety culture have a number of crucial elements, as reported by the Confederation of British Industry in its report, Developing a Safety Culture:

*   importance of leadership and the commitment of the Chief Executive
*   the executive safety role of line management
*   involvement of all employees
*   openness of communication
*   demonstration of care and concern for all those affected by the business.

Researchers at the US Nuclear Regulating Commission NUREG state that the key predictive indicators of safety performance are as follows, in rank order.

1. Effective communication, leading to commonly understood goals and the means to achieve these goals at all levels in the organisation.
2. Good organisational learning, where organisations are tuned to identify and respond to incremental change.
3. Organisational focus: simply the attention devoted by the organisation to workplace health and safety.
4. External factors, including the financial health of the parent organisation, or simply the economic climate within which the company is working and the impact of regulating bodies.

It should be evident from the foregoing that the basic philosophy and elements of workplace incidents (safety) are not dissimilar to those of occupational health, although perhaps, considering the immediacy of workplace incidents, the success (or failure) of intervention of safety management is much more obvious than it is for good occupational health practice.

18.4 Occupational health for health workers

Health workers form the largest occupational group in many countries. In the UK, the health sector is the largest employer of labour, and the National Health Service is probably the largest employer in Europe. The job categories in healthcare are varied. They include:

1. Staff dealing directly with patient care, e.g.
    *   doctors, nurses, midwives
    *   scientific officers
    *   laboratory and physiological measurement technicians
    *   pharmacists
    *   physiotherapists
    *   ambulance crew.
2. Ancillary and support staff, e.g.
    *   administrative and clerical personnel
    *   porters, painters, drivers
    *   laundry, catering and maintenance staff.

There are also trainee grades for some of the above groups. From an occupational health perspective, it is essential to consider health and safety aspects for all staff, including trainees and students, locum grades and patients, visitors and volunteer workers.

The areas of work are also varied, and cover sites within hospitals, clinics, public areas and even patients' homes (e.g. for visits by domiciliary healthcare staff, general practitioners and ambulance staff). It may also be possible for some healthcare facilities to be provided in supermarkets and shopping centres! The traditional work areas include:

*   operating theatres
*   imaging departments
*   outpatient departments
*   wards (e.g. medical and surgical, intensive care, coronary care)
*   laboratories, mortuaries and post-mortem rooms
*   dental surgeries
*   general practice premises
*   offices
*   kitchens.

The range of hazards is considerable.

Physical hazards

*   Ionising radiation is present in radiology departments, and also in clinics and dental surgeries where radiographs are taken. In countries where mobile vans

provide mass miniature radiography, there is a potential for staff to be exposed to ionising radiation. Radioisotopes used for treatment or investigation represent an unsealed source of radiation.

- Nuclear magnetic resonance has become increasingly used in diagnosis. This can affect those who use cardiac pacemakers. The long-term effects of exposure to magnetic fields are, as yet, unknown.
- Radiant heat, wet-bulb temperature and elevated relative humidity (e.g. laundries), noise (e.g. workshops) and other physical hazards are present in parts of healthcare facilities; a comprehensive risk assessment of physical hazards is, therefore, necessary.

Chemical hazards

- Sensitisers and allergens, such as acrylates (used in orthopaedics and dentistry), some pharmaceuticals and latex gloves, have been identified as causes of respiratory and skin problems in healthcare staff.
- Toxic chemicals are used in laboratories, although the amounts employed tend to be in much smaller quantities than in industrial processes. Examples include xylene in histopathology laboratories and formaldehyde in the same laboratories and in post-mortem rooms and mortuaries.
- Narcotic gases include the anaesthetic agents – nitrous oxide, halothane, enflurane and isoflurane are four such agents. In the main, concern is due to the possible effects in recovery room personnel, anaesthetists and anaesthetic assistants, who are exposed daily to exhaled anaesthetic gases from patients and intravenous anaesthesia components. Scavenging devices and improved local and general ventilation in operating theatres and recovery rooms can reduce the exposures to below existing occupational exposure limits. Additionally the increased use of total intravenous anaesthesia (TIVA) reduces both local and environmental pollution. Nitrous oxide is present together with oxygen in Entonox, which is a gas used for analgesia. There are concerns that the availability of Entonox in ambulances may facilitate its abuse as a recreational drug.
- Hazardous drugs that are prepared for or administered to patients can also lead to acute or chronic health effects. In addition, pre-hospital personnel can also be exposed to illegal drugs, such as fentanyl, from both patient contact and associated drug paraphernalia on or near patients.
- Cytotoxic drugs are used for treating patients with cancer. Some of these are alkylating agents; others act as anti-metabolites or inhibit deoxyribonucleic acid (DNA) enzymes. As a result of their action on cellular DNA, contact with these drugs, and sometimes their metabolites, by healthcare staff should be kept to a minimum. Staff at risk of exposure include pharmacists; nurses and doctors, who have to prepare and administer the drugs; and clinical staff and cleaners, who dispose of waste from patients who have been given these drugs and who are also responsible for the removal of soiled and contaminated bedding and linen.
- Asbestos is still found in older facilities in lagging in boiler rooms and in asbestos cement construction materials.

Mechanical and ergonomic hazards

Musculoskeletal disorders, notably low back pain in nurses, is a well-recognised cause of long-term sickness absence in this group of healthcare staff. Part of this may be related to the inappropriate lifting or handling of patients in awkward situations. Contributory factors include the heavy and/or struggling patient, crowded and narrow work areas, lack of lifting aids and poor techniques for lifting and carrying loads. Inadequate supervision of staff to ensure that they follow the manual handling policy has also been cited as an important factor. Training in manual handling may help, and attention to assessment of the task, with the provision of assistance when needed, could reduce the incidence of back pain. Some clinical areas have introduced a strict no lifting policy and have paid greater attention to how moving and handling tasks are undertaken.

Biological hazards

Biological hazards are covered more generally in Chapter 4, the focus here is the healthcare setting. Bloodborne infections, such as hepatitis B, hepatitis C and human immunodeficiency virus (HIV), can be acquired by healthcare staff from contact with infected blood and body fluids. This may occur from needlestick injuries, which are common in medical and nursing staff. Laboratory staff who must process blood samples sent from abroad, or research staff working on specific infectious agents, have been known to develop certain exotic infections such as toxoplasmosis, scrub typhus and Rocky Mountain spotted fever. In high-burden tuberculosis (TB) countries identified in annual World Health Organization (WHO) reports, heath staff are at risk of acquiring TB, including drug-resistant forms, and many studies have shown higher incidences of TB in them than in the general population. Severe acute respiratory syndrome coronavirus 2 (SARS-CoV-2), which is the virus responsible for the coronavirus disease 2019 (COVID-19) pandemic, has demonstrated dramatically the need to protect frontline healthcare workers from infectious diseases.

Occupational health services for healthcare staff should have systems for screening new categories of staff for their immune status before they begin work. The aim of screening is twofold: first, to protect the staff against occupational infections, and, second, to ensure that patients are not put at risk. Immune status for hepatitis B and rubella is usually determined. If staff are not immune, vaccination can confer protection. Where indicated, determination of carrier status and advice on safe systems of work, or redeployment when necessary, will reduce the risk to patients.

Psychosocial hazards

Psychosocial hazards are covered more generally in Chapter 11, the focus here is the healthcare setting.

Stress among healthcare workers is well recognised. Some of the contributing factors are:

- long hours of work, e.g. for junior medical staff
- low control over the pace and nature of work, e.g. junior medical staff
- unsociable hours, e.g. shift system for nurses and interrupted meal or rest breaks (to respond quickly to emergencies) for paramedics and ambulance crew
- dealing with very sick or dying patients and their families, e.g. care assistants and hospice staff
- having to make decisions on matters of life and death, sometimes with inadequate specialist supervision in under-resourced localities
- organisational change
- conflict between ensuring the best care for patients and the costs of treatment
- coping with busy schedules, having to study and prepare for professional examinations, allocating sufficient time for their families and meeting repayment costs of medical school loans, e.g. doctors in training.

As the causes of stress are often multifactorial, efforts to reduce stress may be of limited success, or may only appear to succeed temporarily. The efforts by the occupational health service include trying to eliminate or reduce identified causes and providing counselling and support to help the individual to cope with stress. The former is fraught with difficulties, especially if the management system is thought to be the main contributor to stress in staff. If difficulties with spouses or family, or financial problems, are identified, these factors are outside the influence of the occupational health service and, sometimes, out of the control of the individual.

Violence and assaults on healthcare staff are becoming of increasing concern to occupational health departments in the health service. Certain groups of staff are more at risk from verbal and physical threats. These groups include:

- receptionists
- accident and emergency staff
- ambulance crews
- general practitioners on house calls
- community nurses
- prison services' medical and nursing staff.

The source of these threats may be patients, their relatives or members of the public. The reasons are varied and include:

- frustration from waiting for medical attention when they perceive that they are an emergency and should be attended to immediately
- anger at what they feel is inappropriate or unsuccessful treatment
- attempts to obtain drugs or medicines from the healthcare staff.

Also, staff on shift duties may be vulnerable to assault when going to and from work unaccompanied at different times of the day and night.

Attempts to reduce the likelihood of violence and assault to staff have focused on:

- better training of healthcare staff in dealing with the public, with emphasis on communication skills
- breakaway techniques for coping with physical threats
- improved security in hospitals and at staff quarters
- counselling and support for victims of violence and assaults.

A phenomenon that is attracting increasing attention is the apparently high incidence of 'bullying' in nursing and other healthcare professions. Initial work suggests that there is something in the culture of healthcare that may lead people to behave towards each other in ways that, in other contexts, would be quite unacceptable. Many hospitals and other organisations have instigated anti-bullying strategies at work, such as the introduction of dignity or respect at work policies that encourage staff to report incidents of bullying and set out a process for investigations. Such strategies may be useful in defining clearly what is acceptable behaviour at work and may have a wider benefit in the longer term.

18.5 Audit and quality improvement in occupational health

Audit and quality improvement principles have been successfully introduced in occupational health to improve the delivery of occupational health services. A number of factors have contributed to this development, including economic, professional, social and legal considerations.

Professional audit

Economic
The rising cost of healthcare has focused attention on ensuring that the maximum value is gained from the use of healthcare resources. Pressure on occupational health services to demonstrate that they are providing cost-efficient and cost-effective services is a part of this general trend. In addition, occupational health services often face pressures from their employers to demonstrate that what they do makes a contribution to the economic success of the host organisation. Audit and quality improvement are sometimes used as a means of enhancing the efficiency and effectiveness of services, primarily for economic reasons.

Professional
The wide variation in the ways that occupational health departments undertake common practices has caused occupational health professionals to question the basis of their practice, and to seek evidence on which to base their practice. Audit and quality improvement have been used to identify, investigate and address variations in common practices, such as pre-placement assessment or the management of cases of sickness absence, for the purpose of improving professional performance.

Social

The consumers of healthcare (as individuals or organisations) are now much better informed about choices in healthcare than they were previously and expect to be involved in decision-making. Healthcare professionals are encouraged to become more open and accountable to their clients. Audit and quality improvement processes have been used to widen the involvement of customers in the planning and delivery of occupational healthcare. This approach has been successful in increasing the uptake of services.

Legal

The increasing trend towards litigation in healthcare has led to the need to record and document practice more rigorously than in the past. Clear criteria for the delivery of services, professional standards and records of audit can help to protect the practitioner, as well as the user, of occupational health services.

Development factors

Medical and clinical audit is the systematic, critical analysis of the quality of care, including the use of resources and the resulting outcome and quality of life for the patient. It can involve audit of the structure, process or outcome of care, and commonly is undertaken by setting standards and measuring performance against those standards.

Audit spiral

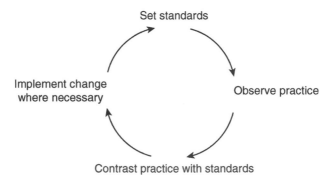

The process of audit is iterative, and opportunities to improve further the quality of care should be sought as a continuous process. Standards that are set by the professionals involved are used to improve services; therefore, it is essential that the standards that are adopted are based upon the best evidence available. Peer-reviewed research papers, guidance documents and evidence of effectiveness should be used to support standard setting. Once standards are set, these must be reviewed regularly and must not be allowed to become obstructions to improvements in the future.

Quality principles

The recipients of healthcare, that is, patients, clients or organisations, expect the professionals delivering healthcare to be trained and competent. How, when and at what cost they deliver healthcare are open to negotiation, and those using or paying for the service expect to have a role in negotiating the type of service with which they are to be provided. While audit confirms the level of current performance against a standard, quality improvement (QI) identifies how to best improve. The principles of quality management can be used to underpin the planning and delivery of services. These principles are described below.

Customer identification
Quality management systems require services to be customer orientated. Customers of an occupational health service will include those who are paying for the service, those who are using the service and those who may be affected by the service. Interactive management presentations, staff surveys and user groups can be employed to help to identify and involve customers of the service.

Needs assessment
A structured needs assessment should be conducted to identify the 'actual' as opposed to the 'perceived' needs of the organisation. A dialogue between service providers', purchasers' and users' needs to be established, so that clear expectations and priorities can be identified. Occupational health professionals may need to educate the customers as part of the process of needs assessment, but must also be prepared to listen and respond to the needs of their clients.

Critical success factors
The occupational health service needs to agree with its customers which factors are critical to its own success, that is, those factors that the service must achieve to meet the customer's expectations. Experience suggests that there should be no more than eight critical success factors which can be used as goals for the service to achieve.

Key processes
Having established what the service is intended to achieve, the key processes that will be used to attain these goals should be identified and reviewed to improve their efficiency and effectiveness. Some practices may have to be curtailed and new ones introduced.

Performance indicators
To manage the delivery of services, it is necessary to have some means of measuring the quantity and quality of services delivered. Performance indicators need to be realistic, clearly defined and capable of being measured objectively. The information provided by the performance indicators can be used to monitor progress and lead to the correction of faults. It is essential that performance indicators are reviewed regularly by providers, purchasers and users of the service.

Some areas of concern

It has been suggested that the quality of an occupational health service may be viewed differently by the different stakeholders. The company (customer) which pays for the service, the employee (client – who may also be a patient in some circumstances) who uses the service and the occupational health professional (provider) who delivers the service may place a different emphasis on different aspects of the services provided. A degree of caution is required when the employer, who controls payment for the service and employs the occupational health professionals delivering the service, has an unconditional dominant role in determining what services should be provided and how. Professional integrity needs to be protected in these circumstances.

Practice guidelines

Increasingly, attention is being paid to the development of evidence-based practice guidelines. Practice guidelines can help to make standards explicit and decision--making more objective. They can be used to help educate professionals, customers and clients as to what is thought to be the best way of dealing with specific conditions.

However, at this point, where the evidence base for some occupational health practices may not be particularly strong, the development of practice guidelines should be viewed with some caution. Where supposedly 'expert opinion' or 'consensus statements' are used to form the basis of the guideline this may simply formalise unsound practices. Practice guidelines may also limit the clinician's choice to an average or standard level of service, which does not necessarily represent best practice in individual circumstances. Practice guidelines may inhibit innovation and could be used in a medicolegal context. However, where the evidence exists to develop high-quality practice guidelines, studies have indicated that marked improvements in clinicians' performance and improved outcomes for patients do occur.

18.6 Occupational, public and environmental health

Although these are three distinct disciplines the reality is that both occupational health and environmental health fall within the broad umbrella of public health, and all are intrinsically linked with similar philosophies and curricula.

Public health can be defined as 'the science and art of preventing disease'; and, by so doing, prolonging life and improving its quality through organised efforts and informed choices of society, organisations, communities and individuals. As with occupational health, public health involves analysing the determinants of health of a population and the threats it faces. The 'population' can be just a handful of people, as large as an entire city or even the whole country; in the case of a pandemic it may encompass several continents. The concept of 'health' takes into account physical, psychological and social wellbeing.

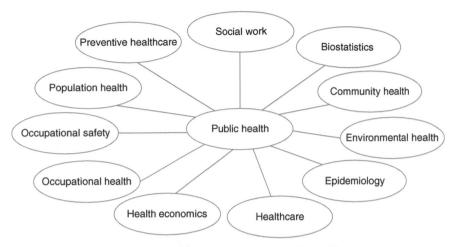

FIGURE 18.7 The various components that feed into/make up public health.

As implied above, public health is an interdisciplinary field with multiple components; for example: epidemiology, biostatistics, social sciences and management of health services are all relevant. Other than occupational health, there are other important subfields, including environmental health, community health, behavioural health, health economics, public policy, mental health, health education, gender issues in health, and sexual and reproductive health (Figure 18.7).

As has been stated repeatedly throughout this text, whether it is occupational health or public health, current practice requires multidisciplinary teams of public health workers and professionals; these teams might include epidemiologists, biostatisticians, medical assistants, public health nurses, midwives, medical microbiologists, economists, sociologists, geneticists, data managers and physicians. Depending on the need, environmental health officers or public health inspectors, bioethicists and even veterinary surgeons, gender experts, or sexual and reproductive health specialists might be called upon.

Environmental health

Environmental health has been defined, in a 1999 document by WHO, as 'those aspects of the human health and disease that are determined by factors in the environment. It also refers to the theory and practice of assessing and controlling factors in the environment that can potentially affect health' (Figure 18.8).

As of 2016, the WHO website on environmental health states:

> Environmental health addresses all the physical, chemical, and biological factors external to a person, and all the related factors impacting behaviours. It encompasses the assessment and control of those environmental factors that can potentially affect health. It is targeted towards preventing disease and creating health-supportive environments. This definition excludes behaviour not related

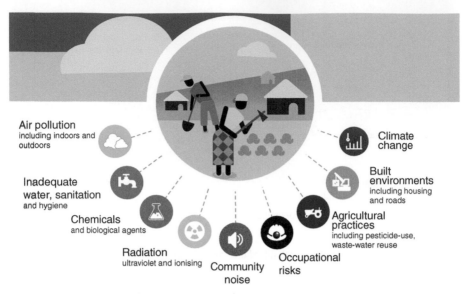

Air pollution
including indoors and
outdoors

Inadequate
water, sanitation
and hygiene

Chemicals
and biological agents

Radiation
ultraviolet and ionising Community
noise

Climate
change

Built
environments
including housing
and roads

Agricultural
practices
including pesticide-use,
waste-water reuse

Occupational
risks

FIGURE 18.8 The elements of environmental health.

to environment, as well as behaviour related to the social and cultural environment, as well as genetics.

WHO has also defined environmental health services as:

...those services which implement environmental health policies through monitoring and control activities. They also carry out that role by promoting the improvement of environmental parameters and by encouraging the use of environmentally
friendly and healthy technologies and behaviours. They also have a leading role in
developing and suggesting new policy areas.

Environmental health is made up of five major contributory components –
each of these disciplines contributes different information to describe problems
and solutions in environmental health. Both within environmental health and
between public/occupational health, there is overlap among all of the disciplines.

1. Environmental epidemiology studies the relationship between environmental exposures (including exposure to chemicals, radiation, microbiological agents, etc.) and human health. Observational studies, which
   simply observe exposures that people have already experienced, are
   common in environmental epidemiology because humans cannot
   ethically be exposed to agents that are known or suspected to
   cause disease.
2. Toxicology studies how environmental exposures lead to specific health
   outcomes, generally in animals, as a means to understand possible health
   outcomes in humans.

3. Exposure science studies human exposure to environmental contaminants by both identifying and quantifying exposures. Exposure science can be used to support environmental epidemiology by better describing environmental exposures that may lead to a particular health outcome, to identify common exposures whose health outcomes may be better understood through a toxicology study or in a risk assessment to determine whether current levels of exposure might exceed recommended levels.

4. Environmental engineering applies scientific and engineering principles for protection of human populations from the effects of adverse environmental factors; protection of environments from potentially deleterious effects of natural and human activities; and general improvement of environmental quality.

5. Environmental law includes the network of treaties, statutes, regulations and common and customary laws addressing the effects of human activity on the natural environment.

Information from epidemiology, toxicology and exposure science can be combined to conduct a risk assessment for specific chemicals, mixtures of chemicals or other risk factors to determine whether an exposure poses significant risk to human health (exposure would likely result in the development of pollution-related diseases). This can in turn be used to develop and implement environmental health policy that, for example, regulates chemical emissions or imposes standards for proper sanitation. Actions of engineering and law can be combined to provide risk management to minimise, monitor and otherwise manage the impact of exposure to protect human health to achieve the objectives of environmental health policy.

Occupational health services contribute to the public health agenda in every country by protecting and promoting the health of the economically active proportion of the general population. In some countries, the contribution made by occupational health services is formally recognised and incorporated into the national policy on health. Preventing occupational injury and disease from occurring in the first place, through an effective risk management strategy at the company level, reduces the potential burden of disease and disability in the population. Of increasing concern is the environmental protection from hazards to the community, including global warming/climate change, arising out of industrial processes or activities, in addition to the wider implications of the use of natural resources, waste disposal, etc. Occupational health services may have a role in identifying potential risks to the wider community and encouraging mitigation measures.

In addition, occupational health services can often attempt to address the risk factors for non-occupational disease by promoting a healthy lifestyle among employees. This may be by improving the healthy choices available to staff in the canteen or by encouraging the employer to provide facilities for exercise, such as subsidised access to sports facilities or an on-site gym. Occupational health staff, in some settings, may also provide individual lifestyle screening, with advice on a healthy diet, weight reduction, exercise programmes, relaxation techniques and improving sleep. Smoking cessation programmes can be run at the workplace, particularly where the employer has introduced a no smoking policy at work. Preventative lifestyle measures also include advice on sensible drinking and where to go for help.

18.7 Occupational health aspects of pandemic disease

A pandemic is a spread of a disease over multiple countries affecting a large number of people. These diseases are infectious, meaning that they are communicable, or caused, by infection. Global disease outbreaks can be caused by a variety of agents and, until SARS-CoV-2, the virus that causes COVID-19, it was commonly believed that most people in economically developed countries would not come into contact with these diseases. The most common communicable diseases include influenza, TB, rhinovirus, norovirus, pertussis and various hepatitis strains. According to the International Labour Organization (ILO), workplace-acquired communicable diseases such as TB are leading to higher rates of work-related deaths in Africa and Asia than for cancer. The 2014 Ebola epidemic affecting multiple nations was a scare that provided a 'wake-up call' for many regional, national and international infection control programmes. However, COVID-19 has provided the most widespread revelation that most places in the world are not prepared for the implementation and sustainability of work-related communicable disease prevention programmes necessary to provide safe workplaces.

It is becoming more apparent that workers bear a heavy burden resulting from widespread, highly communicable diseases. In the midst of a pandemic, it can now be anticipated that the focus of workplace transmission of infectious disease is not only limited to patients and to workers in the healthcare industries, but also among co-workers, between individuals in the general public and throughout so many other types of workplaces. However, even in the face of a pandemic, work must continue. This has reinforced the concept of 'essential workers' that has now expanded to include a broad range of services. Services and operations that must continue to operate to support a critical infrastructure are considered to be essential. However, this umbrella term has gone well beyond encompassing energy, agriculture, emergency services and defence sectors to now include all components of food industries, transportation, package delivery and more. Yet it is rightly the healthcare industry and its essential workers that remain at the forefront of high-risk workplace exposure potential relating to pandemic diseases.

It is not a surprise that emergency healthcare workers are the profession on the front lines and experienced the most immediate effects of the COVID-19 pandemic resulting from providing care to those who have tested positive for the virus. Healthcare professionals' workloads vary by country, region, local population densities and economics within given locations. However, all healthcare workers would agree that they share concerns regarding their personal risk for contracting a pandemic disease and increasing the potential for passing the virus to their fellow workers, friends and family members. Emergency health-care professionals have also had to adapt to unprecedented situations that go well beyond the immediacy of concern in their treatment of patients. Extensive work hours and extended shifts have been further complicated by strained resources that limited critical equipment like ventilators, availability of essential personal protective equipment (PPE) and the reduction of space and capabilities for even admitting some patients. Making life and death decisions for those who might even receive life-saving treatment is also an example of how the potential work-related exposures of healthcare professionals went well beyond the transmission of the virus and into occupational health risks for psychological, physical, ergonomic and psychosocial stressors. Taken collectively, the work-related health impact of the COVID-19 pandemic will take years to assess and to fully understand its impact to the extent that is necessary to prepare appropriately for the inevitable next event. However, unfortunately, muddled among all the data and economic statistics has been the understanding of the science behind the virus, its transmission and the most effective methods for assessing and controlling potential exposures to best protect the workers who are our front line of defence.

Transmission

An important consideration is the modes of transmission for pandemic diseases, especially what has been learnt in relation to SARS-CoV-2. When and how infected people can transmit a given virus will affect the implications for infection prevention and control precautions directly not only within health facilities but also in a growing variety of workplaces. Generically speaking, modes of transmission can include airborne, droplet, contact, fomite, faecal–oral, bloodborne, mother-to-child, animal-to-human and vectorborne transmission. The extent and longevity of a given communicable disease to reach pandemic proportions include the modes of transmission, relative ease of transmission and the acute health effects of a given microbe on its host. The more lethal the virus, the less opportunity for the host to become a migrating vector. Infection with SARS-CoV-2 primarily causes respiratory illness ranging from mild disease to severe disease and death, and approximately one-third of those infected with the virus never develop symptoms. The unique aspect of SARS-CoV-2 is the relatively low percentage of lethality in its hosts and the larger percentages of those with few to no symptoms. This has led to logarithmically increasing numbers of infected hosts that become vectors, some also known as super-spreaders, migrating their potential transmissibility throughout local areas and, with few to no symptoms, the opportunity to travel regionally and internationally.

Transmission of SARS-CoV-2 can occur via indirect, direct or close contact with infected people. Indirect contact transmission for a susceptible host is possible through fomite (objects or materials that are likely to carry infection, such as clothes, utensils and furniture) transmission via surfaces or a contaminated object.

There is strong evidence of virus survival rates for SARS-CoV-2 contamination on multiple surfaces, yet there is a scarcity of reports that can be directly linked to fomite transmissions. This may be the result of susceptible people who come into contact with contaminated surfaces also coming into close contact with infectious hosts, making a distinction between routes of transmission difficult to delineate. However, fomite transmission still remains a viable possibility as other comparable communicable diseases have strong track records for transmission via this mode.

Airborne transmission is a mode that can disseminate an infectious agent within droplet nuclei (aerosols) that remain infectious in air over distance and time. Guidelines for infection control state that airborne transmission can occur via respiratory droplets (typically defined as <10 μm in diameter) when an infected person sneezes, coughs, talks or sings within 1 m of susceptible individuals. These droplets can also be generated from medical procedures or other activities that transmit energy into secretions to generate aerosols that may potentially contain infectious agents. The social (physical) distancing guidelines that are based on general infection control guidelines and that underpin public health recommendations are based on this 1 m principle; however, many national health institutes increased this distance to 2 m relating to their COVID-19 protocol. The terminal settling velocity of aerosols becomes an important concept in this discussion as it reflects the time it takes for an emitted aerosol to lose acceleration and begin falling at a constant speed. When these droplets are less than 5 μm they are considered to be droplet aerosols and can travel longer distances. Several factors determine terminal settling velocity, including size and density, but, as a general rule, aerosols of 1 μm or less do not settle and therefore can remain airborne. Should these respiratory droplets include the virus, they could then reach the mouth, nose or eyes of a susceptible person and result in possible infections. However, as aerosols in the 1 μm range may be expelled by breathing, by talking and through evaporation, a susceptible person may acquire the virus at distances well beyond 2 m from its source. Therefore, the transmission of SARS-CoV-2 may be particularly difficult to control as the spread of aerosols has also been shown to occur within indoor settings as well as in workspaces and common places with poor ventilation.

Another complicating factor for the transmission of SARS-CoV-2 can be attributed to the early build-up of viral load in the infected host. There is now scientific evidence showing that the highest load of this virus's ribonucleic acid (RNA) is detectable in persons one to three days in advance of symptom onset and can continue for up to two weeks in those who are asymptomatic and for up to three weeks in those with mild to moderate symptoms. There is also growing evidence that small aerosol particles in the low- to sub-micrometre size range may be responsible for airborne COVID-19 cases where investigations show that the spread of COVID-19 was not linked to direct or indirect contact. Therefore, the workplace and occupational health professionals have faced unprecedented challenges for the prevention of communicable diseases in the wake of the COVID-19 pandemic. If infected hosts can go about their daily work routines with high viral loads while being asymptomatic for over two weeks, and the spread of small aerosols can remain airborne and increase in concentration with inadequate ventilation, then it becomes essential that all aspects of the hierarchy of controls for protecting workers be put into practice.

Regulatory approach

The US Occupational Safety and Health Administration (OSHA) has put into place an Emergency Temporary Standard as enforceable guidance to inform and protect workers on the steps necessary to reduce the spread of COVID-19. Although intended for US employers and workers, the structure and components of the standard provide a good insight into the direction for both programme development and potential regulatory approach expectations. The hierarchy of controls is applied as measures for worker protection depending on their exposure risk, which varies by the work performed, interaction potential, length of exposure and work environment contamination. The standard is driven towards employers developing prevention and control strategies as an outcome of a workplace hazard assessment to ensure that engineering, administrative, PPE and related controls address infection prevention and to implement safe work practices to prevent worker exposure. Another important component from this US OSHA standard is the requirement for reporting of COVID-19 cases that are related to workplace transmission. The guidance also points to COVID-19 fact sheets on the OSHA website (www.osha.gov) and other OSHA standards that require employers to communicate workplace hazards and control strategies and to ensure that training on PPE, respiratory protection and the like are applied commensurate to the exposure risk presented in work settings. There is also an initiative that would follow this standard for OSHA to perform workplace inspections to ensure that this enforceable guidance has been implemented effectively.

Exposure risk

This standard is aligned with general guidance that had already been promulgated to assist US workers and employers in identifying where their workplace activities fall in OSHA's exposure risk pyramid. The combination of this simplified, graded approach to understanding exposure risk and a workplace hazard assessment is intended to assist employers in identifying exposure risk levels, implementing control strategies and remaining informed and alert for changing outbreak conditions.

- **Very high exposure risk work settings:** examples include aerosol-generating procedures performed on potentially infectious patients or bodies by healthcare or morgue workers. Engineering controls are required here that include using isolation rooms for performing aerosol-generating procedures and ensuring appropriate air-handling systems are installed and maintained in healthcare and postmortem facilities. PPE would include gloves, gown, face shield or goggles, and respirators with a protection factor commensurate to job tasks and exposure risks.

- **High exposure risk work settings:** examples include workplaces with a focus on healthcare delivery and support, medical transport of infected patients, handling or transporting clinical specimens, blood or infectious wastes. Physical barriers are required to control the spread of infectious disease; worker and client management to promote social distancing, adequate and appropriate PPE, hygiene and cleaning supplies. An OSHA fact sheet on exposure risks in healthcare workplaces is available and preparedness for pandemics is on its Emergency Preparedness and Response webpage (https://www.osha.gov/emergency-preparedness).
- **Medium exposure risk work settings:** examples include workplaces with higher frequency interactions with the general public, such as schools, restaurants, retail establishments, travel and mass transport industries and other crowded work environments. Control strategies focus on worker and client management to promote social distancing, adequate and appropriate PPE, hygiene and cleaning supplies.
- **Lower exposure risk work settings:** examples include workplaces with minimal contact with the general public and other co-workers, such as is common in general office work environments. Lower risk work considerations are in line with general cautionary controls. Interim guidance for job tasks in this category is as follows:
  - ¯ Worker tasks not requiring contact with people known to have or suspected of having COVID-19 or close contact frequency (within 6 ft [2 metres] for ≥15 minutes over a 24-hour period) with the general public or other workers are at lower risk of occupational exposure.
  - ¯ Hazard recognition relating to workers' job duties affects their level of occupational risk and such risk may change as workers conduct different tasks or as circumstances change.
  - ¯ Employers and workers with a lower exposure risk are to remain aware of evolving community transmission changes or moving into a higher risk job. Changes that may move employees into higher risk categories may warrant additional precautions.
  - ¯ Employers to monitor public health COVID-19 communications, ensuring worker access to that information, and collaborate with workers to designate effective communication.

There is an overall premise that clear communications between employers and workers reflect that a healthy and safe workplace is provided, increasing reporting of pandemic-related issues to assist in protecting co-workers and reducing absenteeism. Employers need to ensure that their workers understand the difference between seasonal epidemics and global pandemic outbreaks and are aware of job activities that may place workers at increased exposure risk. Programmes should also offer remote work and flexible leave policies, share social distancing strategies, establish clear proper hygiene and disinfection protocols, make readily available proper PPE with instructions on how to wear, use, clean and store it, specify the availability of medical services and afford direct feedback to supervisors. At the most basic level, employers must establish the worker protection principles of consistent social distancing, covering coughs and sneezes, maintaining hand hygiene and frequent cleaning of commonly used surfaces. Employers are to provide all of this information to workers in the form of standardised training. Frequent visual and verbal reminders to workers assist in ensuring overall compliance with programme expectations and reducing rates of infection.

Control strategies to employ include the necessary modifications to the work environment and the adaptation of work practices to maximise worker and client protection. This may include improved ventilation such as increasing ventilation rates and installing high-efficiency air filters, adding physical barriers such as plastic guards, altering business practices such as adding drive-through services, installing hand sanitiser dispensers, providing sanitising wipes and making additional PPE readily available. All of this is part of the response plans utilising the hierarchy of controls that includes elimination, substitution, engineering controls, administrative controls, safe work practices and the final line of PPE. Elimination of the hazard would involve excluding potentially infected individuals from the workplace. Increasing ventilation and installing high-efficiency air filters may be one of the more important, and too often overlooked, engineering controls for higher trafficked work environments, but workplace modifications to assist in programme implementation also fit within this category. With growing evidence of virus transmission outbreaks tied to indoor facilities there are currently widespread efforts to fund and mandate the assessment and upgrading of ventilation systems in public buildings such as schools and in the long-term healthcare industries. Additional efforts to establish minimum ventilation standards for institutions and businesses such as bars, restaurants and gyms are an integral part of reopening guidelines. Administrative controls include limited workforce numbers by shift and location, posting signs reflecting minimum programme expectations, providing training and increasing the frequency of cleaning and disinfection of common work surfaces.

PPE is a common and visible control practice in pandemics; however, it still remains a last step to prevent exposures when the rest of the control hierarchy is deemed insufficient. Early on in the COVID-19 pandemic, the supply of appropriate PPE became an increasingly important issue. What may have been deemed as appropriate PPE may not have been available or was in short supply. Even under these circumstances, both programmes and related trainings should still reflect what is considered appropriate and clarify that modifications and downgrading due to PPE non-availability is considered an interim necessity. In the absence of this clarification, large numbers of workplaces could begin to consider lower levels and increased use of possibly inadequate PPE as the norm rather than the exception. Worker and employer interim guidance for job requirements and the PPE ensemble recommendations for various activities performed include:

- PPE is needed when engineering and administrative controls are insufficient for worker protection even though operations must continue.
- PPE selection is based on results from an employer's hazard assessment and job duties.

- Respiratory-protection options should be based on the best available, including elastomeric respirators and powered air-purifying respirators for frontline healthcare workers. This also assists in increasing filtering facepiece respirator supplies for other affected essential workers with jobs involving medium to higher level risk activities.
- PPE ensembles should reflect exposure risks for droplets or contact as opposed to jobs with higher aerosol-generating potential based on the employer's hazard assessment. Healthcare workers with infected patients, invasive treatment efforts, post-mortem care and laboratories have higher aerosol exposure potential requiring higher level PPE.
- Disposable gloves, typically a single pair of nitrile examination gloves, require doffing and donning of new gloves when torn or visibly contaminated with blood or body fluids.
- Face and eye protection combinations use surgical masks and either goggles or face shields. Personal glasses or cloth face coverings are insufficient with sprays or splashes.
- Tight-fitting respirators, when required, must be used within a comprehensive respiratory protection programme that includes medical examinations, fit testing and training. Surgical and cloth masks are not respirators and do not provide workers with the same level of protection.
- PPE provision, such as respirators or gowns, is to be prioritised for high-hazard activities, especially during shortages.
- Ensure that decontamination and reuse methods for disposable respirators during crises are available.
- After removing PPE, always wash hands with soap and water for at least 20 seconds. Hand hygiene facilities should be made readily available at the point of use.

PPE and items such as uniforms or laboratory coats should have procedures for maintaining, storing, laundering and disposal that also account for potential bloodborne pathogens.

Risk assessment and control

Throughout the initial stages of the COVID-19 pandemic there was a noted over-reliance on respiratory protection as the primary, and at times only, workplace control for exposures. It became evident that the hierarchy of controls was not being applied effectively and when it was considered there was inconsistency in implementation. Occupational health professionals require a systematic approach for risk assessment and control that is based on science, but affording employers an opportunity to similarly assess their workplace risks demands simplicity. The process known as control banding (CB) (see Section 12.5) delivers this balance by providing a qualitative risk assessment to a control process that has been proven to be especially useful in the absence of quantitative information. There are no adequate methods to quantitatively measure inhalable concentrations of infectious organism droplet aerosols that workers are exposed to, there is an utter lack of readily available analytical devices and there is no known infectious dose limit for a wide variety of infectious diseases. Therefore, the existing scientific knowledge and standardised occupational health and hygiene professional protocol become the foundation for developing such a process. The British Occupational Hygiene Society (BOHS) and the Canadian Standards Association (standard Z94.4-2018) employ this CB approach for protecting employees from aerosol-transmissible infectious diseases, such as COVID-19, and BOHS has made it freely available for implementation at workplaces around the world.

With the growing scientific evidence attributing droplet aerosols as an essential component of workplace transmission of SARS-CoV-2, utilising the hierarchy of controls towards eliminating this as a workplace exposure risk is paramount. The BOHS CB model for the prevention of droplet aerosol communicable disease exposure to workers emphasises that PPE as a receptor (worker) control is a last option, focusing first on source and pathway controls. This CB model is built upon the likely assumption that respiratory droplet aerosol communicable disease works on a dose–response function; higher exposure concentrations over longer periods of time increase the likelihood of a work-acquired communicable disease. The BOHS model offers the systematic approach that occupational health practitioners require by presenting a step-by-step process for the identification of source and pathway controls that assist in eliminating or minimising the need for receptor controls. The initial step (Figure 18.9) in this CB process requires a rough assessment of the exposure probability, or likelihood (L0–L4), and an estimated daily exposure duration (D0–D4) to yield a graded approach ranking of exposure (E0–E4). The exposure rank (Figure 18.10) is translated into a colour-coded control band (A–D, lowest to highest controls) with an exposure rank of E0 leading to an outcome of no control band required.

Figure 18.11 emphasises the need to follow the hierarchy of controls and outlines the methods to consider first to last, or best to worst, when addressing the control band outcomes. The first and best to consider are the source controls, the isolation of the disease-infected person or respirable droplet aerosol-generating processes and, if not possible, maximising the distance of this source from other workers. If the aerosol-transmissible infectious disease is not released past its source, then the potential for exposure is eliminated or at least minimised. If

Likelihood	Daily duration		
	D1 (0–3 hours)	D2 (3–6 hours)	D3 (>6 hours)
L0 (No exposure)	E0	E0	E0
L1 (Exposure unlikely)	E1	E1	E1
L2 (Possible exposure)	E2	E2	E3
L3 (Exposure is likely)	E2	E3	E4

FIGURE 18.9 Exposure = likelihood × duration. Source: British Occupational Hygiene Society Covid-19 Working Groups (2020).

Exposure rank	Control band
E0	N
E1	A
E2	B
E3	C
E4	D

FIGURE 18.10 Control band. Source: British Occupational Hygiene Society Covid-19 Working Groups (2020).

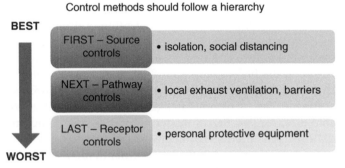

FIGURE 18.11 Control methods. Source: British Occupational Hygiene Society Covid-19 Working Groups (2020).

minimised, the pathway for these aerosols to be carried towards workers or distributed around the workplace can be considered. The pathway controls include engineering control options such as improved ventilation by increasing ventilation rates and installing high-efficiency air filters or adding physical barriers such as plastic guards. Only after these source and pathway control options are decided upon and implemented are the receptor controls of PPE put into consideration for the workers.

The control band exposure reduction protocol outlined in Figure 18.12 further emphasises this hierarchy of controls for the source, pathway and receptor. As the control band elevates with exposure risk from light green (A) to darkest green (D), the control options are prioritised. Recommendations are then given for the source, pathway and receptor control options to determine if and when additional consideration may be required at each step of the process. The higher the risk and the commensurate control band recommendations, the more likely that occupational health and hygiene practitioner assistance may be necessary. The goal is for employers to aim to lower the exposure rank, preferably to E1 levels, by focusing on exposure prevention through the implementation of source and pathway controls to reduce or eliminate the reliance on PPE.

The goal of using CB for protecting workers from respiratory droplet aerosol communicable disease is for the development of comprehensive infection and disease prevention programmes that can be derived effectively from a simplified

	Control band	Control Options
Aim to lower exposure level Goal: Reduce exposure to E1 levels by selecting additional control strategies from the source and pathway categories and reducing reliance on PPE	A	Source–Do these first
		Pathway-Maybe necessary
		Receptor-Not necessary
	B	Source - Do these first, may require multiple options
		Pathway - Do these next, and may require multiple options
		Receptor - Only if source and pathway controls are and effective
	C	Source - Do these first, may require multiple options
		Pathway - Do these next, and may require multiple options
		Receptor-May be prudent
	D	Source - Do these first, may require multiple options
		Pathway - Do these next, and may require multiple options
		Receptor-Probably necessary

FIGURE 18.12 Exposure reduction protocol by control band. PPE, personal protective equipment. Source: British Occupational Hygiene Society Covid-19 Working Groups (2020).

risk assessment and control protocol. In addition to reducing exposure risk by appropriately focusing on the hierarchy of controls, it is also an effective strategy for assisting in the conservation of PPE to ensure that the right protection equipment is available in each workplace at the appropriate time. This aspect of programme development also illustrates how such an approach could be used for future planning for the next pandemic, where we already know it will be highly likely that essential workers must remain at work and that the remaining workforce will be expected to physically return to work.

Lessons learned

Preparation for pandemics and the protection of workers has long been a 'back burner' topic for nations and workplaces alike and probably will be again once related global issues settle down; until it will sadly become a reality once again. The COVID-19 pandemic has had no parallel in modern history. At some level it could be understood that there would be issues, such as PPE shortages and a lack of related controls, with nearly simultaneous national orders to shelter in place coinciding with hospital bed shortages, all approaching near global proportions. There has also been continuous confusion over what is the correct way to protect workers and public health, further exacerbated by conflicting media coverage and topics on the science of the pandemic devolving into political entrench-ments. Occupational health professionals understand the science behind work--related communicable diseases, issues relating to transmissibility, what appro-priate programmes should look like and putting controls into practice to prevent occupational exposure to pandemic diseases. A positive for occupational health is the concept that PPE is now part of the global vernacular. However, under-standing which PPE is the most appropriate choice based on exposure potential and worker tasks performed remains muddled at best and misunderstood at worst. Based on the cumulative lessons to be learned and the essential require-ment to prepare appropriately for whatever comes next, among national insti-tutes of health as well as occupational health and hygiene professionals it must be voiced in unison: 'Never again!'

Over a year after a pandemic was declared the world is still dealing with mul-tiple crises from the state of economies at the larger scale and seemingly unend-ing uncertainty for jobs and incomes on a more local level. Those in charge of policy development must work to ensure that recovery support is far-reaching with a focus on ensuring that jobs and income are available equitably across all cross-sections of society and that the rights of workers and social dialogue are embedded in a recovery process that focuses on individuals and their needs. Policy-makers should strive to support a recovery that is robust and broad-based, focusing on employment, income, workers' rights and a social dialogue that rec-ognises diversity and the adverse effects of unequal outcomes in a pandemic. These policies should also consider assistance to economically developing and transitional countries to ensure that those hardest hit have a partnership path-way to equitable outcomes. Global and local recovery strategies should be based on social dialogue that promotes transition into recovery that is inclusive and sustainable for all workers everywhere.

We have learned that the workers vulnerable to acquiring communicable dis-ease are the expected occupations in the healthcare industries, with nurses among the hardest hit, but also maintenance and manufacturing workers, cleaners, passenger and package vehicle drivers, and childcare and travel atten-dants. The primary focus on infection prevention and control during pandemics is based on practices in healthcare that are concentrated on protecting patients from infectious agent exposures and nosocomial diseases. Although there is much overlap, it is now better understood that infection control does not neces-sarily equate to worker protection. A focus on protecting workers is an essential lesson from the COVID-19 pandemic to ensure both the understanding and the need for staffing and commensurate programmes that require protocol and processes to reduce or eliminate exposures to work-related risks from communi-cable diseases. As we enter into the phase of developing lessons learnt from COVID-19 response activities and transmission prevention programmes, it is also becoming apparent that public health efforts face a comparable predica-ment. The components of protecting the general public are indeed important and also overlap with considerations for workers; however, it is essential for pub-lic health officials to collaborate with occupational health and hygiene profes-sionals to ensure that the protection of workers remains paramount and requires different approaches and considerations. This shift away from the tunnel vision inherent in infection control and public health protocols will require integrating occupational health and safety professions into efforts to develop preventative and responsive risk assessment and control capabilities to protect all workers.

Healthcare professionals are a prime example of workers who are facing additional occupational exposures that have not been considered previously. These include the demands of being consistently required to report to a working environment that is known to be at high risk for communicable disease transmissibility for extended shift lengths that are further exacerbated by co-workers not reporting due to having acquired COVID-19. Tangential, but equally important, issues also emerged in the healthcare industries above and beyond the traditional demands of work overload that included psychosocial stressors from inadequate PPE, unavailable treatment methods, limited bed space and facing decisions of which patients may not receive treatment, all while being required to complete detailed electronic health records for an unending flow of clientele. During the severe acute respiratory syndrome (SARS) outbreak in 2003 it was learnt that this profession, like many occupations reporting to essential high-risk work under high-stress conditions, was susceptible to alcohol abuse, psychological distress and other stress-related disorders. Burnout in the healthcare professions was already identified as a significant issue before COVID-19, so the lack of work-related resources to protect healthcare workers from both physical and mental hazards during a pandemic will inevitably lead to additional work-related illness and injury.

Cumulatively, the lessons described herein make it readily apparent that workers' rights must be further enhanced, widely adhered to and uniformly regulated and protected under law. Workers should be aware of the exposure risk level associated with their job duties. In addition, a pandemic may disproportionately affect people in certain age groups or with specific health histories. Workers with job-related exposure to infections who voluntarily disclose personal health risks should be considered for job accommodations and/or additional protective measures. The disproportionate impact to vulnerable workers, high-hazard worksites and low-income populations must be addressed and opportunities for both protection and recovery should be made readily available on a more level playing field. As a collective society, we must simply ensure that our preparations for the next pandemic are holistic and practicable. We have so many lessons to learn from the COVID-19 pandemic. However, we must also be prepared to consolidate, record, implement and sustain the improvements to preparation and programmes to ensure that the magnitude of these issues, which certainly cost hundreds of thousands of workers' lives globally, are not allowed to happen again.

18.8 Total worker health

The question of balancing the benefits and adverse effects of work on health was addressed by Waddell and Burton in *Is Work Good for your Health and Wellbeing?* in 2006. Their overall finding was that the balance of the evidence is that work is generally good for health and wellbeing for most people, with certain caveats being stated. This report was a key part of the evidence informing the UK Government's health work and wellbeing strategy from 2005, with an outcome being Dame Carol Black's *Working for a Healthier Tomorrow*, which provided widely influential recommendations. Also, in 2005 the World Summit of the United Nations declared the goal of full and productive employment and decent work for all. Good work, or decent work, is described by the ILO as summing up 'the aspirations of people in their working lives'. It involves opportunities for work that are productive and that deliver a fair income, security in the workplace and social protection for families; better prospects for personal development and social integration; freedom for people to express their concerns and to organise and participate in the decisions that affect their lives; and equality of opportunity and treatment for all women and men. More simply, good work encompasses four pillars: employment conditions, social security, rights at the workplace and social dialogue. Decent work is part of many human rights programmes and a large number of countries have adopted Decent Work Country Programmes under the guidance of the ILO (https://www.ilo.org/global/about-the-ilo/how-the-ilo-works/departments-and-offices/program/dwcp/lang--en/index.htm). Besides benefits for individuals, decent work has the potential to promote economic development and to reduce inequality.

As is evident from the ILO formulation, good work goes well beyond controlling workplace hazards and providing individual health-promoting activities in workplaces. This broad conceptualisation means that millions of workers globally are not in good jobs, an occurrence by no means limited to low- and middle-income countries. The US National Institute for Occupational Safety and Health (NIOSH) had also been actively engaged in these questions and in 2011 this resulted in the Total Worker Health® (TWH®) programme. NIOSH defines a TWH approach as 'policies, programs, and practices that integrate protection from work-related safety and health hazards with promotion of injury and illness – prevention efforts to advance worker well-being'. The recognition of work as a social determinant of health is embedded in TWH. This strategy also recognises that in many organisations silos of activity can exist that each impinge on aspects of workers' health, e.g. safety, workers' compensation management, absence management, group health and disability programmes, employee assistance programmes, health promotion, occupational health surveillance and preplacement fitness. The goal is therefore organisational integration with a focus on the prevention of work-related injury and illness, and the advancement of worker health and wellbeing. The issues that should be considered under a TWH programme are listed in Figure 18.13. Recognising the changes that are occurring in workplaces, work and the workforce itself NIOSH developed a Future of Work Initiative that applies the TWH principles to the areas of concern.

The role of the occupational health practitioner in promoting good work in individual companies and enterprises is complex. Many of the drivers of poor jobs are outside the direct influence and scope of occupational health and individual professionals. Casualisation of work in the face of global pressures makes the point. Nevertheless, practitioners and their organisations can bring the evidentiary basis for the health benefits of good work to the attention of

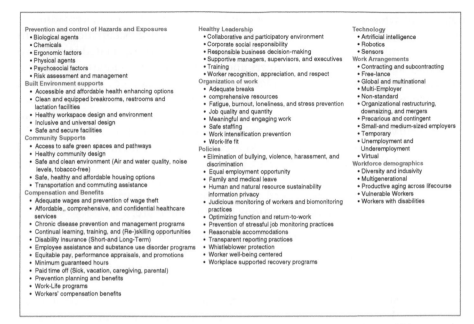

FIGURE 18.13 Issues relevant to advancing worker wellbeing using Total Worker Health® approaches. Source: Centers for Disease Control and Prevention.

employers, employees, organised labour, enforcement agencies and state bodies. Embracing strategies such as TWH can facilitate organisational cross-functional working towards shared goals.

18.9 National occupational health surveillance systems

National data on workplace exposures and the occurrence of occupational diseases and injuries are useful for many reasons, among them planning for occupational health services and inspectorates and the requisite human resources to staff them, adequate funding of workers' compensation and the identification of new causes of disease. The epidemics of silicosis in artificial stone workers is a recent case in point. Enterprises and industries with unacceptable exposures and those in which disease and injury have occurred can be targeted for preventive interventions. The success or otherwise of national regulations and campaigns can be measured and refined, if required, and new activities introduced based on identified needs. The potential benefits of national surveillance systems make them attractive, and there are many worldwide. The ILO encourages countries to have them – but they can achieve the opposite of what they intended: gross under-reporting and under-recording of excessive exposures, diseases and injuries can trivialise occupational health problems, and under-reporting is to be expected. The work-relatedness of diseases may not be recognised – cancers and cardiovascular incidents commonly. Healthcare workers in busy or under-resourced circumstances are reluctant to take time away from patient care to fill in surveillance forms. Even fatal work accidents go unrecorded, notably from the informal economy. Nevertheless, national surveillance is valuable, provided the objectives of it are well thought out. In many countries, attempting to ascertain the numbers of occupational diseases and injuries will fail due to under-reporting, but aiming to identify some enterprises and industries for remedial actions may well be successful. The methods for surveillance need to be tailored to the setting and the objectives. Some methods and considerations in using them are:

- Exposure data from enforcement agency inspections of workplaces. The US OHSA has compiled an extensive database. Only applicable if the inspectors do measurements. May be biased to higher concentrations if inspections are triggered by complaints or suspected over-exposure
- Disease registers. Usually physician reliant. There are several successful registers: those in Scandinavian countries and The Health and Occupation Research (THOR) network in the UK among them. Under-reporting and reporter fatigue over time undermine completeness in many settings, though. Useful for identifying some disease-causing enterprises
- Household surveys. Self-reported disease and injury by participants of routine surveys. Useful, but lack of knowledge of work aetiology of disease is one limitation among many
- Workers' compensation data. Useful but under-reporting particularly of certain disease categories is common, e.g. cancers
- Surveys of a sample of representative enterprises. Exposures and diseases can be measured. Most useful in countries with unreliable recognition and reporting systems. Healthy worker effect (sick workers not at work) a limitation for diseases
- Mortality data. Typically, using death certificates – both cause of death and occupational history are generally unreliable or incomplete. Temporal trends can be scrutinised, though
- Statutory reporting to inspectorates or occupational health institutes by industries. Exposure and disease can be covered. Useful, especially if verified by the inspectorates, e.g. random checks of a small sample of companies.

18.10 Genetic testing

Knowledge has grown substantially over the past several decades on the role of genetics in occupational diseases, and the interaction between the genome and environmental factors encountered at work or emanating from it. A large number of studies have found associations between genes and the ill effects of workplace hazards. New, more affordable and efficient technologies promise many new discoveries in understanding mechanisms and the pre-clinical changes that might portend disease or increased risk. A potential benefit of this knowledge is that diseases can be prevented if harmful exposures are identified and controlled, and if susceptible workers can be identified and then advised to avoid certain exposures. Advocates could thus advance their perspective by using genetic information to play an increasing role in preventing occupational disease. Counter to this advocacy is that the use of genetic information in occupational health practice raises medical, ethical, legal and social issues.

Potentially useful occupational genetic information includes the identification of acquired genetic effects such as changes in DNA caused by chemicals or physical agents. Finding genes that interact with environmental agents to increase or decrease the risk of disease is another example. Direct examination of gene-related material is not the only source of information, as a personal or family history of disease may reveal a possible hereditable vulnerability to certain exposures or circumstances. This type of information could be collected at pre-employment examinations and at life insurance applications, among other procedures.

Single-gene-induced diseases are the exception (haemophilia is such a rarity); mostly, multiple genes are involved in disease causation and the interactions with occupational and environmental factors in the progression to disease are generally complex. Whether or not induced genetic changes or inherited variants (polymorphisms) are expressed phenotypically as susceptibilities or actual diseases is influenced by many internal and external (e.g. occupational) factors. The extent and duration of exposure to a workplace hazard could be one such factor. Thus, finding a genetic variant or genetic damage that has been associated with a negative or positive occupational outcome is usually of uncertain consequence for the individual employee: there may be variable, sometimes small, increases or decreases in risk in a group but typically there is no way of ascertaining the level of risk for a particular employee. Even genes strongly linked to cancer, such as the harmful *BRCA1* variants and breast cancer, only explain malignancies in a proportion of affected women.

In occupational health practice, genetic tests may be used in a variety of ways. Almost all are associated with difficulties, though. Employees mixing anti-cancer drugs have been one target group for monitoring; albeit that many of the changes identified are non-specific (unrelated to workplace exposure) and their predictive value for future disease is uncertain.

Perhaps the most controversial potential use of genetic information is in making decisions about exclusion from certain jobs. Since the implications of genetic findings are usually uncertain for individuals' future risks, many people could be excluded from work without sufficient cause. The concept of the super-worker has been coined to highlight the risk of multiple genetic tests at pre-employment resulting in only the genetically 'sound' having access to some jobs. Employer-provided medical and life insurance cover could be adversely influenced by genetic information: exclusions and increased pricing could follow certain findings. What to tell the employee following a test is also problematic. Since the extent of risk is mostly unclear for individuals, a great deal of

412   **Chapter 18** Special Issues in Occupational Health

lifelong anxiety could unnecessarily result from informing a worker that they have a genetic variant associated (at a group level) with disease. Using genetic information could also divert the primary focus of maintaining a safe and healthy workplace to excluding the vulnerable worker, clearly counter to the spirit of occupational health practice.

Understanding genetics and health and ill health is expected to advance greatly human wellbeing. Occupational health is not excepted from this expectation; however, there are many medical, ethical, legal and social issues that need to be considered before the widespread application of genetic testing at work. For now, positive applications are rare.

18.11 Fatigue and sleep disorders

Fatigue has been defined 'as a result of prolonged mental or physical exertion; it can affect people's performance and impair their mental alertness, which leads to dangerous errors.' Fatigue can occur for many reasons, among them physically demanding work – especially in adverse environmental conditions such as heat – prolonged shifts, insufficient rest, sustained high vigilance and, paradoxically, monotony, or inadequate length or quality of sleep, arising from work circumstances (e.g. shift work) or personal factors.

Fatigue causes not only discomfort but also leads to effects that are potentially dangerous for employees and negative for enterprises. Physical and mental decrements such as slower reactions, reduced ability to process information, memory lapses, absent-mindedness, decreased awareness, lack of attention, underestimation of risk, low motivation and reduced coordination can reduce quality of work and lower productivity. Errors and accidents, at work or on the road, are also increased. Fatigue can be a root cause of major industrial incidents.

Fatigue should not be underestimated as a health and enterprise risk and needs to be managed, like any other hazard. Many jurisdictions place statutory obligations on employers to arrange conditions of work so that the risk of fatigue is reduced; limiting shift duration and scheduling of rest periods are examples. Practitioners should be aware of the jurisdictional stipulations on fatigue management.

As with other hazards, fatigue risk assessments should be undertaken and are also helpful when changes to working hours are introduced and when shift work patterns are changed. Tools are available to estimate the likelihood of fatigue in certain circumstances. A fatigue management policy and methods to enforce it is advisable. Developing the policy in consultation with workplace health and safety committees, or other representative bodies, is sensible, bearing in mind, though, that worker and management preferences may be counter to practices that have been found to reduce fatigue risk; evidence-based practices should be favoured. The policy should take account of local regulation but also enterprise-level practices such as shift-swapping by employees. Adequate staffing levels may be fundamental to managing fatigue, but of course are an unreachable goal in resource-constrained situations. Shift work schedules need to be designed with fatigue reduction in mind.

Sleep disorders

Inadequate duration and quality of sleep are prevalent for many reasons. Because shift work is so common it is often, correctly, emphasised by occupational health services, but underlying medical conditions may explain inadequate sleep, such as anxiety and depression, restless leg syndrome and sleep apnoea, which frequently manifests as daytime somnolence. Domestic environmental factors such as noise also contribute. Night workers are particularly at risk of fatigue because their day sleep is often lighter and shorter and more easily disturbed because of daytime noise, domestic responsibilities and difficulty in sleeping in daylight. Individuals vary in their sleep requirements – both duration and timing. A person's chronotype (circadian preference, morningness/eveningness, colloquially 'owls and larks') influences health problems associated with shift schedules. Importantly, besides cognitive impairment, sleep deprivation has negative mental and physical health consequences, and can reduce quality of life. Sleep disorders, therefore, need to be taken seriously and the causes of them managed. If the explanation for the sleep disorder is not obvious, workers may need investigation; sleep clinics are now commonplace in well-resourced settings.

18.12 Alcohol and drug use and testing in workers

Substance abuse occurs in all segments of society, and affects safety and productivity in workplaces globally, calling for policies and practices to prevent and manage its negative impacts.

The ILO Code of Practice on Management of Alcohol- and Drug-Related Issues in the Workplace is instructive. The complexity of substance abuse is evident in the preamble:

> Problems relating to alcohol and drugs may arise as a consequence of personal, family or social factors, or from certain work situations, or from a combination of these elements. Such problems not only have an adverse effect on the health and wellbeing of workers, but may also cause many work-related problems including a deterioration in job performance. Given that there are multiple causes of alcohol- and drug-related problems, there are consequently multiple approaches to prevention, assistance, treatment and rehabilitation.

Clients and the general population are also at risk: intoxicated professional drivers makes the point.

The provisions of the ILO Code direct employers and practitioners to fair and measured practices. Such as:

- alcohol- and drug-related problems should be considered as health problems, and therefore should be dealt with, without any discrimination, like any other health problem at work and covered by the healthcare systems (public or private) as appropriate

- employers and workers and their representatives should assess the effects of alcohol and drug use in the workplace jointly, and should cooperate in developing a written policy for the enterprise
- the same restrictions or prohibitions with respect to alcohol should apply to both management personnel and workers, so that there is a clear and unambiguous policy
- testing of bodily samples for alcohol and drugs in the context of employment involves moral, ethical and legal issues of fundamental importance, requiring a determination of when it is fair and appropriate to conduct such testing.

The State of Queensland, Australia, has published an informative Framework for alcohol and drug management in the workplace (https://www.worksafe.qld. gov.au/__data/assets/pdf_file/0022/17185/alcohol-drug-management.pdf) with a plan that summarises its approach, as shown in Figure 18.14). The policy should be developed in consultation with workers, health and safety committees and representatives, where these exist. New Zealand's Drugs, Alcohol and Work guide is useful and gives advice about who might reasonably be tested at work (https://www.employment.govt.nz/workplace-policies/tests-and-checks/drugs-alcohol-and-work).

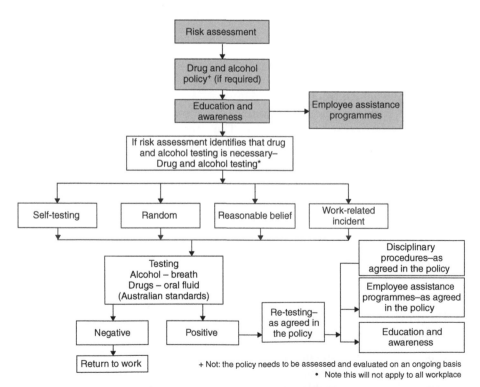

FIGURE 18.14 Development of a drug and alcohol policy. Source: Framework for alcohol and drug management in the workplace. Workplace Health and Safety Queensland.

Employers thinking about drug testing employees should seek legal advice. Testing at the preplacement assessment is recommended with a proviso that the job advertisement alerts applicants of the intention. Consideration should be given to including testing in the employment agreement. According to the guide drug testing may be reasonable if it is done with a view to protecting the safety of employees or the general public, for example:

- if the employee works in a safety critical/sensitive area
- if the employee's work directly impacts the safety of others (e.g. other employees or the public).

Testing a specific employee for a specific purpose may be more reasonable than random 'suspicion-less' testing of all employees. A specific purpose may be where the employee:

- shows signs of being affected by drugs or alcohol
- has recently been involved in a workplace accident or a near-miss.

The ILO Code's provisions and those of the other guides are laudable but difficult to apply in practice; legislation and cultural attitudes towards alcohol and drug use, as well as financial and technical resources, will determine how far it is practicable to follow them.

18.13 Nanomaterials

Nanomaterials present a number of real challenges to occupational health and occupational hygiene practitioners. Nanomaterials are particles that are defined as having two or three dimensions less than 100 nm. In addition, accounting for potential exposure to compounds that approach molecular size presents unique considerations for a combination of the shape, size, surface area and surface activity of particulates presented. Therefore, the challenges faced by practitioners are in one part due to the lack of a clear toxicological basis for setting nanomaterial-specific occupational exposure limits, as nanoparticles can affect a broad range of toxicological end points with their high degree of reactivity, their ability to deposit in various regions of the respiratory tract and their ability to cross normally impenetrable barriers (e.g. blood–brain barrier, skin). The challenges are in another part due to their growing presence in research and development laboratories and in the workplace, as applications for engineered nanoparticles appear endless with both government and private industries investing substantially into researching and developing nanotechnologies. As nanomaterials can be designed at the atomic level, these challenges can also be combined because the same chemical compound can have multiple structural designs that each have different toxicological outcomes for occupational health considerations.

Products utilising nanotechnologies are increasingly commonplace; given the general lack of understanding of their toxicological parameters, there has been an urge for caution as groups of nanomaterials that appear promising in, say, nanomedical applications have themselves been found to be potentially toxic to the patient based on the chemical, physical and synergistic physico-chemical properties of the nanomaterial itself. The potential for worker exposures during the handling of nanomaterials is also very real, as can be seen by worker exposures to polyacrylate nanoparticles in factories, silicon dioxide nanomaterials playing a major role in the development of cardiovascular diseases, nickel nanomaterial powders causing sensitisation, graphene nanomaterials incorporated into facemasks implicated in adverse health effects, etc. These and similar incidents show that it is becoming increasingly clear that the very properties that make nanoparticles technologically beneficial may also make them hazardous to humans and the environment, and news on nanoparticle health effects continues to attract attention from major news outlets. Examples, reflected in many news articles, include reference to the similarity between carbon nanotubes and asbestos, in terms of both their shape characteristics and their pathogenicity. The potential adverse effects of silver nanoparticles on the environment have received criticism, with the UK's House of Lords stating that the food industry is being too secretive about its use of nanotechnology and continuing reports of production line work with nanoparticles being a probable cause for serious health effects in workers.

It is in recognising the power of people to decide which technologies succeed and which do not, whether based on real or perceived risks, where the role of occupational health professionals cannot be over-emphasised in relation to society's ability to reap the full benefits of nanotechnologies. Occupational/industrial hygiene practitioners must establish the appropriate means for assessing and controlling the risks presented by nanomaterials; and occupational health practitioners must be able to understand and screen for these potential work-related exposures and whatever the associated health outcomes may be, as workers represent the first line of people to face possible risks. Only a proper understanding and acceptance of the risks presented by nanomaterials, by both workers and the public at large, will enable nanotechnologies to develop and thrive. This section describes methods for conducting a qualitative risk assessment of nanotechnology operations, applying appropriate controls to minimise risks to workers and occupational health considerations.

Challenges to assessing risk

The traditional occupational hygiene approach to controlling exposures to harmful particles in the workplace (see Section 8.4) is to measure the air concentrations of the particles of interest from the worker's breathing zone, compare those concentrations with exposure limits determined for those particles and implement control measures to reduce concentrations below the exposure limits. This assumes the following: (i) the sampled concentrations are representative of what the worker is actually breathing; (ii) the appropriate index of exposure is known; (iii) analytical methods are available to quantify that index with accuracy/precision and sensitivity/specificity; and (iv) the exposure levels at which those particles produce adverse health effects are known. If any of these is not well characterised, the measurements taken will have limited value as it would be difficult to perform a valid risk assessment. In addressing worker exposures to nanoparticles, the first requirement can be satisfied by obtaining an air sample from the worker's breathing zone using a sampling pump, where forces such as particle inertia and gravity have a minimal impact on the ability of the nanoparticles to follow the sampled air into the sampler since nanoparticles approach molecular size. The second requirement – an appropriate index of exposure – has not yet been satisfied for nanoparticles with no international scientific community consensus on what the relevant index of exposure should be. This lack of consensus directly affects the third requirement, since sampling and analytical methods rely on knowledge of what needs to be measured. The fourth requirement may be the largest barrier to assessing the risk of working with nanomaterials. Very little toxicological data for determining exposure limits for nanoparticles, and virtually no human studies, remain available. This is due to the lack of consensus on the appropriate index of exposure and the relative novelty of nanotechnology and the new materials used in this technology. Nanomaterial issues have been well researched for over a decade, but the barriers remain.

In an attempt to overcome some of these uncertainties, CB (see Section 12.5) was proposed as an alternative to the traditional measurement-based approaches. This strategy would facilitate decisions on appropriate levels of control, based upon product and process information, without complete information on nanoparticle hazards and exposure scenarios. In the pharmaceutical industry, the limited availability of pharmacological and toxicological data of products handled by workers was the main motive to developing control strategies as part of a risk management approach. CB uses categories, or 'bands', of health hazards, which are combined with exposure potentials, or exposure scenarios, to determine the desired levels of control. CB's simplicity is viewed both as a strength and as a weakness, as much of its criticism has focused on issues relating to this qualitative risk assessment approach and how this has forsaken the experts and their traditional, quantitative methods. With nanoparticle exposure and its many toxicological and quantitative measurement uncertainties, however, it is now a viable argument that the CB approach may in fact be superior to the traditional quantitative methods.

The CB concept for nanoparticles was first developed into a usable tool with the creation of the CB Nanotool (https://controlbanding.llnl.gov/), which has garnered considerable international attention from organisations such as WHO, ILO and the International Organization for Standardization (ISO). CB for work with nanomaterials is now recommended by many countries, including Australia, Canada, the Netherlands, France, Switzerland, Germany and South Korea, and the CB Nanotool remains a baseline for their evaluation and validation for national regulatory considerations as well as the primary approach for a qualitative decision matrix for risk assessment that leads to commensurate controls. In January 2014,

ISO issued a new technical specification standard (ISO/TS 12901-2:2014) on the use of CB for managing inhalation risk from engineered nanomaterials. The document proposes guidelines for controlling and managing occupational risk based on a CB approach specifically designed for nano-objects and their aggregates and agglomerates greater than 100nm. The standard provides a description for both proactive and retroactive risk assessment, which are distinguished by whether or not existing controls are used as input variables in determining the control band. The CB Nanotool is described as an example of the proactive approach and Stoffenmanager Nano (https://nano.stoffenmanager.com/) is described as an example of the retroactive approach. Stoffenmanager Nano is an online tool that assesses occupational health risk with inhalation exposure estimates to assist in identifying risk management measures and developing an action plan to manage the risks presented. It is also suggested that the retroactive approach can be considered a means for periodic re-evaluation of the proactive approach.

Applying controls

The CB Nanotool assesses risk by combining engineered nanomaterial composition parameters (shape, size, surface area and surface activity) with their exposure availability (dustiness and amount in use). These indices are linked to bands with four corresponding control approaches. The control approaches are a grouping of three levels of engineering containment, based on sound occupational hygiene principles: (i) general ventilation, (ii) fume hoods or local exhaust ventilation, and (iii) containment. The fourth level is 'seek specialist advice', which is referring to specialist expertise. Through a simplified scoring process, both severity and probability factors are assessed with the outcome based on a CB risk matrix with four risk level outcomes linked to the above approaches. The severity factors include physico-chemical aspects of particle surface chemistry, surface area, solubility, particle number, shape and biological availability for translocation. These factors influence the ability of particles to reach the respiratory tract, their ability to deposit in various regions of the respiratory tract, their ability to penetrate or to be absorbed through skin and their ability to elicit biological responses systemically. The division of severity factor points taken cumulatively is 70% for the nanomaterial and 30% for the parent material. Additional nanomaterial severity factors include carcinogenicity, reproductive toxicity, mutagenicity, dermal toxicity and asthmagen potential. Parent material toxicity of comparable factors is also assessed; however, this information is often more available and can be derived from material safety data sheets. The probability factors determine the extent to which employees may be potentially exposed to nanoscale materials. The probability score is based on the potential for nanoparticles to become airborne. This primarily affects exposure by inhalation; however, it also influences the potential for dermal exposure because the likelihood of skin contact with the nanomaterial increases with more nanoparticles becoming airborne and depositing on work surfaces or the skin. Probability factors scored include the amount of nanomaterial used, the dustiness or mistiness of the operation, the number of employees performing the task, as well as the frequency and duration of the task. For the element of uncertainty, especially with nanomaterial severity factors, 75% of the point value of a high score would be assigned to a given factor with 'unknown information'. The CB Nanotool has now been quantitatively validated and this research, the latest version of the Nanotool, an instructional sheet and additional resources are available at http://controlbanding.llnl.gov.

Role of occupational health

Occupational/industrial hygiene practitioners need to engage in risk assessment together with occupational hygiene colleagues in determining the action to take for workers potentially exposed to nanomaterials. Consideration of the health effects of a nanomaterial requires the known toxicology of the bulk of material to be first assessed and then any anticipated effects of the nanoform of the material. The main routes of exposure are the respiratory tract and skin. Following nasal inhalation direct translocation via the olfactory nerves is an unusual but potential route for nanomaterials. These routes may also be the target organs of the effect; however, as discussed, nanomaterials may access other compartments more readily, thereby causing target organ effects remotely. Analogy may be made to combustion-derived ultrafine particles, which are associated with increased cardiovascular risk despite an inhaled exposure.

There is no one health effect specific to nanomaterials which have been attributed as the cause of a new-onset nickel contact allergy, a toxic epidermal necrolysis from dendrimers, which are nanoscale macromolecules, metal fume fever with nano-zinc oxide nanomaterials, pulmonary effusion and fibrosis with nano-polyacrylates or bronchiolitis obliterans organising pneumonia with nano-titanium dioxide. In some circumstances it may be reasonable to consider nanobiomonitoring for exposure rather than effect, and where there is toxicological evidence to support the strategy. Health surveillance for the effects of nanomaterial exposure may not be appropriate unless the principles of screening (see Section 5.4) are met. It is more likely that health surveillance would be applicable for the known effects of the bulk material and that the fact of exposure to a nanomaterial was recorded and kept for an appropriate period of time. The time period would depend on the considered outcome, which might be 40 years or so after the first exposure, where concerns of long latency effects such as cancer may exist, dependent on the applicable legislation. This would constitute a form of local registry of nanomaterial workers and there has been some thought given to setting up national schemes. Such records would facilitate subsequent epidemiological studies should these become appropriate. The recording of untoward occurrences such as spills with the potential for heavier exposure might be important information to note. It is often the case with emergent disease that sporadic cases arise; journal case reports can usefully highlight the occurrence. Occupational disease-reporting schemes such as the UK's THOR scheme, USA's Sensor, France's rnv3p and Australia's SABRE provide the opportunity to detect early signals of new causes of occupational disease.

Considerations for the nanotechnology industry

The need for standardisation of toxicological parameters has been emphasised by researchers in nanotoxicology to afford better utility and consistency of research with nanomaterials as their use and exponential growth in application continue. A standardised database of toxicological research findings harnessed and presented in a format, preferably captured in material safety data sheets, which are currently woefully lacking for nanomaterial-specific information, that can feed directly into the CB Nanotool's severity and probability risk matrix would be an important step towards achieving this standardisation. Making the latest research available for experts and practitioners alike in this manner would play an important role in the protection of workers in the nanotechnology industries. The CB Nanotool's structure, weighting of risks, utility for exposure mitigation and improvements place the CB Nanotool in the middle of directing the research still to come, maximising its effectiveness for all those involved in the nanotechnology industries. At the scientific level, the CB Nanotool's approach has been found by numerous researchers to have the potential to offer the greatest utility to nanomaterial producers at both the micro- and macro-levels. However, it should be recognised that CB toolkits must always be used with some degree of caution. The different factors considered, weighted and that influence the overall risk levels and control bands are determined as educated 'guesses' as to factor importance and range delineation. Any qualitative risk assessment requires frequent use, validation and evaluation of recommended control effectiveness. It is therefore strongly encouraged that the use of a wide range of applications will undoubtedly improve and refine assessments.

18.14 Medically unexplained illnesses

Today, certainly in high-income countries occupational physicians see more illness but less disease. Although musculoskeletal disorders and stress-related complaints dominate, they too are interrelated and both are subject to 'somatising tendencies' (presenting as physical symptoms related to different target organ systems). Thus, the new 'age of existentialism' is dominated by conditions such as those listed below, the last two of which are covered in this section:

- stress
- non-specific effect modifiers
- diffuse pain syndromes
- electromagnetic or electrical sensitivity
- a combination of psychological, neurological and immunological issues
- chronic fatigue syndrome (CFS)
- multiple chemical sensitivity (MCS)
- damp- and mould-associated symptoms.

In some parts of the world the term idiopathic environmental intolerance (IEI) has replaced MCS but in others IEI is used to encompass a broader group of unexplained conditions characterised by heterogeneous symptoms provoked by environmental triggers such as chemicals, biological agents (mould among them) and electromagnetic fields. MCS in this usage is one of several conditions under the general term IEI.

Multiple chemical sensitivity

Like CFS, MCS is controversial but also very problematic and disruptive when it occurs. Individuals report intolerance to a variety of chemicals at exposure levels far below those that would be expected to affect most people. Sufferers report a wide range of symptoms affecting many different target organs, for which there is often no alternative consistent medical, biological or toxicological explanation. MCS is relatively rare, and the incidence has stabilised or declined globally. The condition may be triggered by (perceived) over-exposure to one specific chemical (not necessarily in a workplace setting), which can then generalise to other substances and chemicals. As with CFS, psychosocial factors are believed to have a major role in the development and continuation of this condition, but the pathophysiology is under investigation, notably mechanisms involving smell and the olfactory system. Treatment is usually difficult and requires specialist help. The prognosis is poor, and many patients avoid chemicals (low levels of perfumes and fragrances included) as their primary therapy, resulting in social isolation and inability to work. Some jurisdictions provide disability grants for MCS so application for this financial support should be considered.

Dampness and mould-associated symptoms

Moulds (filamentous fungi) are commonly found in homes, workplaces and other buildings. This is particularly so when there is dampness and the ventilation is poor, sometimes because of buildings having been sealed to preserve heat. There are thousands of mould species and they require water to grow, hence their occurrence with dampness in structures. Moulds contribute to indoor air pollution and a 2009 WHO review on dampness and moulds found sufficient evidence of associations (not causation, though) between exposure and several respiratory symptoms and conditions: cough, wheeze, asthma exacerbation and upper respiratory symptoms most confidently, but asthma development and respiratory infections also. What is controversial is the situation in which patients report a range of non-specific symptoms when experiencing contact with mould, typically visible mould in a home or worksite. Symptoms include joint or muscle pain, itchy skin, forgetfulness and poor concentration, headaches, fatigue and weakness and those related to the gastrointestinal tract. They can be very troubling for the patient but there is little or no sound evidence that they arise directly from mould toxicity. Removing visible mould, treating damp in affected areas of buildings and improving ventilation are usually indicated but the non-specific symptoms may persist despite these interventions. Generally, identification of the offending mould species is not helpful as the non-specific symptoms have not been shown to be associated with particular moulds. Immunological tests (e.g. immunoglobulin E) also offer little help because there are very many moulds and *in vitro* tests have been developed for only a small fraction. False-positive and false-negative tests frequently complicate interpretation of these tests.

18.15 Military populations

The ability and capability of those joining and working in a country's military is paramount. Applicants joining a national defence force are usually screened not only for aptitude and fitness but also medically, given the unique environments in military work and the physical and psychological demands that can be present both at home and when deployed abroad.

To understand the occupational risks in many militaries, the traditional categorisation of hazards, which includes physical, chemical, biological, ergonomic and psychological, applies; however, there are also unique hazards associated with each component (i.e. army, navy, air force).

Among the physical hazards impacting all components, exposure to noise is highly prevalent because of the difficulty in controlling it. Many strategies for noise control are difficult to implement in military settings. Processes cannot be enclosed nor is it possible to engineer them out, resulting in uptake of PPE developments such as noise-cancelling technologies in communication headsets and custom-moulded earplugs. Special attention to venting of custom-moulded plugs (often with a pinhole) is required to prevent barotrauma in environments where noise exposure occurs in conjunction with pressure changes, e.g. in aircrew trades. Compensation related to noise exposure is common, and, as a result, early integration of annual surveillance audiogram results in electronic medical records has occurred. Unilateral hearing loss because of exposure to weapon firing/detonation is a peculiarity found less frequently outside of military settings.

Another common physical hazard is that of temperature extremes. Heat exposure relates to not only the nature and amount of equipment required to be worn but also some of the environments in which it is worn. However, in military settings, cold exposure is also common; for example, military divers can spend hours in deep cold water, even undertaking 'ice dives' – diving under frozen bodies of water.

In terms of vibration, segmental exposure resulting from the use of tools, as is common in many non-military trades, can occur. In the military, whole-body vibration exposure can occur through both airborne transmission and contact transmission. Trades at particular risk for the latter include armoured vehicle drivers and rotary wing aircrew, who are particularly prone to neck pain as a result. Prevention efforts have included alterations to aircraft seat design and implementation of pre-flight physiotherapy-supported muscle-stretching pro-grammes. The combination of common physical exposures in military environments such as noise, vibration and pressure (e.g. low-level flying) can not only exacerbate the effects of each exposure but also contribute to compounding systemic health effects, both acute (e.g. motion sickness) and chronic (e.g. cardiovascular disease). Performance degradation because of increased fatigue, distraction and decreased situational awareness can also result.

Exposure to radiation can occur in multiple settings; the impacts of laser strikes is important and difficult to eliminate with protective gear, especially eye-wear, because prevention requires knowledge of the nature of the specific laser, e.g. wavelength, Q-switched versus pulsed. As a result, some military members may be classified as 'radiation workers' and require occupational dose monitoring. Radiation is also one of the components of CBRN (chemical, biological, radiological and nuclear) defence. Prevention programming for CBRN as a whole may include pre-treatments, pre-exposure vaccinations or individually issued medications such as atropine, pyridostigmine bromide (pre-treatment for nerve agents), diazepam or antibiotics, among others, in order to manage possible exposures associated with a particular operation.

Chemical exposures of particular relevance in day-to-day operations include fuels (which include diesel, jet fuels such as JP-8 and nitrated fuels) and metals such as cadmium, beryllium (avionics, air weapons systems and aircraft structures) and leaded ammunition. Carbon fibre exposure from degrading or burning vehicle structures has emerged as vehicle compositions change. The health impacts of exposure to products of combustion from various substances and complex structures are increasingly understood in trades that undertake not only firefighting but also clean-up thereafter. Like the compounding effects of physical exposures, this is also possible for chemical exposures. There have been numerous reports of complex, multisystem disorders with constellations of difficult-to-categorise symptoms emerging after various military operations over the years (e.g. Gulf War Syndrome), which can be, at the same time controversial and concerning, and for which ongoing research continues.

Exposure to pressure in hypobaric flight environments and hyperbaric diving environments is common, and many navy and air-force trades have specific medical selection as well as training considerations as a result. Although not unique to military environments, exposures in confined spaces (submarines) to blast (breaching) and high G-force (high-performance aircraft) occur, as do musculoskeletal injuries from demanding physical tasks. Ergonomic hazards are related to body-worn equipment and helmet-mounted gear (e.g. night vision goggles), awkward positioning (para-jumping with gear), repetitive activities, etc. Indeed, research on gear design is focused not only on comfort, fit and protection, but also on integration with other gear or equipment. Gear integration is important both for ergonomics and for intrinsic safety (a design concept related to managing ignition potential related to electrical and thermal energies).

Exposure to biological hazards is often a deployment-related concern, as endemic illnesses including vector-borne illnesses may differ from those at home, thus pre-deployment medical screening includes vaccination review. Psychological hazards resulting in PTSD are present not only on deployment but also on humanitarian missions and rescue work as well. Programming to assist those with operational-stress injuries (OSI) has emerged – substance use programmes also exist for these individuals. Fatigue risk management programmes have emerged not only to prevent fatigue but also to manage circadian dyssynchrony.

Areas of research in military medicine related to combat casualty care have increasingly enabled adoption of high-tech solutions. Aeromedevac and patient transport capabilities are increasingly enabled by artificial intelligence (AI) with tools that support clinical decision-making and patient monitoring among others.

Assessment of occupational risk in military settings considers not only individual health but also 'operational effectiveness', with medical screening and surveillance focused on capacity and the risk of subtle or sudden incapacitation. This requires an understanding of the range of occupational hazards across the defence force, and with each specific component.

18.16 eHealth/Occupational digital health

The SARS-COV-2 pandemic of 2019 provided the impetus to accelerate the application of digital technologies to workplaces, especially in the healthcare field. These changes were implemented rapidly in many organisations, but they are likely to stay and become ever more pervasive. Digital health is the field of knowledge and practice associated with the development and use of digital technologies to improve health; this includes interconnected health systems, smart devices, computational analysis techniques and communication media to aid healthcare professionals and their clients manage illnesses and health risks, as well as promote health and wellbeing.

Terminology

The components of digital health include:

AI. Uses algorithms that may be fixed or updated automatically and iteratively (adaptive algorithms).

- Narrow AI: focuses on a specific task or works within a small number of parameters, such as reading radiological images or speech recognition and dictation.
- Strong or general AI: learns to do various tasks, e.g. control of prosthetic upper limbs.

Big data. Four dimensions – volume, velocity, variety and veracity – characterise this concept, which embraces the analysis of 'data lakes'; a goal might be developing effective clinical decision support (CDS) systems or predictive analytics.

Blockchain. Simultaneous use and sharing of an incorruptible database within a large decentralised, accessible network, as implemented in some electronic health record systems.

eHealth. The use of information and communications technologies in support of health and health-related fields, including healthcare services, health surveillance, health literature and health education, knowledge and research.

Health data. The European Union (EU) refers to personal information (also called personal data) that relates to the health status of a person. This includes both medical data (doctor referrals and prescriptions, medical examination reports, laboratory tests, radiographs, etc.) and administrative and financial information about health (the scheduling of medical appointments, invoices for healthcare services, medical certificates for sick leave management, etc.).

Internet of Things (IoT). Consists of identifiable, interrelated computing devices, physical devices or sensors with the ability to connect to the Internet; these may be embedded into objects or people and the ability to transfer data, e.g. blood pressure, blood sugar and coagulation-level measuring devices.

Mobile health or mhealth. Uses mobile wireless technologies such as apps for public health surveillance during epidemics.

Telemedicine. Medical information exchanged from one site to another through electronic communications with the purpose of improving the health status of patients, e.g. telephone or video consultations.

Telepresence. The use of virtual presence technology to allow remote observation or action by a distant observer, e.g. remote surgery presence.

Practical considerations

It is likely that occupational health physicians and nurses are using digital health daily either explicitly or sometimes without overt recognition, although all will be aware of the data protection principles enacted in different jurisdictions such as the EU's General Data Protection Regulation (GDPR). In common with other areas of medical practice occupational health has embraced telemedicine with many organisations undertaking telephone consultations and more recently video consultations. With the wide variety of contexts in which occupational medicine is delivered the field was a relatively early adopter of telemedicine, particularly in the offshore oil and gas sector as well as in seafaring and other remote work. In the discipline of ergonomics, an early system of telephone consultation and Web-based assessments combined with photographs and videos has been used for assessing workstations. More recently, there has been some limited usage of mobile technologies for distance assessment of workplaces with mobile phones and also with bespoke telepresence technology. In France real-time teledermoscopy for skin cancer among agricultural workers has been used with results suggesting that in the context of occupational medicine it is feasible and could be useful for improving skin cancer screening in at-risk populations while avoiding face-to-face examinations by a dermatologist in over half of cases. The use of electronic health records for migrant farm workers was implemented in California in 2003 and a similar system exists in Spain. Such systems facilitate continuity of care from the resident country and have advantages over manual personally held records.

Much of the work of occupational health surveillance might be delivered through Web-based technology and subject to analysis or screening. Work as a health outcome and the impact of work on health is not always easily assessed, not least because occupational information is lacking in health records. The advent of algorithms to allow automated coding of job titles in large data sets or in real time will permit analysis and add utility to data collection. Teaching and training in occupational health are also likely to see increased usage of e-learning, which will have the benefit of widening access.

Digital health technologies are envisioned by WHO as using health data to promote health and wellbeing, and to achieve the health-related sustainable development goals and WHO's 'triple billion targets' (Figure 18.15). Such aims will also help the further implementation within occupational health, a specialty that works within countries and across international boundaries through multinational private sector organisations.

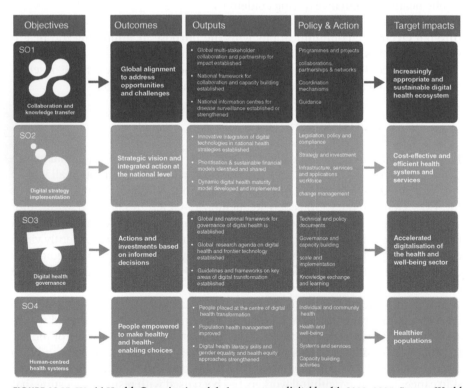

FIGURE 18.15 World Health Organization global strategy on digital health 2020–2025. Source: World Health Organization Draft global strategy on digital health 2020–2025. https://www.who.int/docs/default-source/documents/gs4dhdaa2a9f352b0445bafbc79ca799dce4d.pdf.

Barriers to adoption

Infrastructure has been a problem, although in some locations it is well developed; for example, the Ontario Telemedicine Network in Canada, which is one of the world's largest, supporting two-way video conferencing to provide patient care at hundreds of healthcare sites throughout Ontario. Technology use was higher and therapeutic areas of care were more diverse in more rural areas than in other parts of Ontario, showing that it led to improved access to medical care services, especially in sparsely populated regions. In 2017, it was estimated that 76% of US hospitals connected their patients and doctors through telemedicine. The widespread use of mobile phones and the roll out of 5G connectivity further increase the reach of such technologies. The technology has at times been ahead of the law or professional guidance, and occupational health practitioners need to be sure of the applicable regulations for their jurisdiction of practice and those of any place where a patient may be consulted via telemedicine.

18.17 Mild traumatic brain injury/concussion

Annually, around 1.4 million people attend emergency departments in England and Wales with a recent head injury; of these, up to 50% are children aged under 15 years. Ninety-five per cent of people who have sustained a head injury present with a normal or minimally impaired conscious level (Glasgow Coma Scale greater than 12/15). Concussion is perhaps best considered as a mechanism of injury rather than a diagnosis and it may lead to a varying severity of traumatic brain injury (Box 18.1). The estimated annual incidence of mild traumatic brain injury (mTBI) is 500/100 000 in the USA, with similar figures for Canada. Causes of concussive brain injury for adults include motor vehicle accidents, sports, falls, assault, explosive blasts and workplace injury; in the latter case, it is the circumstance rather than the mechanism of injury that is of particular interest. Full recovery occurs for most people within three months of mTBI, although around 15% have persistent symptoms.

Clinical presentation

The diagnosis of mTBI is a clinical diagnosis having excluded a neurological condition that requires urgent specialty consultation. Currently, there is no good evidence to support the routine use of brain imaging, serum biomarkers or electroencephalography (EEG) in patients with a history of mTBI. Most symptoms occur soon after the event and those only arising after 30 days or more are unlikely to be related to mTBI and appropriate assessment should take place. The symptom severity shortly after mTBI is reported to be the most reliable predictor of recovery.

Box 18.1 | Mayo Clinic Traumatic Brain Injury (TBI) Severity classification system

A. Classify as moderate–severe (definite) TBI if one or more of the following criteria apply:

1. Death due to this TBI

2. Loss of consciousness of 30 minutes or more

3. Post-traumatic anterograde amnesia of 24 hours or more

4. Worst Glasgow Coma Scale full score in first 24 hours <13 (unless invalidated upon review, e.g. attributable to intoxication, sedation, systemic shock)

5. One or more of the following present:
   - Intracerebral haematoma
   - Subdural haematoma
   - Epidural haematoma
   - Cerebral contusion
   - Haemorrhagic contusion
   - Penetrating TBI (dura penetrated)
   - Subarachnoid haemorrhage
   - Brainstem injury

B. If none of criteria A apply, classify as mild (probable) TBI if one or more of the following criteria apply:

1. Loss of consciousness of momentary to <30 minutes

2. Post-traumatic anterograde amnesia of momentary to <24 hours

3. Depressed, basilar or linear skull fracture (dura intact)

C. If none of criteria A or B apply, classify as symptomatic (possible) TBI if one or more of the following symptoms are present:

   - Blurred vision
   - Confusion (mental state changes)
   - Dazed
   - Dizziness
   - Focal neurological symptoms
   - Headache
   - Nausea

Source: Adapted from Malec et al. (2007).

The focus of a medical history should be on: current symptoms (Box 18.2) and the patient's concerns; the context and mechanism of the injury; change in consciousness – severity, duration and timing; any coincident injuries; previous medical and mental health; and psychosocial factors. Psychosocial factors can be inherent in the workplace and may impact the health and mental wellbeing of workers. An appropriate physical examination should be completed, especially of the neurological system and of mental health status. The use of standardised assessment tools that can be repeated to track progress is recommended, e.g. the Rivermead Post-Concussion Symptom Questionnaire, Post-Concussion Symptom Scale, Sport Concussion Assessment Tool 5th Edition (SCAT5).

Occupational management

Early education of patients about expectations of symptoms and the likelihood of resolution together with treatment reduces the chances of persistent symptoms. A brief period of rest for 24–48 hours post injury is appropriate and patients can be encouraged to become gradually and progressively more active as

Box 18.2 | Possible post-mild traumatic brain injury (mTBI)-related symptoms

Physical symptoms	Cognitive symptoms	Behaviour/ emotional symptoms
Headache, dizziness, balance disorders, nausea, fatigue, sleep disturbance, blurred vision, sensitivity to light, hearing difficulties/loss, tinnitus, sensitivity to noise, seizure, transient neurological abnormalities, numbness, tingling, neck pain	Problems with attention, concentration, memory, speed of processing, judgement, executive control	Depression, anxiety, agitation, irritability, impulsivity, aggression

Source: Adapted from VA/DoD Clinical Practice Guideline for the Management of Concussion-mild Traumatic Brain Injury Version 2.0 – 2016.

tolerated. However, prolonged periods of complete rest exceeding 48–72 hours may slow recovery. Avoid work activities with a likelihood of further mTBI exposure risk in the first 7–10 days. Encourage gradual and progressive activity at home and work. Assess whether the worker's medical impairments might cause harm for the worker or third parties when performing their work activities.

Advise the worker and, with consent, the employer of any medical restrictions so that any reasonable work adjustments can be accommodated. Among the difficulties for workers with a history of mTBI is the 'invisible' nature of their condition and that cognitive problems are those that most often affect return to work. Where there are persistent symptoms or a decline in function patients should be considered for early referral to a multidisciplinary treatment programme, ideally with a physician who has expertise in mTBI. The aim is to allow the earliest return to work within the worker's capacity (physical and mental) so as not to exacerbate their symptoms while recognising that workers with mTBI who remain employed have better health outcomes.

18.18 The measurement of critical wellbeing components

The modern world, and especially that part that constitutes work, is now one of ever-changing technology, mobile telecommunication devices 'welded to your side' and a significant blurring of the work–home boundary with never any true 'off-time', with significantly extended working hours and more exacerbating the issue. The result of this is an increasingly stressed workforce with burgeoning levels of fatigue and compromised physical/cognitive capabilities as the norm; where draconian sickness absence policies/processes/procedures exist, rising levels of presenteeism and plummeting individual wellbeing and organisational wellness result. The following provides the latest insights into, and technology available to measure, these factors for the first time and provides integrated metrics to empower individuals to make whatever personal changes they can and to inform organisations to make insightful data-driven strategic changes – both sustainably.

Historically, almost none of the elements described above have ever been measurable (objectively and quantitatively) because they are a physiological reaction – for example, stress is a *reaction* to a situation and not about the actual situation itself. As a result, the occupational health professional has always had to rely on self-completed questionnaires – with all of the inherent inaccuracies, biases and opportunities for a lack of honesty, such as exaggeration or denial.

For many years cardiologists have measured an aspect of the beat of the heart called heart rate variability (HRV), which, in simple terms, is a measure of the variation in time between each heartbeat. It is measured from the 'R' component of the 'PQRSTU complex' of one heartbeat to the 'R' of the next (Figure 18.16). A normal healthy heart does not beat evenly like a metronome, but instead there

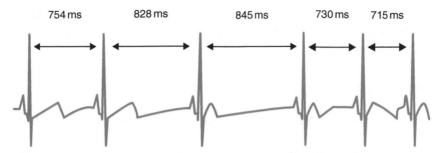

FIGURE 18.16 The variability in time intervals between the 'R' component of a heartbeat.

are constant variations when the number of milliseconds between heartbeats is investigated. This variation is controlled by a part of the nervous system called the autonomic nervous system (ANS). It works regardless/independently of our desire and regulates our heart rate, blood pressure, breathing, digestion and the like. The ANS is subdivided into two large components, the sympathetic branch activates stress hormone production (also known as the fight-or-flight mechanism) whereas the parasympathetic branch slows heart rate and restores our balance after stress passes (the relaxation response).

The brain is processing information in a region called the hypothalamus constantly, and, through the ANS, sends signals to the rest of the body either to stimulate or to relax different functions. It responds not only to poor sleep, or a negative interaction with a manager or colleague, but also to positive stimuli, such as a promotion/pay rise or a fabulous meal. Our bodies can handle all kinds of stimuli daily and day after day – yet 'life goes on'. However, if one or more stimuli persist, such as stress, poor sleep, unhealthy diet, dysfunctional relationships (work, personal and domestic), isolation or solitude (social connectivity), compromised finances and lack of exercise, then this balance may be disrupted, and the individual's fight-or-flight response can move into 'overdrive'.

What measure of heart rate variability is important to evaluate stress?

In short, HRV increases during periods of relaxation and recovery activities and decreases during periods of stress. Therefore, typically HRV is higher when the heart is beating slowly and decreases as the heart beats more quickly – this is best described as heart rate and HRV having a generally inverse relationship. Unsurprisingly, HRV changes from day to day based on activity levels and the amount of work-related stress. In addition to these external stress factors, there are internal stress factors that cause daily variation in HRV levels – which include poor nutrition, alcohol use, illness, etc. To supplement this, it is known that higher fitness levels usually result in increased HRV compared with people with lower fitness levels. A high HRV is commonly viewed as an indicator of a healthy heart.

HRV can be measured with, for example, time and frequency domain methods for evaluating sympathovagal balance (i.e. the balance between sympathetic and parasympathetic activity).

Measurement of heart rate variability

One key component in the ability to measure stress is access to quality real-time HRV data as they offer granular detail within the heart's normal rhythms, providing individual trends in response to various stimuli. Recent advances in technology, including wearable devices, data capture and processing, have presented the opportunity to measure stress and other important metrics that relate to wellbeing in the workplace. Much of this progress has been driven in sport and military environments – where analysing physical performance data plays a major part – but there is also a continual quest to understand better how pressure impacts athletic and cognitive performance. These recent advances mean that HRV can be measured with a chest band or through a wrist-based device – although the former is more accurate, the latter is less invasive to the user and hence its usability ensures derivation of much more data over a much longer period.

Heart rate variability stress and fatigue indicators

HRV then forms the basis of stress measurement and occupational health professionals can investigate these further responses using algorithms and software to understand what is going on in much greater detail. For instance, the ANS response can show whether an individual responds to a stimulus with a 'threat' or 'challenge' mindset and distinguishes between an emotional or rational response. By blending other data such as activity it is also possible to build models that offer an insight into the 'mental cost' of a task and, therefore, to understand the mental demands and potential fatigue risk. Monitoring over time provides the occupational health professional with the opportunity to build biorhythm models and predict how individuals, teams and organisations will respond to different situations and needs (Figure 18.17).

Stress in the workplace

Although sport presents a comparatively easy environment in which to harvest data, advances in GDPR, data security and data architecture mean that this technology and expertise can be applied to organisational occupational health and safety strategies. Mental health and total worker wellbeing (see Section 18.10) and stress are already key items on the agenda for businesses, often down to the increase in demand on our attention by different forms of technology and data at increasing pace (Figure 18.18). The ability to monitor how stress is impacting performance and wellbeing, together with the potential to perform proactive

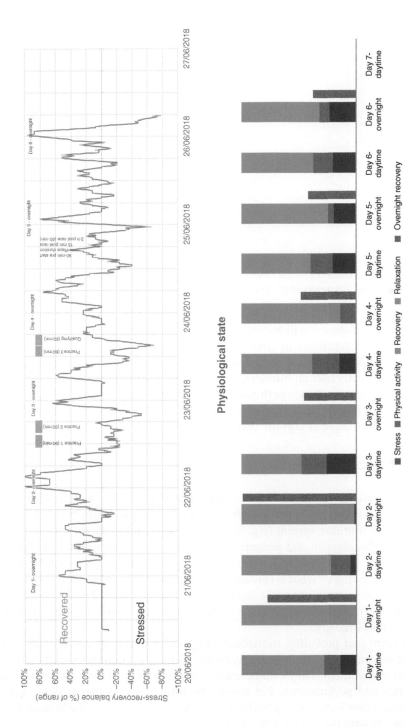

FIGURE 18.17 Time-series heart rate variability analysis, mapping the recovery (above 0%) and stress (below 0%) balance. Source: Courtesy of IHP-Analytics Ltd.

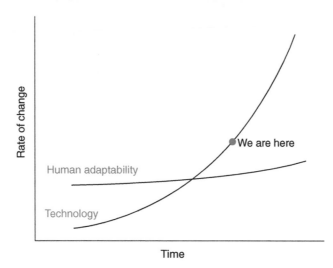

FIGURE 18.18 Graph to demonstrate Moore's law – how technology is evolving at a far greater rate than our ability as humans to adapt. Source: Moore, G.E. (1965). Cramming more components onto integrated circuits. *Electronics* 38 (8): 114–117.

intervention strategies, will become a necessity for modern organisations looking for agility and resilience in current times. It is worthy of note that, although stress is increasingly documented as a bad thing, stress response through the ANS is a perfectly normal human response mechanism. Stress, seen as an occurrence or as a preparation to perform (for instance), should be seen as good as well as normal. It is only when stress falls outside of an individual's 'norms' and/or becomes cumulative or chronic that it should become a cause for concern.

Workplace context

HRV data offer a wealth of insight into both the performance and wellbeing of individuals and teams, with a well-published example being how stress can weaken the immune system (e.g. Segerstrom and Miller, 2004) with considerations for absenteeism and presenteeism statistics. It is important to factor in a way of determining what environmental and contextual factors are influencing the stress responses – what is causing the symptoms? This is where a true picture of workplace stress requires the biometric data to be blended with job and task data such as calendars, technology usage or perhaps vehicle telematics data in the transport industry.

Far from just providing individual insight, HRV data in combination with other data can be used to inform leadership about team dynamics, cultural strategy and engagement. They could even provide feedback on their own leadership attributes and performance. Put simply, by integrating biometric data such as HRV with other factors it is possible to turn previously intangible human workforce behaviours into tangible metrics.

Workforce data in this format have the ability to empower organisations with agile, tangible and potent human resources and occupational health strategies. They provide robust quantitative data rather than the traditional subjective self-completed questionnaire-type data so commonly deployed currently and provide a new level of objective assessment that has the potential to connect employee to employer and provide benefit to both parties in unison. Additionally, comparison of subjective responses with biometric indicators provides an excellent opportunity to challenge innate biases and perceptions that naturally detract from cohesion, engagement and team dynamics, and can form the basis for optimised and truly individualised development programmes. Depending on the data capability they can also provide this assorted information in real time, breaking the mould on outdated 6–12-month retrospective appraisals – this could be so potent for those individuals in safety-critical roles such as nuclear, emergency services and similar response activities.

Driving positive interventions

Once stress, fatigue and more can be quantitatively measured and occupational health professionals understand the work-related factors influencing individuals and/or groups, then they can begin to look at ways of improving wellbeing and performance. In almost every instance, quantum gains can be made in focusing on the core physiological basics that interplay with stress and that are readily affected by technological advances: sleep, activity, rest and recovery. It is likely that an improvement in one of these basic human functions will change the individual's ability to manage the stress more effectively. Conversely, cumulative stress can impact upon our ability to perform the others well too; hence, it is better to provide a holistic viewpoint with an idea of what change will provide the greatest impact (Figures 18.19 and 18.20) to facilitate simple indications for change.

Providing accurate, work-specific data to individuals, teams and organisations in itself can be a major instigator for change. A combination of bringing a metric to a previously 'unknown known' together with direct context that relates to the user is a powerful motivator in comparison with a theoretical model or generic training. This breeds 'self-awareness', a conscious rational understanding that quashes our previous beliefs directly. An example would be our internal perception of stress, i.e. 'I feel stressed/under pressure', which is a normal emotional response. Real-time data quantify that response and provide (in most instances) a realisation that perception is greater than actual stress, both initiating a natural internal 'thermostatic' response that modifies the reaction and a basis for instigating a coping strategy such as deep breathing exercises.

Fundamentally, HRV data, with stress and fatigue as the leading occupational health indicators, can now form the basis of accurate, optimised performance and wellbeing strategies, enhancing the agility and resilience of an organisation and potentially allowing it flex (and particularly its workforce) within an increasingly turbulent workplace. For the first time, it is feasible for occupational health

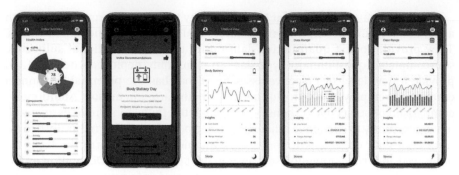

FIGURE 18.19 Illustrative dashboard of real-time user feedback on the basics of sleep, rest, recovery, stress and activity. Source: Graphics reproduced by kind permission of IHP-Analytics Ltd. (My Work Life Analytics™; http://www.ihp-analytics.com).

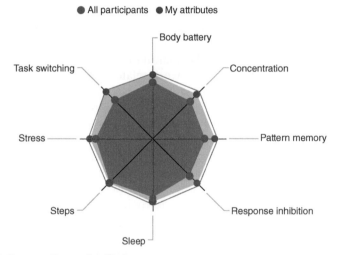

FIGURE 18.20 Some attributes of wellbeing.

professionals to assist a business to see itself as a living organism and hence make data-driven decisions to optimise its performance and wellbeing.

Sleep

Although a great deal of research into sleep has been undertaken, its individual nature means that currently it is difficult to identify which components (HRV currently identifies duration, deep, light and rapid eye movement sleep) would improve the overall quality and restorative function. Attention, therefore, should rightly begin with improving sleep hygiene, such as identifying the individual's natural chronotype preference and adjusting 'sleep time' and 'awake time' to suit this, along with room temperature and natural light. As with most natural cycles occurring within the human body, consistency of routine also positively impacts quality. Using a wearable device, the individual is able to monitor longitudinal sleep components and experiment with different elements to understand their natural preferences better. For organisations, the impact of a wide-scale improvement in sleep quality, while largely out of their control, should not be underestimated.

Rest/recovery

The traditional framework of 9 a.m. to 5 p.m. work hours combined with a greater intensity of technological communications and a need to ensure productivity has meant that individuals can seriously neglect a natural need for breaks and rest. Furthermore, there is a difference between 'taking a break' and creating a period of sustained and effective 'recharge' or restoration of energy and other mental/physical resources. An occupational health practitioner should give careful consideration as to how work patterns could be altered to allow for this, with even short durations of 10 minutes being beneficial. Many meditation or sleep apps now facilitate short recharge sessions, closing the individual out from the surrounding environment and increasing the quality of the short restorative effort.

Although there are challenges to collecting personal data from a GDPR and data security perspective in addition to the occasional misguided user and/or dissenter incorrectly using the capability or trying to create a negative perspective/reputation that could be attached to the perspective of overtly 'monitoring' employees for the good of the organisation, this certainly does not have to be the case. When programmes are designed and driven by occupational health and human science professionals (wherein the individual is empowered to drive their own change journey) there is a significant value and benefit to the employee in using data to understand how to optimise their work–life balance, and from the organisational perspective to assist the organisation strategically to hone its human resource and wellbeing functions accurately. With careful application of the technology, human analytics has the potential to greatly enhance the employee's experience and thus positively impact productivity, engagement and mental health (among other things). As with other areas of technological growth, the more data that can be collected, the greater the ability of organisations to refine and optimise their commitment to wellbeing, with the potential to use predictive analytics to support their workforce proactively rather than dealing with expensive reactive intervention.

Further Reading

Black, C. (2008). *Dame Carol Black's Review of the Health of Britain's Working Age Population. Working for a Healthier Tomorrow*. London: The Stationery Office https://www.gov.uk/government/publications/working-for-a-healthier-tomorrow-work-and-health-in-britain.

Confederation of British Industry (1990). *Developing a Safety Culture: Business for Safety*. London: CBI.

Malec, J.F., Brown, A.W., Leibson, C.L. et al. (2007). The Mayo classification system for traumatic brain injury severity. *Journal of Neurotrauma* 24 (9): 1417–1424. https://doi.org/10.1089/neu.2006.0245.

National Institute for Occupational Safety and Health (2020). *Total Worker Health Program*. https://www.cdc.gov/niosh/twh.

Ontario Neurotrauma Foundation (2018). *Guideline for concussion/mild traumatic brain injury & prolonged symptoms*, 3e. https://braininjuryguidelines.org/concussion/fileadmin/pdf/Concussion_guideline_3rd_edition_final.pdf.

Segerstrom, S.C. and Miller, G.E. (2004). Psychological stress and the human immune system: a meta-analytic study of 30 years of inquiry. *Psychological Bulletin* 130 (4): 601–630. https://doi.org/10.1037/0033-2909.130.4.601.

The Topol Review (2019). *Preparing the healthcare workforce to deliver the digital future. Health Education England*. https://topol.hee.nhs.uk.

World Health Organization (2021). *Global Strategy on Digital Health 2020–2025*. Geneva: WHO https://www.who.int/docs/default-source/documents/gs4dhdaa2a9f352b0445bafbc79ca799dce4d.pdf.

CHAPTER 19

Expert and Medicolegal Report Writing

19.1 Introduction

There are many situations in occupational health that require a legal remedy when interested parties disagree. For instance, the attribution of illness to work or a product, or a disagreement on fitness for work, or the degree of disability and its relationship to work. The various stakeholders in litigation may be employers and employees, or employers and clients, or groups of current and former employees and industries or corporations, even governments. Consequently, occupational health practitioners – occupational therapists, psychologists, physicians and hygienists among others – may be asked or required to provide an expert opinion, sometimes as a formal medicolegal document. In most jurisdictions the duty to uphold patient confidentiality is subordinate to the duty to give evidence to a court; practitioners have no privilege against disclosure of relevant client information, as lawyers do. These expert opinions can be fundamental to the legal matter or a substantial contributor to it. Writing them is no small task and defending them in legal environments can be intimidating, excepting the 'professional' expert report writers who have done it numerous times. This chapter provides some guidance to expert report writing and points out some pitfalls to avoid. It should be borne in mind, though, that many jurisdictions and specific legal matters have particular requirements for expert reports; these need to be identified, usually while taking instruction from the legal representative requesting the report.

Pocket Consultant: Occupational Health, Sixth Edition. Kerry Gardiner, David Rees, Anil Adisesh, David Zalk, and Malcolm Harrington.
© 2022 John Wiley & Sons Ltd. Published 2022 by John Wiley & Sons Ltd.

19.2 The role of an expert

Before providing an expert opinion, you should be satisfied that you have the necessary expertise and no conflicts of interest. It can be expected that expertise will be scrutinised and any conflicts of interest should have been declared to the engaging lawyer. Experts write a report, and come to court should this be necessary, to pass on the benefits of their specialised knowledge and experience. There are limits to an expert's role. Dennis Davis, a well-known South African judge, had this to say on the issue:

> Agreed, an expert is called by a particular party, presumably because the conclusion of the expert, using his or her expertise, is in favour of the line of argument of the particular party. But that does not absolve the expert from providing the court with as objective and unbiased opinion, based on his or her expertise, as is possible. An expert is not a hired gun who dispenses his or her expertise for the purposes of a particular case. An expert does not assume the role of an advocate, nor give evidence which goes beyond the logic which is dictated by the scientific knowledge which that expert claims to possess.

The key task of an occupational health expert is, thus, to guide the court to a correct decision on questions falling within their specialist field. According to the Medical Protection Society an expert should aim to produce a report that is free-standing, which means that the reader must be able to glean the central issues of the case, understand the evidence available and reach a clear under-standing of the range of expert opinion, without needing to look at any other document, on the issues addressed by the expert. A crucial role is to cover the evidence undermining your opinion and explain why it is insufficiently persua-sive to alter your evaluation.

Knowledgeable, unbiased and independent experts can legitimately differ on many aspects of a case – attribution of disease to exposures at work is a notable one. For a small number of agents a threshold of exposure above which a disease is likely (>50%) to have been caused by the exposure is generally accepted. Such a threshold for asbestos and lung cancer is 25 fibres per millilitre-years. However, these determinations are the exception and so opinions on causation will vary. A naval employee who presented with liver disease caused by hepatitis B infection after cleaning the sewerage storage tanks of a ship returning from sea makes the point. One expert's opinion was that it was probable that the task resulted in the infection because sewerage can be contaminated by blood, the main medium of transmission of the virus, and because the person was healthy before undertak-ing the task. Another expert disagreed because it was not established that the employee was free of the virus prior to doing the work, and because he had had sex with several women around the time of the task – hepatitis B can be sexually transmitted. (In passing, the court found that on the balance of probability the disease should be attributed to his work.) In a case such as this it can be helpful for the writer of an expert report to try and put themselves in the shoes of the adjudicators, usually not occupational health experts. Our role is to give a clear opinion, noting that an opinion that states that there is insufficient evidence to reach a conclusion is a clear one. The opinion should take account of the legal test for the association under question: the balance of probability (>50%); a material contributor to the outcome; or beyond reasonable doubt (more demanding) are typical levels of stringency to be applied. A detailed justification for the opinion should be given in terms accessible to a non-specialist. The evidence both for and against your opinion should be presented. Research, *authoritative* textbooks, personal experience with similar cases and the views of other specialists (written or objectively established) can all be used.

Importantly, the role of an expert should be restricted to the specialist domains of the person providing the opinion. This seems obvious, but the temptation to drift into the domains of others, or to be persuaded to do it by the instructing lawyer, can be strong. For instance, the difficulties that arose in the case of *General Medical Council vs Meadow* (2006) are salutary. An eminent paediatrician quoted a statistic he had erroneously calculated, resulting in professional misconduct charges and a long legal process.

Experts may be asked to declare that the facts in the report are within his or her own knowledge and that the opinions and views expressed are complete and truly those of the writer.

In summary, an expert opinion should be independent, unbiased, clear, supported by evidence and understandable by non-experts (but not simplistic, of course).

19.3 The content and format of reports

The content of expert and medicolegal reports differs according to the jurisdiction, the nature of the legal matter and the requirements, or preferences, of the instructing counsel. A case of possible negligence will need different information from one of work attribution of a disease and its impact on fitness for a particular job. Detailed instruction on the format and content of the report should thus be obtained in writing from the legal representatives in the matter. The expected content outside the competence of the expert under instruction should be made clear at this point.

The professional indemnity organisations, occupational health-related professional societies, law societies and others have published guides on expert and medicolegal reports. Some are jurisdiction and profession specific and should be consulted. This section, therefore, just covers some general features.

- Cover page. Depending on the context this may be extensive with a curriculum vitae, documents examined, medical examinations and tests, a list of references, etc. or it may simply concern patient/client particulars, dates of evaluations and identification and qualifications of the report writer. Preferably, the instructing lawyer should provide a template for this (and other aspects of the report).

- The salient information on the matter. What is salient varies greatly according to the issue at hand. Occupational hygiene, occupational therapy and medical reports have different aims and content. For hygiene reports the validity of the measurement data may be key, possibly covering sampling strategies and instrumentation and laboratory quality assurance, even over some years. In patient reports, the basis and certainty of the diagnosis, whether sufficient exposure occurred to cause the disease and the expected duration of unfitness (complete or partial) for work are usually central.
- Disability (impairments, activity limitations and participation restrictions). Assessment of potentially vocational and life-limiting impairments and their consequences is important and is best done in a multidisciplinary manner. For the doctor reporting on current impairment, expected response to optimal treatment and likely duration of the incapacity are usually necessary. Use of an accepted impairment determination method is recommended and may be required, sometimes specifying older versions than current – the *American Medical Association Guides to the Evaluation of Permanent Impairment* are widely used.

  Fitness to work at 'own job' and in the open labour market are often central to the magnitude of the benefits awarded to the injured party. So, fitness to work needs to be ascertained reliably. Sometimes it is easy: a person with lung function tests poor enough to seriously impede travel to and from the job is unfit for work in the open labour market; confined space workers with paralysis that prevents easy egress will not be able to work in their usual role. But most cases are more complex and occupational therapists are usually more valuable than other practitioners in making the determinations on work capacity. Psychological sequelae can contribute substantially to the negative impacts of disease and injury. The effects of paraplegia are far more than physical and vocational, and so are lung diseases that limit participation in sport and leisure activities like gardening and hiking. Families may need to fundamentally change their lives to care for the disabled members, causing reduced income and conflict in the family. A psychological assessment may, thus, be material in assessing losses sustained as a result of occupational disease and injury. It should be noted, though, that most workers' compensation systems proscribe claims for psychological sequalae – 'excluding pain and suffering' is a typical phrase – unless there are special circumstances, such as negligence on the part of the employer.
- The future. Not infrequently experts are asked to provide information on the likely future course of the client's condition, as this will usually influence the calculation of benefits sought. Considerations typically include one or more of:
  - Response to prolonged optimal treatment.
  - Prognosis, future impairment and life expectancy (partly so that loss of earnings due to the condition can be estimated). Life expectancy is usually very uncertain for an individual patient with a chronic condition. It is sensible to state this uncertainty using words such as: 'Studies have found increased mortality in groups with the condition so the client probably has reduced life expectancy but the extent of loss for any individual cannot be

estimated with any confidence.' Life insurance companies may be able to aid lawyers on life expectancy more than occupational health experts.

- Medical complications and their expected frequency in similar settings to the client's. There may be many complications and their incidences can be determined by the setting. Silicosis illustrates the broad scope of potential complications, which include tuberculosis (common in high-burden countries), progression of small opacities (common), the development of massive fibrosis (quite common), lung cancer (uncommon in silicosis alone but co-exposures to other workplace carcinogens and smoking will increase occurrence), pneumothorax (uncommon but difficult to treat) and cor pulmonale (uncommon). Relevant literature should inform the estimates of frequency: for instance, silicosis has been found to progress in 20–90% of subjects in different studies depending to some extent on the length of follow-up; the mode is around a third.
- Future medical care. Unless you are experienced in this aspect it is wise to consult standard guides, the treating physician and possibly colleagues in a variety of disciplines because future medical requirements may not be obvious when considered within one discipline. Patients with silicosis make the point. Besides the routine consultations for the diseases, patients with silicosis require annual influenza vaccinations and pneumococcal vaccination depending on their individual history. In high-income countries computed tomography (CT) scanning is probably indicated to detect early lung cancer in long-term smokers with the pneumoconiosis. Isoniazid preventive therapy is recommended for those with latent tuberculosis. Frequent tuberculosis screening is necessary in high-burden countries, but the nature of the screening will vary.
- Future medical costs. In the authors' experience it is prudent to consider carefully the advisability of contributing to this aspect especially if distant future costs need to be estimated.
- Disclaimer. In some cases, it is advisable to note areas of the report where you have concerns about the reliability of the available information or tests done, and how your opinion could change should new facts be provided to you.
- Comments on other experts' reports. You might also be asked to critique the opinions of other experts, especially if they do not concur with yours. Advice on how to go about this generally includes:
  - note areas of agreement and disagreement, especially those material to the matter
  - give evidence that both supports and counters the contrary views given by the other expert
  - restrict your critique to the scope of your instructions and your own expertise
  - views of another expert not relevant to your instruction probably do not need comment
  - distinguish clearly between facts, opinions (e.g. based on experience) and assumptions made (e.g. about the extent of exposure to a hazardous agent in the absence of objective measurements).

19.4 Some pitfalls

This section covers some pitfalls in writing the reports but not those when appearing in court or quasi-judicial environments, which are matters beyond the scope of this chapter.

The main point made by Judge Davis on the role of experts (see Section 19.2) should be front of mind: an objective and unbiased opinion must be given; experts are not 'hired guns'. Failure to adhere to this injunction not only risks damaging the expert's reputation and integrity, but also places them at risk of a civil claim or complaint to the agency governing their professional conduct.

Accepting payment on the contingency that 'your side wins' is inadvisable. If known to the other party or the court, should it get to one, the independence and objectivity of the expert would reasonably be called into doubt. The report and the expert are likely to be subjected to greater scrutiny than would otherwise have been the case.

Stay within the scope of expertise that is evident from your qualifications and experience. 'Straying outside your lane' is likely to lead to questions on competence and could discredit the whole report.

Confidentiality needs to be respected regarding the details of the matter, and sometimes even the expert's involvement in it. The client may be prohibited from seeing the report. Before discussing the matter with colleagues, which can be useful, it is advisable to seek guidance from the instructing lawyers so that they and their client can consent or not to disclosure. In some jurisdictions the client's treating physician needs to be informed of important medical conditions identified during compiling the expert opinion.

Bear in mind the perils of relying on 'facts' ingrained by your own long-held views or those of esteemed teachers. They may be out of date. Evidence accumulates over time and can then quite quickly overturn previously accepted knowledge. Systematic reviews and the synthesis of data from several studies using techniques such as meta-analyses are commonplace, and their findings can strongly influence practice and establish associations between exposures and diseases. Clearly, reference to recent published literature is advisable in preparing an expert report. A common mistake is to cherry pick articles from among the body of literature that support a cherished or preferred view. Far better to rely on systematic reviews, recent statements and updates from professional societies and authoritative textbooks, provided they are not outdated.

Perceived conflicts of interest may be a concern if doctors or occupational therapists routinely attending to a patient or client compile a report, or company-associated hygienists write expert reports using company exposure data. Possible conflicts of interest should be disclosed and discussed with instructing lawyers.

Reference

General Medical Council vs Meadow, EWCA Civ 1390 (2006). http://www.bailii.org/ew/cases/EWCA/Civ/2006/1390.html

CHAPTER 20

Ethical Aspects of Occupational Health

The intention of the sixth edition of this book was to provide a broader and more international context. Rather than a focus on legal issues, which vary between jurisdictions, we here consider ethical issues – the ones that challenge us all in our everyday practice. Since extant widely respected principles are available, it was considered appropriate simply to replicate here the excellent International Commission for Occupational Health's 2014 *International Code of Ethics: For Occupational Health Professionals*.

As has been described in Chapter 1, the aim of occupational health practice is to protect and promote workers' health, to sustain and improve their working capacity and ability, to contribute to the establishment and maintenance of a safe and healthy working environment for all and to promote the adaptation of work to the capabilities of workers, taking into account their state of health.

On the basis of the principle of equity, occupational health professionals should assist workers in obtaining and maintaining employment notwithstanding health status or any 'lack of ability'. It should be duly recognised that there are particular occupational health needs of workers as determined by factors such as sex, gender, age, physiological condition, social aspects, communication barriers, or other factors. Such needs should be met on an individual basis with due concern to protection of health in relation to work and without leaving any possibility for undue discrimination.

For the purpose of this Code, the expression 'occupational health professionals' is meant to include all those who, in a professional capacity, carry out occupational safety and health tasks, provide occupational health services

Pocket Consultant: Occupational Health, Sixth Edition. Kerry Gardiner, David Rees, Anil Adisesh, David Zalk, and Malcolm Harrington.
© 2022 John Wiley & Sons Ltd. Published 2022 by John Wiley & Sons Ltd.

or are involved in an occupational health practice. The term 'employers' means persons with recognised responsibility, commitment and duties towards workers in their employment by virtue of a mutually agreed relationship (a self-employed person is regarded as being both an employer and a worker). The term 'workers' applies to any persons who work, whether full time, part time or temporarily for an employer; this term is used here in a broad sense covering all employees, including management staff and the self-employed (a self-employed person is regarded as having the duties of both an employer and a worker). The expression 'competent authority' means a minister, government department or other public authority having the power to issue regulations, orders or other instruction having the force of law, and who is in charge of supervising and enforcing their implementation.

As there is a wide range of duties, obligations and responsibilities as well as complex relationships among those concerned and involved in occupational safety and health matters it calls for a clear view about the ethics of occupational health professionals and standards in their professional conduct. When specialists of several professions are working together within a multidisciplinary approach, they should endeavour to base their action on shared sets of values and have an understanding of each other's duties, obligations, responsibilities, and professional standards.

Basic requirements for a sound occupational practice include a full professional independence, i.e. that occupational health professionals must enjoy an independence in the exercise of their functions which should enable them to make judgements and give advice for the protection of the workers' health and for their safety within the undertaking, e.g. a business, in accordance with their knowledge and conscience. Occupational health professionals should make sure that the necessary conditions are met to enable them to carry out their activities according to good practice and to the highest professional standards. This should include adequate staffing, training and retraining, support and access to an appropriate level of senior management.

Further basic requirements for acceptable occupational health practice, often specified by national regulations, include free access to the workplace, the possibility of taking samples and assessing the working environment, making job analyses and participating in enquiries and consulting the competent authority on the implementation of occupational safety and health standards in the undertaking. Special attention should be given to ethical dilemmas which may arise from pursuing simultaneously objectives which may be competing such as the protection of employment and the protection of health, the right to information and confidentiality, and the conflicts between individual and collective interests.

Basic principles
The following three paragraphs summarise the principles of ethics and values on which is based the International Code of Ethics for Occupational Health Professionals.

A. *The purpose of occupational health is to serve the health and social wellbeing of the workers individually and collectively. Occupational health practice must be performed according to the highest professional standards and ethical principles. Occupational health professionals must contribute to environmental and community health.*

B. *The duties of occupational health professionals include protecting the life and the health of the worker, respecting human dignity and promoting the highest ethical principles in occupational health policies and programmes. Integrity in professional conduct, impartiality and the protection of the confidentiality of health data and of the privacy of workers are part of these duties.*

C. *Occupational health professionals are experts who must enjoy full professional independence in the execution of their functions. They must acquire and maintain the competence necessary for their duties and require conditions which allow them to carry out their tasks according to good practice and professional ethics.*

Duties and obligations of occupational health professionals
Aims and advisory role

1. *The primary aim of occupational health practice is to safeguard and promote the health of workers, to promote a safe and healthy working environment, to protect the working capacity of workers and their access to employment. In pursuing this aim, occupational health professionals must use validated methods of risk evaluation, propose effective preventive measures and follow up their implementation. Occupational health professionals must provide competent and honest advice to employers on fulfilling their responsibility in the field of occupational safety and health as well as to the workers on the protection and promotion of their health in relation to work. Occupational health professionals should maintain direct contact with safety and health committees, where they exist.*

Knowledge and expertise

2. *Occupational health professionals must continuously strive to be familiar with the work and the working environment as well as to develop their competence and to remain well informed in scientific and technical knowledge, occupational hazards and the most efficient means to eliminate or to minimise the relevant risks. As the emphasis must be on primary prevention defined in terms of policies, design, choice of clean technologies, engineering control measures and adapting work organisation and workplaces to workers, occupational health professionals must regularly and routinely,*

whenever possible, visit the workplaces and consult the workers and the management on the work that is performed.

Development of a policy and a programme

3. *Occupational health professionals must advise management and the workers on factors at work which may affect workers' health. The risk assessment of occupational hazards must lead to the establishment of an occupational safety and health policy and of a programme of prevention adapted to the needs of undertakings and workplaces. The occupational health professionals must propose such a policy and programme on the basis of scientific and technical knowledge currently available as well as of their knowledge of the work organisation and environment. Occupational health professionals must ensure that they possess the required skill or secure the necessary expertise in order to provide advice on programmes of prevention which should include, as appropriate, measures for monitoring and management of occupational safety and health hazards and, in case of failure, for minimising consequences.*

Emphasis on prevention and on a prompt action

4. *Special consideration should be given to the rapid application of simple preventive measures which are technically sound and easily implemented. Further evaluation must check whether these measures are effective or if a more complete solution must be sought. When doubts exist about the severity of an occupational hazard, prudent precautionary action must be considered immediately and taken as appropriate. When there are uncertainties or differing opinions concerning nature of the hazards or the risks involved, occupational health professionals must be transparent in their assessment with respect to all concerned, avoid ambiguity in communicating their opinion and consult other professionals as necessary.*

Follow-up of remedial actions

5. *In the case of refusal or of unwillingness to take adequate steps to remove an undue risk or to remedy a situation which presents evidence of danger to health or safety, the occupational health professionals must make, as rapidly as possible, their concern clear, in writing, to the appropriate senior management executive, stressing the need for taking into account scientific knowledge and for applying relevant health protection standards, including exposure limits, and recalling the obligation of the employer to apply laws and regulations and to protect the health of workers in their employment. The workers concerned and their representatives in the enterprise should be informed and the competent authority should be contacted, whenever necessary.*

Safety and health information

6. *Occupational health professionals must contribute to the information for workers on occupational hazards to which they may be exposed in an*

objective and understandable manner which does not conceal any fact and emphasises the preventive measures. Occupational health professionals must co-operate with the employer, the workers and their representatives to ensure adequate information and training on health and safety to the management personnel and workers. Occupational health professionals must provide appropriate information to the employers, workers and their representatives about the level of scientific certainty or uncertainty of known and suspected occupational hazards at the workplace.

Commercial secrets

7. *Occupational health professionals are obliged not to reveal industrial or commercial secrets of which they may become aware in the exercise of their activities. However, they must not withhold information which is necessary to protect the safety and health of workers or of the community. When needed, occupational health professionals must consult the competent authority in charge of supervising the implementation of the relevant legislation.*

Health surveillance

8. *The occupational health objectives, methods and procedures of health surveillance must be clearly defined with priority given to adaptation of workplaces to workers who must receive information in this respect. The relevance and validity of these methods and procedures must be assessed. The surveillance must be carried out with the informed consent of the workers. The potentially positive and negative consequences of participation in screening and health surveillance programmes should be discussed as part of the consent process. The health surveillance must be performed by an occupational health professional approved by the competent authority.*

Information to the worker

9. *The results of examinations, carried out within the framework of health surveillance must be explained to the worker concerned. The determination of fitness for a given job, when required, must be based on a good knowledge of the job demands and of the worksite and on the assessment of the health of the worker. The workers must be informed of the opportunity to challenge the conclusions concerning their fitness in relation to work that they feel contrary to their interest. An appeals procedure must be established in this respect.*

Information to the employer

10. *The results of the examinations prescribed by national laws or regulations must only be conveyed to management in terms of fitness for the envisaged work or of limitations necessary from a medical point of view in the assignment*

of tasks or in the exposure to occupational hazards, with the emphasis put on proposals to adapt the tasks and working conditions to the abilities of the worker. General information on work fitness or in relation to health or the potential or probable health effects of work hazards, may be provided with the informed consent of the worker concerned, in so far as this is necessary to guarantee the protection of the worker's health.

Danger to a third party

11. *Where the health condition of the worker and the nature of the tasks performed are such as to be likely to endanger the safety of others, the worker must be clearly informed of the situation. In the case of a particularly hazardous situation, the management and, if so required by national regulations, the competent authority must also be informed of the measures necessary to safeguard other persons. In giving advice, the occupational health professional must try to reconcile employment of the worker concerned with the safety or health of others that may be endangered.*

Biological monitoring and investigations

12. *Biological tests and other investigations must be chosen for their validity and relevance for protection of the health of the worker concerned, with due regard to their sensitivity, their specificity and their predictive value. Occupational health professionals must not use screening tests or investigations which are not reliable, or which do not have a sufficient predictive value in relation to the requirements of the work assignment. Where a choice is possible and appropriate, preference must always be given to non-invasive methods and to examinations, which do not involve any danger to the health of the worker concerned. An invasive investigation or an examination which involves a risk to the health of the worker concerned may only be advised after an evaluation of the benefits to the worker and the risks involved. Such an investigation is subject to the worker's informed consent and must be performed according to the highest professional standards. It cannot be justified for insurance purposes or in relation to insurance claims.*

Health promotion

13. *When engaging in health education, health promotion, health screening and public health programmes, occupational health professionals must seek the participation of both employers and workers in their design and in their implementation. They must also protect the confidentiality of personal health data of the workers and prevent their misuse.*

Protection of community and environment

14. *Occupational health professionals must be aware of their role in relation to the protection of the community and of the environment. With a view to*

contributing to environmental health and public health, occupational health professionals must initiate and participate, as appropriate, in identifying, assessing, advertising and advising for the purpose of prevention on occupational and environmental hazards arising or which may result from operations or processes in the enterprise.

Contribution to scientific knowledge

15. *Occupational health professionals must report objectively to the scientific community as well as to the public health and labour authorities on new or suspected occupational hazards. They must also report on new and relevant preventive methods. Occupational health professionals involved in research must design and carry out their activities on a sound scientific basis with full professional independence and follow the ethical principles attached to research work and to medical research, including an evaluation by an independent committee on ethics, as appropriate.*

Conditions of execution of the functions of occupational health professionals
Competence, integrity and impartiality

16. *Occupational health professionals must always act, as a matter of prime concern, in the interest of the health and safety of the workers. Occupational health professionals must base their judgements on scientific knowledge and technical competence and call upon specialised expert advice as necessary. Occupational health professionals must refrain from any judgement, advice or activity which may endanger the trust in their integrity and impartiality.*

Professional independence

17. *Occupational health professionals must seek and maintain full professional independence and observe the rules of confidentiality in the execution of their functions. Occupational health professionals must under no circumstances allow their judgement and statements to be influenced by any conflict of interest, in particular when advising the employer, the workers or their representatives in the undertaking on occupational hazards and situations which present evidence of danger to health or safety.*

Equity, non-discrimination and communication

18. *The occupational health professionals must build a relationship of trust, confidence and equity with the people to whom they provide occupational health services. All workers should be treated in an equitable manner, without any form of discrimination as regards their condition, their convictions or the reason which led to the consultation of the occupational health professionals. Occupational health professionals must establish and maintain clear channels of communication among themselves, the senior management responsible for decisions at the highest level about the conditions*

and the organisation of work and the working environment in the under-
taking, and with the workers' representatives.

Clause on ethics in contracts of employment

19. *Occupational health professionals must request that a clause on ethics be*
    incorporated in their contract of employment. This clause on ethics should
    include, in particular, their right to apply professional standards, guide-
    lines and codes of ethics. Occupational health professionals must not accept
    conditions of occupational health practice which do not allow for
    performance of their functions according to the desired professional stan-
    dards and principles of ethics. Contracts of employment should contain
    guidance on the legal, contractual and ethical aspects and on management
    of conflict, access to records and confidentiality in particular. Occupational
    health professionals must ensure that their contract of employment or ser-
    vice does not contain provisions which could limit their professional
    independence. In case of doubt about the terms of the contract legal advice
    must be sought and the competent authority must be consulted as
    appropriate.

Records

20. *Occupational health professionals must keep good records with the appro-*
    priate degree of confidentiality for the purpose of identifying occupational
    health problems in the enterprise. Such records include data relating to the
    surveillance of the working environment, personal data such as the
    employment history and occupational health data such as the history of
    occupational exposure, results of personal monitoring of exposure to
    occupational hazards and fitness certificates. Workers must be given access
    to the data relating to the surveillance of the working environment and to
    their own occupational health records.

Medical confidentiality

21. *Individual medical data and the results of medical investigations must be*
    recorded in confidential medical files which must be kept secured under the
    responsibility of the occupational health physician or the occupational
    health nurse. Access to medical files, their transmission and their release
    are governed by national laws or regulations on medical data where they
    exist and relevant national codes of ethics for health professionals and
    medical practitioners. The information contained in these files must only be
    used for occupational health purposes.

Collective health data

22. *When there is no possibility of individual identification, information on*
    aggregate health data on groups of workers may be disclosed to management
    and workers' representatives in the undertaking or to safety and health
    committees, where they exist, in order to help them in their duties to protect

the health and safety of exposed groups of workers. Occupational injuries and work-related diseases must be reported to the competent authority according to national laws and regulations.

Relationships with health professionals

23. *Occupational health professionals must not seek personal information which is not relevant to the protection, maintenance or promotion of workers' health in relation to work or to the overall health of the workforce. Occupational health physicians may seek further medical information or data from the worker's personal physician or hospital medical staff, with the worker's informed consent, but only for the purpose of protecting, maintaining or promoting the health of the worker concerned. In so doing, the occupational health physician must inform the worker's personal physician or hospital medical staff of his or her role and of the purpose for which the medical information or data is required. With the agreement of the worker, the occupational health physician or the occupational health nurse may, if necessary, inform the worker's personal physician of relevant health data as well as of hazards, occupational exposures and constraints at work which represent a particular risk in view of the worker's state of health.*

Combating abuses

24. *Occupational health professionals must co-operate with other health professionals in the protection of the confidentiality of the health and medical data concerning workers. Occupational health professionals must identify, assess and point out to those concerned procedures or practices which are, in their opinion, contrary to the principles of ethics embodied in this Code and inform the competent authority when necessary. This concerns in particular instances of misuse or abuse of occupational health data, concealing or withholding findings, violating medical confidentiality or of inadequate protection of records in particular as regards information placed on computers.*

Relationships with social partners

25. *Occupational health professionals must increase the awareness of employers, workers and their representatives of the need for full professional independence and commitment to protect medical confidentiality in order to respect human dignity and to enhance the acceptability and effectiveness of occupational health practice.*

Promoting ethics and professional audit

26. *Occupational health professionals must seek the support and co-operation of employers, workers and their organisations, as well as of the competent authorities, for implementing the highest standards of ethics in occupational health practice. Occupational health professionals must institute a*

programme of professional audit of their activities to ensure that appropriate standards have been set, that they are being met and that deficiencies, if any, are detected and corrected and that steps are taken to ensure continuous improvement of professional performance.

Occupational health professionals should also make themselves familiar with any jurisdictional professional guidance such as that from national specialty societies. A broader professional duty would be to promote the adoption of the above or similar ethical guidance for the benefit of all workplace stakeholders.

Further Reading

International Commission on Occupational Health (2014). *International Code of Ethics: For Occupational Health Professionals*, 3e. http://www.icohweb.org/site/multimedia/code_of_ethics/code-of-ethics-en.pdf.

INDEX

Page numbers: Figures given in *italics* and Tables in **bold**

Pocket Consultant: Occupational Health, Sixth Edition. Kerry Gardiner, David Rees, Anil Adisesh, David Zalk, and Malcolm Harrington.
© 2022 John Wiley & Sons Ltd. Published 2022 by John Wiley & Sons Ltd.

F_2

Printed and bound by CPI Group (UK) Ltd, Croydon, CR0 4YY

27/10/2024

14580352-0002

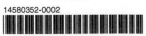